Grant's DISSECTOR

TENTH EDITION

Eberhardt K. Sauerland, M.D.

**Professor of Cellular and Structural Biology
and Associate Professor of Psychiatry
The University of Texas Health Science Center
San Antonio, Texas**

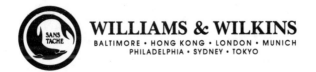

WILLIAMS & WILKINS
BALTIMORE · HONG KONG · LONDON · MUNICH
PHILADELPHIA · SYDNEY · TOKYO

Editor: John N. Gardner
Associate Editor: Victoria M. Vaughn
Copy Editor: Shelley Potler
Designer: Norman Och
Illustration Planner: Lorraine Wrzosek
Production Coordinator: Barbara J. Felton
Cover Designer: Amy Sweet

Copyright © 1991
Williams & Wilkins
428 East Preston Street
Baltimore, Maryland 21202, USA

Accurate indications, adverse reactions, and dosage schedules for drugs are provided in this book, but it is possible that they may change. The reader is urged to review the package information data of the manufacturers of the medications mentioned.

Printed in the United States of America

By J. C. B. GRANT AND H. A. CATES
First Edition, 1940
  Reprinted 1942

Second Edition, 1945

Third Edition, 1948
  Reprinted 1951

Fourth Edition, 1953
  Reprinted 1956, 1957

By J. C. B. GRANT
Fifth Edition, 1959
  Reprinted 1961, 1965

Sixth Edition, 1967
  Reprinted 1968, 1970

By E. K. SAUERLAND
Seventh Edition, 1974
  Reprinted 1974, 1975, 1976

Eighth Edition, 1978
  Reprinted 1979, 1980 (twice), 1982 (twice), 1983

Ninth Edition, 1984

Library of Congress Cataloging-in-Publication Data

Sauerland, Eberhardt K., 1933-
    Grant's dissector. — 10th ed. / Eberhardt K. Sauerland.
      p.   cm.
    Includes index.
    ISBN 0-683-03707-2
    1. Human dissection—Laboratory manuals. I. Title. II. Title:
Dissector.
    [DNLM: 1. Dissection. QS 130 S255g]
    QM34.S27   1991
    611'.0028—dc20
    DNLM/DLC   91-15336
    for Library of Congress   CIP

Grant's DISSECTOR

TENTH EDITION

A portion of the royalties from this *Dissector* has been donated to establish the **J.C.B. GRANT ANATOMY SCHOLARSHIP** in honor of the late John C. Boileau Grant (1886–1973), Professor Emeritus of Anatomy at the University of Toronto. This award will be given annually to an exceptional medical, dental, physical therapy, or occupational therapy student who wishes to pursue advanced anatomical studies at the University of Toronto.

PREFACE

This *Dissector* is a manual intended to facilitate and guide human anatomical dissections. It is **not** a replacement for a textbook. It is **not** an atlas. The first edition of *Grant's Dissector* appeared 50 years ago in 1940. During the following six editions in three decades, this manual became an almost indispensable item for American and Canadian students engaged in human anatomical dissections. In 1972, Professor J.C. Boileau Grant asked me to prepare the seventh and subsequent editions of the *Dissector* and to adapt this manual to the ever-changing needs of medical school curricula.

Over the past 15 years, it has become apparent that students tend to view and use *Grant's Dissector* and *Grant's Atlas* as a functional unit. This successful tradition has been maintained and the present tenth edition of the *Dissector* has been closely coordinated with the new and expanded ninth edition of *Grant's Atlas*. The chapters in both books follow the same sequence, and the *Dissector* contains numerous references to appropriate and applicable *Atlas* illustrations including diagrams, radiographs, and MRI/CT images.

Since recent medical curricula have reduced the number of hours available for gross anatomical studies, it was our objective to save time whenever possible. Consequently: (1) The text is concise. (2) Illustrations and diagrams quickly convey information and concepts. (3) As stated, the text contains numerous references to appropriate illustrations in *Grant's Atlas*. These references ensure the most efficient and complete use of the *Atlas* during anatomical dissections or review. (4) Since rapid and competent dissections often depend on thorough knowledge of pertinent bony reference points, a brief discussion of relevant bony landmarks is included.

Each anatomical region under consideration for dissection is introduced by brief GENERAL REMARKS and DEFINITIONS. Following that, the student is encouraged to study applicable IMPORTANT LANDMARKS. Subsequently, the objectives for the contemplated dissection are stated under the heading, "Before you begin . . .". Only then, and with this background and orientation in mind, will the student embark on the actual DISSECTION.

The chapter sequence of the *Dissector* has been correlated with that of the *Atlas*. However, each chapter stands alone as an independent unit. Thus, anatomical dissections may be carried out in any sequence desired and as specified by the instructor. The teaching staff may choose to delete certain parts of this manual from the class assignment. This is often necessary because many gross anatomy courses across the nation are under severe time constraints. On the other hand, additional dissection projects may be desirable, particularly for students on special assignment or on elective rotations. These projects have been grouped together in the *Appendix* and include such topics as the dissection of smaller joints, the bull's eye, and the lumbar approach to the kidney.

Studies in gross anatomy are more meaningful to students if they are aware of the clinical significance of various structures. Clinically relevant comments complement the regular text whenever indicated. These clinically oriented correlations are set in smaller type and screened for special attention and quick referral.

For this tenth edition of the *Dissector*, hundreds of comments from various reviewers have been carefully considered. There has been general consensus that the approach to the perineum and pelvis should be more traditional; as a result, Chapter 3 has been changed considerably to accommodate the current needs of our students.

The chapter is divided into two separate sections, taking into account the differences between male and female specimens. The chapters on the upper and lower limbs have been simplified in that the limbs will be skinned entirely in initial effort, thus allowing a comprehensive examination of the deep fascia, superficial veins, and cutaneous nerves. The sections on clinically relevant comments have been expanded. In addition, all line drawings have been improved by providing uniform labels. Every effort has been made to make the references to *Grant's Atlas* as complete as possible.

I am greatly indebted to a number of family members and friends, whose understanding and support was essential during the preparation of this manual. In particular, I wish to thank my son, George, and his wife for their personal time and their expertise concerning computer operation. My good friends at "Laughing Waters" provided shelter from distractions that would have otherwise delayed publication of this tenth edition.

In addition to the late Professor J.C.B. Grant, I am most grateful to a number of colleagues who have provided excellent ideas and suggestions for the improvement of various editions of this manual. Their names are cited here in alphabetical order: Doctors Susan L. Abbondanzo, Erle K. Adrian, G. Callas, J. Collins, Donald Duncan, R.V. Gregg, Craig S. Hammes, R.M. Harper, W.J. Hild, Linda Johnson, R.D. Laurenson, G.F. Lewis, R.G. MacKenzie, D.S. Maxwell, R.R. Peterson, B.A. Tracey Sauerland, C.H. Sawyer, M.F. Teaford, K. Thibodeau, J.S. Thompson, and Robert Trelease. Many other anatomists have contributed anonymously by providing comments to the Editorial Staff at Williams & Wilkins; their constructive ideas are greatly appreciated. I especially thank Anne Agur, the new Editor of *Grant's Atlas*, for her dedication and efforts to maintain and improve the functional unity of both the *Dissector* and the *Atlas*. At Williams & Wilkins, the cast of dedicated contributors to every aspect of the book publishing business is most impressive. In particular, I am grateful to John N. Gardner, Vice President and Publisher.

E.K. SAUERLAND

CONTENTS

4 THE BACK

5 THE LOWER LIMB

6 THE UPPER LIMB

7 THE HEAD AND NECK

I   APPENDIX
LUMBAR APPROACH TO KIDNEY

II   APPENDIX
JOINTS

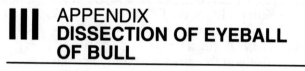

III APPENDIX
**DISSECTION OF EYEBALL
OF BULL**

INTRODUCTION TO DISSECTION

Purpose of Dissection. There is no substitute for dissection, i.e., a three-dimensional approach to the structures of the human body. Observe and palpate the topographic relations of various structures to each other. Feel the texture of blood vessels, nerves, and various tissues. Test the rigidity of bones and the strength of ligaments. Explore and appreciate the three dimensions of anatomical structures. This will prepare you well for an intelligent approach to physical examination and surgery.

The Cadaver. When the student is assigned to a cadaver or subject, he or she assumes responsibility for its proper care. The student will find the body already preserved or embalmed, the arteries occasionally injected with a (red) coloring matter, the veins sometimes full of clotted blood, and sometimes empty. The whole body has been kept moist by adequate wrappings or by submersion into suitable preservative fluid. Uncover only those parts of the body to be dissected. Inspect every part periodically, and renew and moisten wrappings as the occasion demands. No part must ever be left exposed to the air needlessly. Special attention must be given to the face, hands, feet, and external genitalia. Once a part is allowed to become dry and hard, it can never be fully restored, and its proper dissection is impossible. Plastic bags are particularly useful to prevent drying.

The student must always remember that former living persons have donated their bodies for medical studies benevolently and in good faith. Therefore, the cadaver must be treated with respect and dignity. Improper behavior in the dissecting laboratory (such as eating, drinking, making crude jokes, playing entertaining music, taking photographs without permission, illegally removing body parts from the laboratory, mutilations, or grave robbery—for example, by enriching oneself with the gold teeth of the deceased) cannot be tolerated.

Working Conditions. Be sure that the light falls on the part under investigation. Adequate light is essential for efficient dissection. Work in a position that is comfortable and not tiring. Make use of blocks to stabilize parts of the cadaver and to maintain its most suitable posture. Protect clothing by wearing a long laboratory coat or apron. Wearing protective gloves has become common practice for anyone handling human material (dead or alive). You may be required to wear disposable latex gloves. When cutting bony structures, protect your eyes with glasses or goggles against flying chips.

Instruments

Usually, the student will be provided with a list of dissecting instruments preferred by the faculty or individual instructors. If in doubt, procure the following (Fig. I.1):

1. **Two pairs of forceps** with transversely ridged handles to prevent slipping. The ends should be blunt and rounded and the gripping surfaces should be corrugated. The second pair is needed for distracting the tissue. Many students find it advantageous to use one big and one small pair of forceps. The small one, mouth-toothed or sharp-pointed, is used to hold on to delicate structures.
2. **A seeker or probe** consisting of rigid steel with a bent, blunt tip. In addition, a flexible blunt probe is useful for insertion into vessels or ducts (e.g., during exploration of such structures as coronary arteries, uterine tubes, urethra, etc.). Pointed needle-like seekers, as well as abruptly hooked instruments are dangerous and should not be used.
3. **A scalpel** designed for detachable knife blades. The scalpel handle should be made of metal (not plastic). The blade should be about 3.5 to 4 cm long. The cutting edge must have some convexity near the point. The blade must be sharp at all times. No one can do good work with a dull knife. Therefore, a sufficient supply of blades will be needed. The rounded end of the handle can be conveniently used to separate soft tissues.
4. **Two pairs of scissors**, a larger, heavy dissecting scissors about 15 cm in length, and a fine pair of scissors with two sharp points for the dissection of delicate structures. Consult the instructor.

Dissecting Techniques. Keep in mind that a variable amount of subcutaneous fat lies immediately deep to the skin. That fat contains superficial nerves and vessels, particularly veins. Therefore, in removing skin, all fat should be left behind (unless instructed otherwise). In those sub-

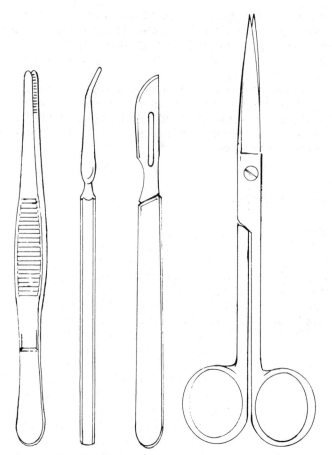

Figure I.1. Examples of useful dissecting instruments.

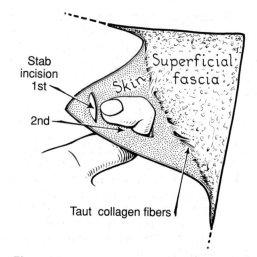

Figure I.2. When removing skin, apply traction.

jects nearly devoid of fat, one needs to exercise special care in order not to go too deep. The thickness of skin varies from region to region. For example, the skin is relatively thin in the anterior region of the forearm; in contrast, it is considerably thicker in the area of the back. Generally, incisions should be made cautiously and not exceeding the thickness of the skin. If, during removal of skin, you see

brownish muscular fibers shining through the filmy deep fascia, your cut is too deep. Always remember to put *traction on the skin* as it is being removed, to keep the sharp knife directed against it, and to leave the fat in place (unless specified otherwise). In this manner, you will work faster and encounter fewer difficulties (Figs. I.2 and I.3).

The unnecessary destruction of many soft structures can be avoided and a great deal of time can be saved by employing the method of *blunt dissection*, utilizing one's fingers or the blunt handle of the scalpel to separate various structures gently from each other. Delicate structures (e.g., fine blood vessels and nerves adhering to each other) can be efficiently separated by utilizing the *scissor technique*. As illustrated in Figure I.4, use a fine pair of scissors of the sharp-sharp type and gently force the blades apart in a direction parallel to the structures of interest.

Efficiency. Time is immensely valuable. Learn as much as possible in the shortest possible time. The following suggestions will help increase efficiency:

1. Acquire a *theoretical concept* of the area under investigation *before* attempting to dissect it. Do not "dig

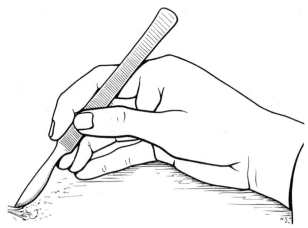

Figure I.3. When dissecting, rest the hand. Eliminate unsteady movements.

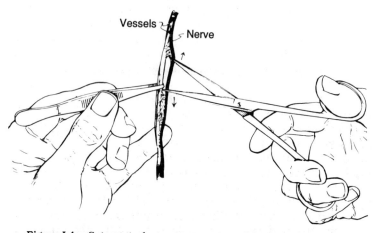

Figure I.4. Scissor technique: separating delicate structures.

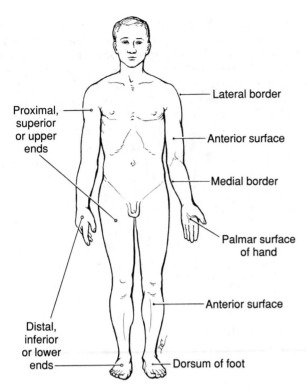

Proximal, superior or upper ends

Lateral border

Anterior surface

Medial border

Palmar surface of hand

Distal, inferior or lower ends

Anterior surface

Dorsum of foot

Figure I.5. Anatomical position (except for right forearm).

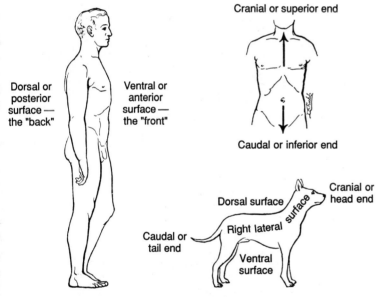

Dorsal or posterior surface — the "back"

Ventral or anterior surface — the "front"

Cranial or superior end

Caudal or inferior end

Dorsal surface

Cranial or head end

Right lateral surface

Caudal or tail end

Ventral surface

Figure I.6. Essential terms for orientation.

around" and happen to find "something interesting." You must deliberately search for certain structures.

2. Make full use of a good *atlas*.
3. Always palpate *bony landmarks* because they are keys in search for related soft structures. It is mandatory to have a skull available when dissecting the head.
4. *Use your time wisely.* To spend an hour tracing the terminal twigs of a cutaneous nerve when the general skin area supplied by the nerve is obvious is spending an

hour for little gain. To spend 3 minutes to define the exact fiber direction of a ligament is to spend 3 minutes for great gain; you will understand why and how that ligament restrains or prevents certain movements of bony structures.

5. Demonstrate the *essential features* of a given anatomical region with *clarity*. Remove fat, connective tissue, and smaller veins. If a clear-cut display of arteries is obtained, the general arrangement of the companion veins will be obvious.

Terminology

Anatomical Position (Fig. I.5). Anatomists have agreed to relate everything they describe to a universally approved and accepted position of the body. It is that position in which the body stands erect with the feet together, arms by the side, and the palms facing forward. That the dissector is (on most occasions) working with the cadaver lying on its back makes not the slightest difference. The statement that a given structure is inferior to another one is clearly understood by anatomists and surgeons: it means that this given structure is nearer to the feet.

Figure I.6 illustrates such essential terms as *superior (cranial), inferior (caudal), anterior (ventral),* and *posterior (dorsal).* The terms *coronal, sagittal,* and *transverse (horizontal)* are explained in Figure I.7.

Descriptions

Anatomical structures can be precisely described. Learn and practice to give an *accurate account* of each important structure in an *orderly* and *logical fashion.* Always project self into a future professional situation: Remember, you must give orderly and logical accounts when reporting on radiological findings, on performed surgery or autopsies, etc.

When encountering a *muscle* during dissection or review, be aware of its size and shape, its origin and insertion, its function and its nerve supply. Usually, muscles act on *joints.* You should be able to describe the type of joint and the extent of its movements. When studying *blood vessels,* be cognizant of their proximal and distal connections. In any region under consideration, you should know the origin and destination of encountered *nerves* as well as their functional composition (motor, sensory, mixed, autonomic).

Variations

No cadaver will conform in all details of its anatomical construction to the patterns outlined in the pages of this book. This manual describes the most common patterns encountered in the adult. Minor and even major variants frequently occur: arteries may arise from sources other

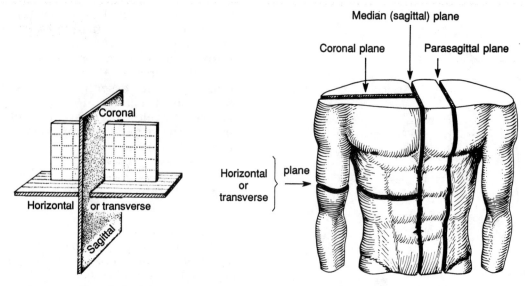

Figure I.7. Fundamental planes in the body: sagittal, coronal, transverse.

than those indicated or may pursue different courses. Muscles may have extra heads of origin or be absent entirely. Organs may vary from their usual shape and/or be found in other than "normal" positions. There may be accessory organs. The usual anatomical relations may be distorted by disease processes (e.g., cancer) or by prior surgical intervention. This is particularly true for the abdomen and thorax.

Regard the cadaver you are working on as a "typical example." By all means, examine as many different subjects as possible. Only in this manner will you be able to familiarize yourself with the accepted "normal" and with variations and anomalies. Variations, particularly in arteries and nerves, will be emphasized in this manual whenever appropriate.

Illustrations

The line drawings and schemata shown in this book are intended to orient the dissector and to facilitate the approach to a given anatomical region. They are designed to offer explanations, increase comprehension, and attract attention to a useful point of reference. The additional use of a good *ATLAS* is highly desirable.

Students who are using **GRANT's ATLAS OF ANATOMY** will find throughout the text of this manual references to appropriate plate numbers in the 9th edition of the *Atlas*. For example: (*Atlas*, 3.17).

CHAPTER 1

THE THORAX

Thoracic Wall

Bony Landmarks and Surface Anatomy

Refer to individual bones or to an articulated skeleton. Study the following:

Vertebra (*Atlas*, 4.7). It consists of a weight-bearing **body** and a protective vertebral arch which is made up of two rounded pedicles (roots) and two flat plates or laminae. At the junction of the **pedicle** and **lamina**, a **transverse process** projects laterally, and **articular processes** project superiorly and inferiorly. At the junction of the two laminae, a **spinous process** projects posteriorly in the median plane. The bodies and transverse processes of the thoracic vertebrae have facets for the ribs (Fig. 1.1).

> Place your index finger in the **vertebral foramen** of a vertebra (Fig. 1.2). Observe that the size of the vertebral foramina differs from vertebra to vertebra (*Atlas*, 4.8, 4.17B). In the articulated vertebral column, the vertebral foramina collectively form a bony tube, the **vertebral canal**. This canal encloses and protects the important spinal cord.
>
> Abnormal curvatures of the spine (kyphosis, with convexity backward; scoliosis, lateral curvature or deformity) may be seen in the dissecting laboratory. These clinical conditions may be related to altering the shape and volume capacity of the thoracic cavity.

Rib (Fig. 1.3; *Atlas*, 1.9A). Identify **head, neck, tubercle,** and **body**. On the external surface, observe the angle where the body takes a bend and also a twist; therefore, a rib will not lie flat on a table. The lower border of a typical rib is sharp and flange-like to shelter a **costal groove** for the intercostal nerve and vessels. Note the distinctly different shape of the 1st rib. It is a superlative in being the highest, shortest, broadest, and most curved (*Atlas*, 1.9B). On occasion, there may be a cervical rib which is usually due to an enlarged costal element of the 7th cervical vertebra (*Atlas*, 1.10A). A bicipital rib occurs when there is partial fusion of two adjacent ribs (*Atlas*, 1.10B).

Sternum (*Atlas*, 1.11). Identify the wide upper segment, the **manubrium**. The **body** is made up of four distinguishable bony segments. The pointed lower extremity of the sternum is the **xiphoid process** (Gr. *xiphos*, sword). It is cartilaginous in youth, but ossified in the middle-aged and older person. Occasionally, the body of the sternum may be perforated. This hole may be mistaken as a bullet wound when, in fact, it is the result of a relatively common defect in the ossification process of the sternum (*Atlas*, 1.11C).

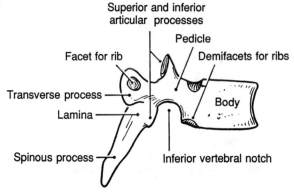

Figure 1.1. Typical thoracic vertebra, lateral view.

Superior and inferior articular processes

Facet for rib

Pedicle

Demifacets for ribs

Transverse process

Body

Lamina

Spinous process

Inferior vertebral notch

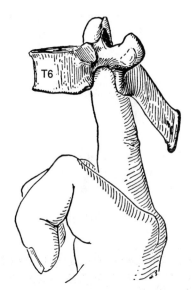

Figure 1.2. A vertebral foramen is not larger than a finger ring.

T6

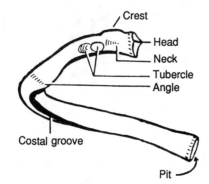

Figure 1.3. Typical left rib, posterior view.

Refer to an articulated skeleton and understand the following (Fig. 1.4; *Atlas*, 1.13A through 1.14B):

1. Two adjacent vertebral bodies are united by a fibrocartilaginous intervertebral disc. This is a joint of the symphysis variety.
2. Two adjacent vertebral arches are united by their articular processes.
3. An **intervertebral foramen** is completed between the pedicles of two adjacent vertebrae. It transmits the spinal nerve of the corresponding segment (Fig. 1.4) and associated spinal vessels.
4. The head of a rib articulates typically with two vertebral bodies and the intervening disc. The tubercle of a rib articulates with the transverse process of the vertebra with the same segmental number. Example (Fig. 1.4): The head of rib 5 articulates with vertebral bodies T4 and T5. The tubercle of rib 5 articulates with the transverse process of T5.
5. The anterior extremity of each rib is connected to the sternum by means of a bar of hyaline cartilage. These costal cartilages become progressively longer from 1st to 7th rib (*Atlas*, 1.8). Costal cartilages 8, 9, and 10 reach only as far as the cartilage next superior.
6. Ribs 11 and 12 have free pointed ends; therefore, they are also known as "floating ribs" (*Atlas*, 1.8).

In addition, identify the following bony structures or landmarks related to the dissection of the thoracic wall (Fig. 1.5; *Atlas*, 6.21).

1. **Jugular notch** (suprasternal notch).
2. **Sternal angle** marking the junction of manubrium with body of sternum. At this level, the 2nd rib can be palpated.
3. Medial end of **clavicle** marking the sternoclavicular joint (*Atlas*, 1.12B).
4. Lateral end of clavicle marking the acromioclavicular joint.
5. **Acromion** of scapula forming the point of the shoulder.
6. **Coracoid process** of scapula.

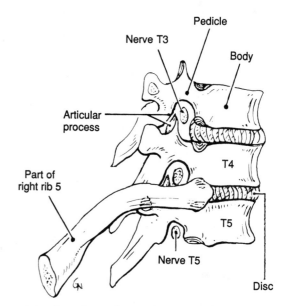

Figure 1.4. Part of vertebral column, thoracic region: intervertebral disc; intervertebral foramen with spinal nerve; rib attachments.

As a useful practical exercise for the student's future activities in **physical diagnosis**, the following study is recommended (Fig. 1.6): With a grease pencil, mark the subject's sternum, clavicle, and ribs 2 through 6. Identify and number the intercostal spaces (ICS). The 2nd ICS is located between ribs 2 and 3. The mammary papilla (nipple) lies at the level of ICS 4 in the male, more inferiorly in the female. Outline the **borders of a normal heart** (Fig. 1.6; *Atlas*, 1.47): The apex lies in ICS 5 and about 8 to 10 cm to the left of the midsternal line. Mark the right border by a vertical line 2.5 cm (1 inch) lateral to the right sternal margin. The inferior border crosses the junction between xiphoid process and body of sternum. The left border curves superiorly from the apex to ICS 2, about 2.5 cm from the left sternal margin. Part of the aortic arch projects on ICS 1, just to the left of the manubrium. In the living person in erect posture these borders will shift. Identify the borders of the heart in a radiograph of the chest (*Atlas*, 1.24).

Every physician must be familiar with the **auscultation points of the heart.** These are locations on the thoracic wall where sounds from specific heart valves may be heard most distinctly through a stethoscope (*Atlas*, 1.47).

Outline the **borders of the lungs:** The apex of each lung extends up into the neck for about 2.5 cm (cupula). The anterior borders of both lungs approach the midsternal line. The left lung deviates laterally at the level of ribs 4 and 5 to form the cardiac notch. Mark the approximate position of the horizontal fissure that begins near the right midaxillary line and extends forward along the right 4th costal cartilage. The oblique fissures of both lungs extend inferiorly and end near the 6th costochondral junction.

Review the projections of the heart and lungs on the thoracic wall (*Atlas*, 1.23). Once more, correlate your observations with a normal radiograph of the chest (*Atlas*, 1.24).

Before you begin . . .

Prior to dissection of muscles, due consideration must be given to the superficially positioned mammary gland. The thoracic wall is covered anteriorly with muscles that

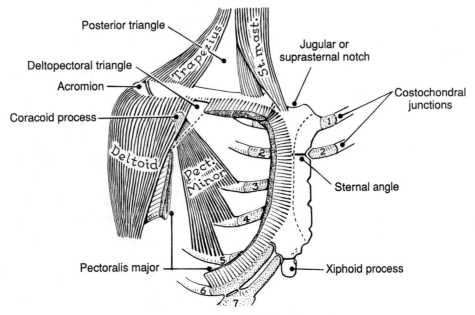

Figure 1.5. Landmarks of thoracic region.

belong to the upper limb. If you have already covered the UPPER LIMB, these muscles (pectoralis major and minor; subclavius) have already been dissected. If you are beginning your cadaver dissection with this first chapter (thorax), these muscles must be dissected and reflected before the intercostal spaces and their contents can be approached. Subsequently, the anterior thoracic wall will be removed to provide access to the thoracic cavity.

Skin Incisions

Do not cut too deep. You may inadvertently damage superficially positioned nerves. Disregard the following instructions for skin incisions if you have already dissected the UPPER LIMB. If you are beginning your cadaver dissection with the THORAX, make the following skin incisions now (Fig. 1.7):

1. From jugular notch *A* along the clavicle and across the acromion *B* to point *E*, about 10 cm distal to the acromion.
2. From *A* to the xiphisternal junction *C*.
3. From *C* horizontally lateralward until stopped by the table *D*.
4. From *C* superiorly and laterally and along the anterior axillary fold to point *E*. Avoid the nipple.
5. From *E* halfway around the medial side of the arm to point *F*.

Reflect the outlined flaps and discard them.

Dissection

Note: If you have already dissected the mammary gland, platysma, pectoralis major, pectoralis minor and subclavius as part of a previous assignment of the UPPER LIMB, skip these sections and continue with the INTERCOSTAL MUSCLES (p. 9). Otherwise, proceed with the sequence as outlined below.

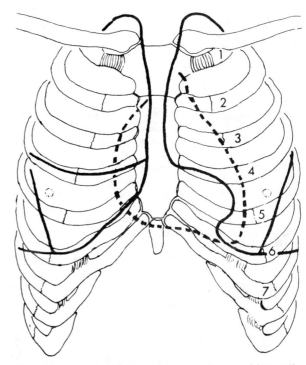

Figure 1.6. Projections of heart (*broken line*) and lungs (*heavy solid lines*) on anterior chest wall.

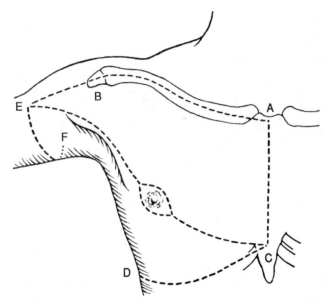

Figure 1.7. Skin incisions for dissection of thoracic wall.

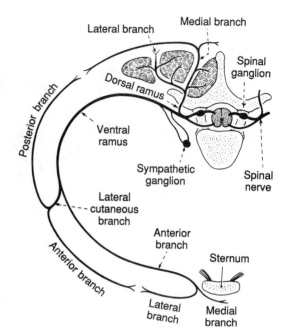

Figure 1.8. Typical spinal nerve.

Mammary Gland (*Atlas*, 1.3, 1.4). Since it is a modified skin gland, it lies in the superficial fascia. The rounded contour of the female breast is due to the superficial fat lying in compartments bounded by areolar septa, the **suspensory ligaments of Cooper**. These septa pass from the deep fascia to the deep layer of the skin. With the rounded handle of the knife, scoop collections of fat out of their compartments. Subsequently, trace some of the **lactiferous ducts** that converge on the tip of the **nipple**. Note that the nipple rises from the center of the pigmented **areola**.

Try to identify an orifice of one of the 15 to 20 lactiferous ducts (*Atlas*, 1.4). Probe through the fat under the nipple and find the ducts as they approach the nipple. You may wish to attempt to pass a bristle or fine wire into a duct, and trace it to the corresponding lobe of glandular tissue. Finally, remove the entire mammary gland and observe that it can be easily separated from the fascia of the underlying pectoralis major muscle.

In advanced carcinoma of the breast, the tumor may invade the underlying pectoralis major muscle and its fascia. Understand that this condition leads to a fixation of the malignant breast lesion to the chest wall.

Cancer of the breast (and its accompanying fibrosis) also has a tendency to shorten the suspensory ligaments of Cooper. Understand that the resulting traction of Cooper's ligaments on the skin leads to a characteristic dimpling of the skin.

Although the **lymphatic drainage** of the breast is difficult to demonstrate during routine dissection, it must nevertheless be thoroughly understood by any physician. Refer to *Atlas*, 1.5 and familiarize yourself with the arrangement of lymph channels and lymph nodes draining the breast tissue. Cancer has a tendency to spread along these lymph passages. Occasionally, cancer will block the lymphatic system on the side of the malignant lesion. In that case, lymph drainage (including transportation of cancer cells) may go to the opposite breast and its lymphatic drainage. Study a **lymphogram** of the nodes involved in the lymphatic drainage of the breast (*Atlas*, 1.6). Pay particular attention to the important axillary nodes. Also, study a normal lateral **mammogram** (*Atlas*, 1.7).

Platysma (*Atlas*, 1.2). Since the platysma is in the superficial fascia, it may have been inadvertently removed with the skin. If it is still present, look for its brownish-red muscle fibers as they cross the clavicle. The platysma is no thicker than a sheet of paper. You may not be able to find the thin platysma inferior to the clavicle. In that case, you will see it later during dissection of the neck. Do not attempt to search for the platysma in the neck region superior to the clavicle. If you find the platysma, turn it superiorly. Observe one or more of the distal ends of the supraclavicular nerves. These nerves cling to the deep surface of the platysma and send twigs through it to the skin. They are cutaneous nerves from C3-C4 (*Atlas*, 8.4). The supraclavicular nerves do *not* supply the platysma. The muscle fibers of the platysma are innervated by a branch of cranial nerve VII (facial nerve).

Cutaneous Branches of Spinal Nerves (*Atlas*, 1.2). The dissection of these branches can be intelligently performed only if the student is familiar with the disposition of a typical spinal nerve (Fig. 1.8; *Atlas*, 1.20). **Anterior cutaneous twigs** emerge from the intercostal spaces just lateral to the sternal margin. Be familiar with the area of their distribution, but do not dissect these very small nerves. The **lateral cutaneous branches** are substantially larger, and one representative (segments 4, 5, or 6) should be dissected: Make a vertical cut through the superficial fascia just lateral to the sternum. Make a horizontal cut corresponding to the lower horizontal skin incision. Reflect the flap of superficial fascia lateralward. Identify an intercostal space by fingertip palpation between two ribs. Search for the lateral cutaneous branch where it leaves its intercostal space and passes between the digitations of the **serratus anterior** (Fig. 1.9; *Atlas*, 1.2). Free the nerve. Trace its anterior and posterior branches for a short distance. Next, identify the lateral cutaneous branch of T2,

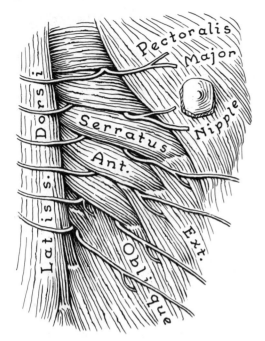

Figure 1.9. Anterior and posterior branches of lateral cutaneous nerves.

the **intercostobrachial nerve** (*Atlas,* 1.2). This nerve supplies the skin and subcutaneous tissue on the back and medial side of the arm (*Atlas,* 6.10A and **B**). If you have already dissected the UPPER LIMB, establish the continuity of the intercostobrachial nerve. If you are beginning with the THORAX, follow the nerve into the subcutaneous tissue of the posterior axillary fold.

> The **intercostobrachial nerve** is often involved in the phenomenon of "referred pain" in cases of angina pectoris. Referred pain is perceived in an area other than its actual origin. In cases of angina pectoris, the actual problem resides in the insufficiently perfused heart, but the resulting visceral pain is also referred to upper thoracic nerve segments, i.e., to an area of the anterior chest wall, often extending to the left arm. Understand that sympathetic nerves supplying the heart also carry afferent cardiac pain fibers back to the upper 4 or 5 thoracic segments of the spinal cord. Thus, the intercostobrachial nerve (T2) becomes involved in the phenomenon of referred cardiac pain.

Pectoralis Major (*Atlas,* 1.2). Clean its whole anterior surface. Identify the **clavicular part** and the **sternocostal part** (on rare occasions absent). With blunt dissection (handle of knife), separate the clavicular and sternocostal parts. Trace the tendon of the muscle to its insertion in the humerus. Observe that: (a) the anterior lamina of the tendon belongs to the clavicular head; (b) the posterior lamina is folded on itself and belongs to the sternal head. Superior to the clavicular head, and between it and the adjacent deltoid muscle, lies the **deltopectoral triangle**. It contains the **cephalic vein**, which is a superficial vein of the upper limb (*Atlas,* 6.4). Realize that the pectoralis major constitutes the most important part of the anterior wall of the axilla

(*Atlas,* 6.18). Palpate your own anterior axillary fold, and activate its muscular components.

Near the clavicle, insert a finger into the previously established gap between the sternocostal and clavicular parts of the pectoralis major muscle. Gently push the finger underneath the *clavicular head* superiorly and laterally until you feel strands of tissue entering the deep (posterior) surface of the muscle. These are the strands of the **lateral pectoral nerve.** Now, detach the clavicular head close to the clavicle, and reflect it toward the arm. You may want to preserve nerve and blood vessels to the muscle. These structures can be severed later if necessary.

Relax the *sternal head* of the pectoralis major by flexing and adducting the arm of the cadaver. Gently insinuate your fingers posterior to the sternal head. Your fingers are now in the space between the posterior surface of the pectoralis major and the **clavipectoral fascia,** which envelops the pectoralis minor (*Atlas,* 6.15). Palpate the vessels and nerves entering the deep surface of the pectoralis major. The pectoralis major and minor are two separate muscles which must *not* be reflected together. Use the clavipectoral fascia as a dividing plane between these two muscles. Next, reflect the **pectoralis major.** Detach the sternal head from its sternal and costal origins (Fig. 1.5), and reflect it toward the arm. Note that the **medial pectoral nerve** pierces the **pectoralis minor** before it enters the sternal head of the pectoralis major (*Atlas,* 6.19B, 6.22). Leave arterial branches and nerves attached to the muscle for subsequent identification.

Pectoralis Minor and Subclavius. After reflection of the pectoralis major, the **clavipectoral fascia** is exposed. It encloses the subclavius (a slender muscle immediately inferior to the clavicle) and the pectoralis minor (*Atlas,* 6.15). Clean and trace the cephalic vein as it crosses the pectoralis minor tendon anteriorly and pierces the clavipectoral fascia (*Atlas,* 6.14). Piercing the clavipectoral fascia with the vein are the thoracoacromial artery and the lateral pectoral nerve. Clean these structures and maintain them. Detach the pectoralis minor from its costal origin and reflect it superiorly. Leave the muscle attached to its insertion in the coracoid process of the scapula. Remove the remains of the clavipectoral fascia and any fat that might exist between the pectoralis minor and the rib cage. Now, the **thoracoacromial artery** can be conveniently traced to its origin from the axillary artery (*Atlas,* 6.6, 6.22). Note that the thoracoacromial artery has several branches: a pectoral branch to the pectoralis major and minor, a deltoid, a clavicular, and an acromical branch. Lateral to the pectoralis minor identify the **lateral thoracic artery.** To obtain a clearer view of this vessel, free it from surrounding fat. Remove small veins. Trace the cephalic vein to the axillary vein. Do *not* disturb or destroy the contents of the axilla.

Intercostal Muscles (*Atlas,* 1.15, 1.18). Define the **external intercostal muscles** that run obliquely in an anterior-inferior direction between the adjacent borders of two ribs. Note that the muscles do not extend forward beyond the ends of the bony ribs. More anteriorly, the muscles are replaced by the **external intercostal membrane.** Incise this membrane at the 4th intercostal space (ICS 4), i.e.,

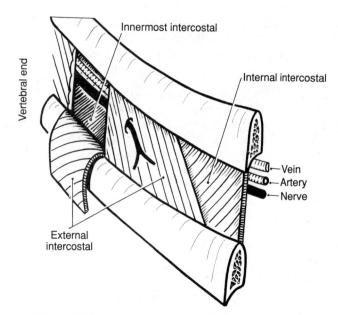

Figure 1.10. Intercostal space and related structures.

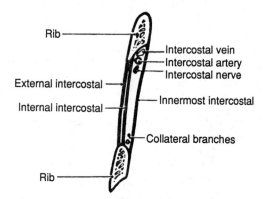

Figure 1.11. Intercostal space on coronal section: intercostal muscles; intercostal nerve; intercostal vessels.

the space between ribs 4 and 5. Insert the flat handle of the knife or forceps deep to the membrane. Push the handle along ICS 4 into the areolar tissue deep to the external intercostal muscle. With the handle as a guide, cut the muscle from the rib above and turn it inferiorly (Fig. 1.10). Follow the external intercostal muscle laterally until you reach the digitations of the serratus anterior. Observe the external intercostal becoming progressively thicker posteriorly.

The fibers of the **internal intercostal muscles** run at right angles to the external intercostal fibers (*Atlas*, 1.15, 1.18). The internal intercostals extend from the most anterior portion of the intercostal space laterally as far as the angles of the ribs. In ICS 4, carefully detach the internal intercostal from the inferior margin of rib 5 and reflect it superiorly. Now, with the aid of a probe, locate the 4th intercostal nerve just inferior to rib 4 (Figs. 1.10, 1.11). Subsequently, identify the intercostal vessels. (The innermost intercostal muscles are posteriorly located and do not reach as far anterior as the external intercostals; Fig. 1.12. They will be seen later).

Remove, additionally, the intercostal muscles from ICS 1 through 5. Resect the muscles as far as the posterior axillary line, elevating the digitations of the serratus anterior. Be careful not to damage the subjacent costal pleura.

About 1 cm from the margin of the sternum, notice the **internal thoracic** (internal mammary) **vessels** (*Atlas*, 1.15). Realize that these vessels are attached to the anterior thoracic wall by numerous fine arterial branches, venous tributaries, and by muscle slips of the **transversus thoracis** (Fig. 1.12; *Atlas*, 1.16).

The next objective is to remove the anterior thoracic wall, but to leave the internal thoracic vessels behind and intact. You must really understand the anatomy of the anterior chest wall before carrying out this procedure (*Atlas*, 1.15, 1.16). Great care must be taken, or the internal thoracic vessels will be inadvertently destroyed. Proceed as follows: on both sides of the cadaver, free ribs 2 to 5 from the subjacent pleura. Use your fingers or a blunt instrument. The pleura must be moist. If it is not, moisten it. Gently tear the transversus thoracis from the internal surface of the ribs so that the internal thoracic vessels may be freed. Next, with a small hand saw, cut ribs 2 through 5 at a right angle to each rib in the posterior axillary line.

Note: Some instructors prefer to have the ribs cut as far posteriorly as possible (i.e., as close to the table as possible) to allow greater freedom in exploring the thorax. This approach also diminishes the hazard of injury to the dissector's hands and fingers due to sharp edges of ribs. Use a hand saw to prevent splintering of the bones. Some instructors suggest that cloths or paper towels be placed on the jagged edges of the ribs in order to protect the dissectors from injury. Ask your instructor as to the preferred method of rib removal.

Next, cut through the sternum at ICS 5. With a saw, carefully (not too deep!) cut across the manubrium sterni at ICS 1. Now, gently elevate the inferior part of the sternum together with the attached portions of severed ribs. Reflect the anterior chest wall upward and remove it. Store the isolated anterior chest wall for future studies and reference.

In the removed and isolated anterior thoracic wall, examine one of the **sternocostal joints** (*Atlas*, 1.12A). Cut through fine ligaments and the joint capsule, and open the synovial cavity. Understand that slight gliding movements occur in the sternocostal joints during (respiratory) movements of the ribs.

Clean the **internal thoracic artery** (*Atlas*, 1.15, 1.16). Follow the vessels toward the diaphragm. To facilitate dissection, remove the costal cartilage of rib 6. Observe that the internal thoracic artery ends in ICS 6 by dividing into the **superior epigastric artery** (medially located) and the **musculophrenic artery**. Later, the superior epigastric artery will be dissected in the sheath of the rectus abdominis where it anastomoses with the inferior epigastric artery (*Atlas*, 2.6). The musculophrenic artery supplies the lower intercostal muscles and the adjacent part of the diaphragm.

Note: The origin of the internal thoracic artery from the subclavian artery will be displayed after removal of the lungs.

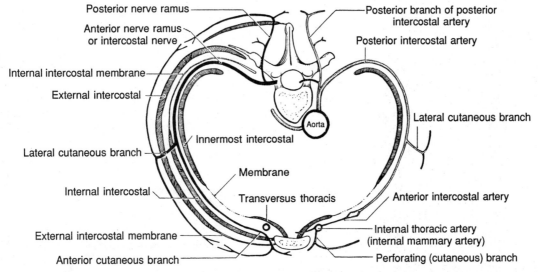

Figure 1.12. Schematic transverse section through thorax. Intercostal muscles, intercostal nerve, and intercostal artery.

Pleural Cavity

General Remarks and Definitions

The thoracic cavity contains two **pleural sacs** and the **mediastinum** (*Atlas*, 1.21A). The mediastinum (L. *quod per medium stat*, which stands in the middle) is the median space between the two pleural cavities. It contains the heart and many other important structures such as the aorta, trachea, and esophagus. The two pleural cavities occupy the lateral parts of the thoracic cavity. During development, the lungs invaginate the pleural cavities (Fig. 1.13 or *Atlas*, 1.21C). Each **lung** is completely covered with a smooth glistening membrane, the **pulmonary or visceral pleura**. Each lung is attached to the mediastinum by an isthmus through which the airways and blood vessels enter or leave the organ. This area of attachment to the mediastinum is known as the **root of the lung**. Here, the visceral pleura is continuous with the parietal pleura that lines the walls of the pleural cavity.

Parietal Pleura (Fig. 1.13; *Atlas*, 1.21B).   The parietal pleura can be subdivided into the following portions: **costal** pleura (lining the rib cage); **mediastinal** pleura (lining the mediastinum); **diaphragmatic** pleura (lining the diaphragm); and **cupola** (cervical pleura, extending into the neck).

The lines along which costal pleura becomes diaphragmatic and mediastinal are known as **pleural reflections** (see Fig. 1.15). At *three sites*, these reflections are so acute that the two portions of the parietal pleura are not only continuous but also *in actual contact with one another* by their inner or serous surfaces. No lung tissue with its visceral pleura intervenes between the apposing pleural layers. These sites of reflections of parietal pleura are known as **pleural recesses** (Figs. 1.14, 1.15). The **right and left costodiaphragmatic recesses** are found at the most infe-

rior limits of the parietal pleura. Here the diaphragm lies so close to the costal wall as to bring costal and diaphragmatic surfaces of the parietal pleura into apposition. During ordinary inspiration, the thin inferior margin of the lung does not extend into the costodiaphragmatic recess. The **costomediastinal recess** is defined as the parietal pleural reflection from the anterior portion of the thoracic wall to the mediastinum. Rib cage and parietal pleura are separated from each other by a small amount of loose connective tissue which provides a cleavage plane for surgical (and other manipulative) separation of the pleura from the thoracic wall. This tissue plane is known as the **endothoracic fascia** (Fig. 1.15).

Understand that the two pleural cavities are two separate and closed *potential spaces*. Normally, there is only a small amount of serous lubricating fluid in the pleural cavity. This substance reduces friction between parietal and visceral pleura during respiratory movements.

Under pathological conditions, the *potential space* of the pleural cavity may become a real one. If air is allowed to enter the pleural cavity (pneumothorax), the lung collapses due to its elasticity (compare Fig. 1.13). If blood is accumulated in the pleural cavity, we speak of "hemothorax."

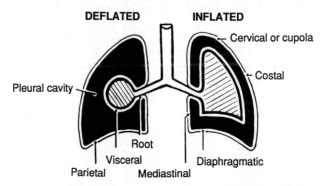

Figure 1.13. Schema of pleural membranes (pleurae) and pleural cavity.

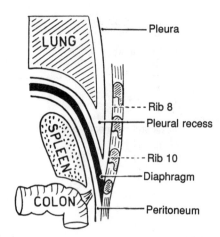

Figure 1.14. Left costodiaphragmatic pleural recess.

> Pleurisy is an inflammation of the pleurae. It usually leads to the formation of pleural adhesions between parietal and visceral pleura. You may encounter such adhesions in the cadaver. These adhesions must be broken down before the lung can be completely mobilized.
>
> The parietal pleura, particularly the costal pleura, is exquisitely pain sensitive. In contrast, the visceral pleura is not sensitive to pain. This fact has obvious clinical implications.

Before you begin . . .

The right and left pleural cavities must be explored. This should be done both before and after removal of the lungs. Subsequently, the right and left sides of the mediastinum will be examined, and nerves and vessels related to the posterior thoracic wall will be dissected.

Dissection

Incise both pleural sacs (if not already damaged), and place your hand into the **pleural cavity**. Palpate the root of the lung. Verify that it is attached to the mediastinum. All other portions of the lung are free within the pleural cavity. However, you may encounter pleural adhesions in various places as a result of old pleurisy. Sever these adhesions with your fingers. Explore with your hand the various parts of the **parietal pleura: costal, diaphragmatic, mediastinal, and cupola**. Place your fingers into the **costomediastinal recess**. Find it on the left side in the region where the heart lies close to the anterior thoracic wall. Palpate the extensive and deep **right and left costodiaphragmatic recesses**. In addition, study the three recesses in a suitable transverse section (*Atlas*, 1.45).

Study the lungs *in situ* (*Atlas*, 1.28). Observe the **oblique fissure** in both lungs. Identify the **horizontal fissure** of the right lung. Note that the right lung has three **lobes** (*superior, middle, and inferior*) whereas the left lung has two lobes (*superior and inferior*). Identify the still closed pericardial sac that contains the heart and that is part of the classic middle mediastinum.

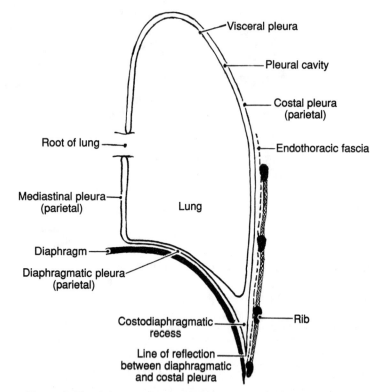

Figure 1.15. Schema of parietal pleura, line of pleural reflection, recess, and pleural cavity. At the root of the lung, the parietal pleura is continuous with the visceral pleura. The costal parietal pleura is separated from the thoracic wall by endothoracic fascia.

Root of Lung. The mediastinal pleura becomes visceral pleura at the root of the lung. The connecting portion between parietal and visceral pleurae is a tube or sleeve of pleura. In its *upper half* lie all the structures that pass from and to the lung (*Atlas*, 1.31, 1.32). This is the actual **root** of the lung. The *lower half* of the sleeve is empty (except for a few lymph vessels). It is collapsed and known as the **pulmonary ligament** (*Atlas*, 1.31, 1.32). This ligament reaches caudally nearly to the diaphragm. It is difficult to see or to palpate at this time.

Removal of Lung. Remember that the phrenic nerves pass anterior to the roots of the lungs whereas the vagus nerves course posteriorly. These nerves must **not** be damaged during removal of the lungs. Identify these nerves and then proceed as follows: Place your hand into the pleural cavity between lung and mediastinum. With one hand push the lung laterally, thereby stretching and exposing the root of the lung. With a scalpel in the other hand, carefully transect the root in the middle between lung and mediastinum. Take care *not* to cut into the mediastinum. Remove both lungs and store them for future studies, using the storage method required by your instructor. In many cases, a plastic bag is convenient for this purpose.

Pleural Cavity and Reflections. Explore again the extent of the **costodiaphragmatic recess**. Push your fingers deep into it. In the midaxillary line, identify ICS 9. Pass a probe or needle horizontally through the thoracic wall at ICS 9. The probe should appear in the costodiaphragmatic recess, close to the line of reflection between costal and di-

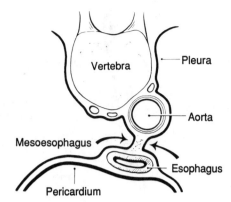

Figure 1.16. Mediastinal layers of pleura forming a "mesoesophagus."

aphragmatic pleurae (see Fig. 1.14). Review the extent of the pleura (*Atlas*, 1.25, 1.26).

Follow the right and left layers of the **mediastinal pleura** dorsally. Posterior to the pericardial sac, they pass to the sides of the esophagus. Posterior to the esophagus, the two layers come together (Fig. 1.16) to form a "mesoesophagus." This structure passes posteriorly to the descending aorta where the two layers separate to reach the sides of the vertebral bodies. Subsequently, each layer becomes costal pleura. Verify these facts. Place one hand in each pleural cavity and bring the fingertips together posterior to the inferior portion of the esophagus (Fig. 1.16).

Note that certain structures are conspicuous through the mediastinal pleura. With the pleura intact, identify on the *right side* (*Atlas*, 1.43): superior vena cava; azygos vein and tributaries; phrenic nerve running anterior to root of lung; sympathetic trunk; and intercostal nerves and vessels. The esophagus is subpleural except where it is crossed by the arch of the azygos vein. Superior to this venous arch, palpate the elastic trachea. It lies anterior to the esophagus. On the *left side* identify (*Atlas*, 1.44): large bulge of heart; phrenic nerve; aortic arch; descending aorta; sympathetic trunk; and intercostal nerves and vessels. The esophagus is subpleural at both ends: (a) above the aortic arch; and (b) just before it pierces the diaphragm.

Removal of Costal and Mediastinal Pleura. Peel off the parietal pleura from the rib cage, starting at the level of the

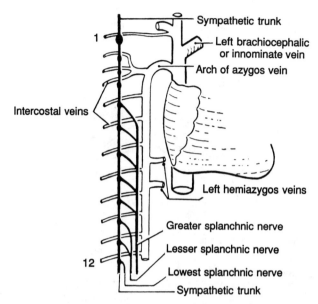

Figure 1.17. Schema of right sympathetic trunk and splanchnic nerves.

cut ribs 2 to 5. Realize that the **endothoracic fascia** provides a natural cleavage plane for manipulative separation of pleura from the adjacent thoracic wall. Next, gently remove the pleura where it covers the vertebral column, aorta, esophagus, and pericardium (Fig. 1.16). Be careful not to injure the **phrenic nerve**. This nerve is positioned between mediastinal pleura and pericardium about 1.5 cm anterior to the root of the lung (*Atlas*, 1.43, 1.44).

With the pleura removed, demonstrate the following structures (*Atlas*, 1.43, 1.44): the **phrenic nerve**, which is immediately subpleural throughout its course in the thorax. Superior to the cupola, identify the **subclavian artery**, and trace the **internal thoracic artery** to it. Observe a long and slender branch of the internal thoracic artery, the **pericardiacophrenic artery**. This artery accompanies the phrenic nerve toward the diaphragm. Clean one intercostal nerve, artery, and vein.

Sympathetic Trunk (Fig. 1.17; *Atlas*, 1.43, 1.44, 1.83). It is bilateral. Find it on the neck of rib 1. Follow it inferiorly. It crosses successively the heads of ribs 2 to 9. Subsequently, it lies on the sides of the lower thoracic vertebrae. Note that the sympathetic trunk has a series of swellings, the **sympathetic ganglia**, one for each segment. Find the following branches:

1. **Rami communicantes.** At each segment, a **white ramus communicans** (preganglionic) passes from intercostal (spinal) nerve to sympathetic ganglion. A **gray ramus communicans** (postganglionic) passes from sympathetic ganglion to intercostal nerve. You may not be able to distinguish white from gray rami. However, demonstrate the fact that *two rami communicate* with each intercostal nerve and its corresponding sympathetic ganglion. Understand the functional significance of these rami (*left half* of Fig. 1.18).

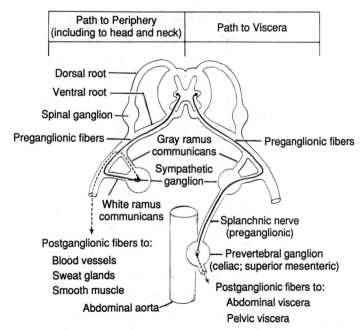

Path to Periphery (including to head and neck)	Path to Viscera

Figure 1.18. General plan of sympathetic nerve distribution.

2. **Splanchnic nerves.** Identify the largest of the three splanchnic nerves, the **greater splanchnic nerve.** Demonstrate that it receives contributions from several sympathetic ganglia (Fig. 1.17). The nerve carries preganglionic sympathetic fibers to the abdomen. Understand the functional significance of the splanchnic nerve (*right half* of Fig. 1.18).

Explore the inner aspect of ICS 4. Note that the **innermost intercostal muscles** are posteriorly located and do not reach as far anterior as the external intercostals (*Atlas,* 1.17, 1.19). Observe that the intercostal nerve and vessels are positioned between the planes of intercostal muscles (Fig. 1.19). Review the vascular and nervous structures related to the intercostal space (*Atlas,* 1.20).

Lungs

Refer to the two isolated lungs (*Atlas,* 1.30 through 1.32). Identify the surfaces and borders. The **surfaces** are **costal, medial** (having a mediastinal and vertebral part), and **basal or diaphragmatic.** The **borders** are anterior and inferior. They are thin and sharp. The **apex** of the lung rises as high as the neck of the 1st rib, but not higher. The right lung is shorter but more voluminous than the left. Each lung is divided into a **superior** and an **inferior lobe** by an **oblique fissure.** Identify these lobes and observe that most of the inferior lobe occupies the posterior part of the thoracic cavity while most of the superior lobe occupies the anterior part. The superior lobe of the right lung is further subdivided by a **horizontal fissure,** thereby producing anteriorly a small **middle lobe.** This lobe reaches lateralward only as far as the midaxillary line.

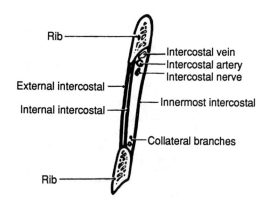

Figure 1.19. Position of intercostal nerve, intercostal artery, and intercostal vein in relation to ribs and intercostal muscles.

In the well-embalmed and hardened lung, **contact impressions** from topographically related structures can be observed. On the mediastinal surface of the *right lung* (*Atlas,* 1.31) identify the **cardiac impression** and the **groove for the esophagus.** On the mediastinal surface of the *left lung* (*Atlas,* 1.32) identify the **cardiac impression** and the continuous **groove for aortic arch and descending aorta.**

Examine the **hilus** of both lungs. Observe the relative positions of **bronchus, pulmonary artery, and pulmonary veins** (*Atlas,* 1.31, 1.32). Generally, the bronchus lies posterior, the artery superior, and the veins inferior. The **right superior bronchus** has a special location. It is higher than any other bronchus, and even higher than the pulmonary artery (Fig. 1.20 or *Atlas,* 1.35). Therefore, this bronchus has also been named "eparterial bronchus." The **pulmonary trunk** and its branches can be demonstrated radiographically in the living person by injecting contrast material into the right side of the heart (*Atlas,* 1.36). In this manner, radiographically visible branches of the pulmonary arteries can be followed into individual pulmonary segments.

There are additional structures at the hilus: bronchial arteries that are nutrient vessels for the lung tissue; lymph nodes and lymph vessels; autonomic nerve fibers. Be aware of these structures, but do not make a special effort to dissect them.

Dissection

The fat-free lung tissue is readily forced apart with the blunt ends of two pairs of forceps. Use this technique. Identify the **main bronchus.** If the root of the lung was cut close to the lung tissue, the main bronchus was left behind in the mediastinum. In this case, only the subsidiary bronchi can be seen at the hilus. In the *left lung,* identify the **superior (upper) and inferior (lower) lobar bronchi** (Fig. 1.20; *Atlas,* 1.37). In the *right lung,* identify the **superior, middle, and inferior bronchi.**

Next, identify the **segmental bronchi** (*Atlas,* 1.37, 1.39, 1.40). Verify by palpation that they contain pieces of cartilage. Pass a probe into each segmental bronchus. Follow each structure for 2 to 3 cm into the lung tissue. Remove

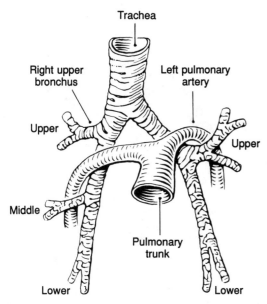

Figure 1.20. Topographic relations of pulmonary arteries and bronchi.

These vessels are distributed together with the bronchial tree. Bronchioles and arterioles are intrasegmental. In contrast, the tributaries to the pulmonary veins lie at the periphery of any pulmonary unit, e.g., at the periphery of a segment; i.e., they are intersegmental (*Atlas*, 1.33). The pulmonary veins carry oxygenated blood.

Realize that the lungs have a rich nerve supply via the anterior and posterior pulmonary plexuses (*Atlas*, 1.41). Sympathetic contributions are received from the right and left sympathetic trunks, while parasympathetic contributions are received from the right and left vagus. Note and verify that branches of these nerves are applied to bronchi and pulmonary vessels on their way to every part of the lungs.

Knowledge of the segmental bronchial distribution is a necessary prerequisite for pulmonary radiology, surgery, and medicine. Frequently, a specific diseased segment is identified and surgically removed.

Obstruction of a bronchus prevents proper ventilation to the lung peripheral to the obstruction. The air trapped peripherally is absorbed slowly with time, resulting in volume loss of the concerned lung tissue (atelectasis; collapse).

The trachea and bronchi (tracheobronchial tree) can be visualized by endoscopic examination using a flexible bronchofiberscope. Thus, endobronchial inflammatory processes, tumors, or aspirated foreign bodies can be visualized and photographed. In the management of pulmonary diseases, fiberoptic bronchoscopy may be combined with lavage of individual bronchi. The concerned bronchus is irrigated with saline. Subsequently, thick mucus plugs or inspissated bronchial secretions can be suctioned and removed. As a result, the corresponding pulmonary segment receives better ventilation.

The bronchial tree can also be demonstrated radiographically by injecting contrast material into the various parts of the air passages (*Atlas*, 1.38).

intervening (black) lymph nodes. Cut away some lung tissue near the hilus. Identify:

Right Lung (*Atlas*, 1.37):

Superior lobe
 1. apical
 2. posterior
 3. anterior
Middle lobe
 4. lateral
 5. medial
Inferior lobe
 6. superior
 7. medial basal
 8. anterior basal
 9. lateral basal
 10. posterior basal

Left Lung (*Atlas*, 1.37):

Superior lobe
 1. + 2. apical-posterior
 3. anterior
 4. superior lingular
 5. inferior lingular
Inferior lobe
 6. superior
 7. + 8. anterior-medial basal
 9. lateral basal
 10. posterior basal

Select one segmental bronchus. Open it with a pair of scissors, and follow it and its ramifications far into the lung tissue. Identify the **pulmonary artery** and its branches (*Atlas*, 1.34) which carry deoxygenated blood.

Mediastinum

Definitions and Subdivisions

The median region between the two pleural sacs is the mediastinum (*Atlas*, 1.21A). It extends from the superior aperture of the thorax to the diaphragm, and from the sternum to the bodies of the 12 thoracic vertebrae. Purely for descriptive purposes, this extensive region is arbitrarily subdivided into subsidiary parts (Fig. 1.21).

A horizontal plane at the level of the sternal angle cuts the intervertebral disc between thoracic vertebrae 4 and 5. Above this imaginary plane lies the superior mediastinum (S in Fig. 1.21). This plane is especially convenient since it indicates the level of the superior border of the fibrous pericardium and the level of the bifurcation of the trachea, i.e., the superior border of the root of the lung.

The remaining portion of the mediastinum (inferior to the superior mediastinum) is divided into three parts: (a) **anterior mediastinum** (A in Fig. 1.21), the small and relatively unimportant portion between sternum and pericardium; (b) **middle mediastinum** (M in Fig. 1.21), contain-

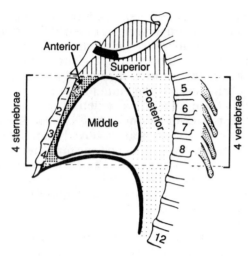

Figure 1.21. The four classic anatomical subdivisions of the mediastinum.

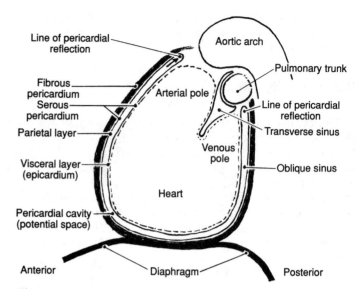

Figure 1.22. Schema of pericardium and heart in sagittal section. Pulmonary trunk (with subsequent bifurcation into right and left pulmonary arteries).

ing the pericardium with the enclosed heart and the roots of the great vessels; (c) **posterior mediastinum** (*P* in Fig. 1.21), the portion posterior to the pericardium and anterior to the bodies of the lower 8 thoracic vertebrae. Certain structures traversing the length of the mediastinum (e.g., esophagus, vagus, phrenic nerve, thoracic duct) lie, of course, in more than one mediastinal subdivision.

The foregoing definition of the divisions of the mediastinum is the classic anatomical description. However, clinicians often use a more simple and pragmatic description in an attempt to aid in differential diagnosis. For example, the noted radiologist Benjamin Felson finds the divisions of the mediastinum, as defined by the great anatomists, not suitable for roentgen diagnosis of mediastinal lesions. Therefore, he uses radiographic subdivisions as follows: The 'anterior' and 'middle' mediastinum are divided by the line extending along the posterior aspect of the heart and anterior to the trachea. The 'middle' and 'posterior' mediastinal compartments are separated by the line connecting a point on each thoracic vertebra about a centimeter behind its anterior margin. Using these pragmatic subdivisions, the 'anterior' mediastinum contains the classic anterior and middle mediastinal compartments. The 'posterior' mediastinum delineates the thoracic paravertebral space with its characteristic neurogenic lesions. The 'middle' mediastinum is the area between the 'anterior' and 'posterior' mediastinum. It includes all the longitudinal structures with their characteristic pathological lesions. The classic anatomical term "superior mediastinum" becomes superfluous. Unfortunately, the medical profession does not use a consistent definition for subdivisions of the mediastinum. The student should be aware of these circumstances and be ready to adapt to different definitions later in the clinical years. At this time, and during this gross anatomy course, the student will use and be responsible for the **classic anatomical descriptions of the mediastinum.**

It must be stressed that, in the living person, the mediastinum is a highly mobile region. Observe the loose fat and areolar tissue of the mediastinum. Recognize that it is perfectly suited to accommodate movements and volume changes in the thoracic cavity (e.g., movements of trachea during respiration; pulsations of great vessels; volume changes of esophagus).

Radiologists and clinicians are often confronted with a "widening of the mediastinum" seen on a chest film. Conceptually, any structure located in the mediastinum can contribute to this pathological widening. Often it is seen after trauma resulting in hemor-

rhage into the mediastinum from one or more lacerated great vessels (e.g. aorta or superior vena cava). Commonly, lymphoma leads to vast enlargement of lymph nodes in the mediastinum with resulting widening. Tumors of the esophagus or of the thymus as well as inflammatory processes in the mediastinum can lead to a "widening of the mediastinum." A thorough knowledge of the mediastinum and its contents is a prerequisite for a logical diagnostic approach.

Middle Mediastinum

The **middle mediastinum** contains the pericardium (with adjacent phrenic nerves), the **heart,** and the roots of the great vessels passing to and from the heart. The **pericardium** or pericardial sac (Fig. 1.22; *Atlas,* 1.29, 1.60A) is a sac enclosing the heart and pierced by the roots of eight vessels (two arteries, two caval veins, four pulmonary veins). Its outer surface, now fully exposed, is fibrous, tough, and it appears dull. Refer to Figure 1.22 and understand the following:

1. The inferior part of the tough, fibrous pericardium is densely attached to the tendinous part of the diaphragm. Thus, the function of the heart is influenced by diaphragmatic movements.
2. The inner surface of the fibrous pericardium is covered with the *parietal layer* of smooth, **serous pericardium.**
3. At the roots of the eight great vessels connecting to the heart, the serous pericardium is reflected onto the heart as the *visceral layer* of **serous pericardium.** This smooth visceral layer is also known as **epicardium.**
4. Between the opposing surfaces of parietal and visceral layers of serous pericardium is a potential space, the **pericardial cavity.**
5. The transverse sinus is a transversely running passageway between venous and arterial poles of the heart.

6. Posteriorly, the oblique sinus is a blind recess of the pericardial cavity between pulmonary veins and inferior vena cava.

Before you begin . . .

The pericardial sac must be opened to provide access to the heart. After manual exploration of the pericardial cavity and its two sinuses, the heart should be skillfully detached from its eight great vessels. Subsequently, the isolated heart can be dissected. However, prior to removal of the heart, the student is encouraged to examine as much as possible the vascular connections to the heart and the three-dimensional relationships between heart and major vessels. This should be done in the beginning of the next section.

Inspection of Great Vessels and Related Structures

Prior to opening of the pericardial sac, identify the **superior vena cava**, the **aortic arch**, and the **pulmonary trunk or artery** (*Atlas*, 1.43, 1.44). Gently probe in the interval between aortic arch and pulmonary trunk and identify the **ligamentum arteriosum.** This structure passes from the root of the left pulmonary artery to the arch of the aorta. With a probe, identify the left vagus nerve and also a small initial portion of one its important branches: the left recurrent laryngeal nerve, passing inferior to the aortic arch and just lateral and posterior to the ligamentum arteriosum. The right pulmonary artery is difficult to trace at this time; however, be aware that it passes inferior to the aortic arch on its way to the right lung. Make sure that the previously described structures are not disturbed during the removal of the heart from the pericardial sac.

The Pericardial Sac: Opening, Inspection, and Manual Exploration

With a pair of forceps, pinch up a fold of the pericardial sac where it overlies the right atrium. With scissors nick the fold and enter the pericardial cavity. Open the pericardial sac widely. Remove the entire anterior portion of the pericardial sac to ensure sufficient access to the heart. Sponge the interior of the pericardial sac with water.

Examine the **pericardium.** Notice the contrast between the outer, rough and dull **fibrous pericardium** and the inner *parietal layer* of smooth, glistening, **serous pericardium.** Observe that the smooth *visceral layer* of pericardium, the **epicardium,** intimately invests the heart.

Establish the extent of the **pericardial cavity.** Push a probe anterior to the ascending aorta to the superior limit of the cavity (*arrow* in Fig. 1.22). Establish that the superior limit corresponds approximately to the level of the sternal angle (i.e., where the second costal cartilage is attached to the sternum; *Atlas*, 1.49, 1.50).

With your fingers, explore the lines of reflection from the visceral to the parietal pericardium (*Atlas*, 1.61 illustrates these lines of reflection). With the heart still in the pericardial cavity, insinuate your *left* index finger between the superior vena cava and ascending aorta. Then, push the finger posterior to the pulmonary artery. Now, your finger lies in a serous-lined tunnel known as the **transverse pericardial sinus.** Leave your finger in the sinus. Next, with your *right* hand, lift up the apex of the heart and push two fingers posterior to the heart into the **oblique pericardial sinus** (*Atlas*, 1.61). It is a serous-lined cul-de-sac bounded on the right by (a) the inferior vena cava; and (b) the right inferior and superior pulmonary veins. On the left, the sinus is bounded by (a) the left inferior pulmonary vein; and (b) the left superior pulmonary vein. Palpate and observe that your right and left fingers are separated by (two layers of) serous pericardium.

Review the projection of the heart on the anterior chest wall (Fig. 1.6; *Atlas*, 1.47). Study the surfaces of the heart in situ (*Atlas*, 1.50): Note that the **right ventricle** makes up the largest part of the anterior surface of the heart. The **right border** consists of the **right atrium.** The **left border** is formed by the **left ventricle,** which is responsible for the **apex** of the heart. At the superior end of the left border, the **auricle of the left atrium** can be seen. The **inferior border** belongs to the **right ventricle,** except for a small portion on the extreme left that belongs to the left ventricle. Correlate these observations with a radiograph of the chest (*Atlas*, 1.24).

The pericardium and the pericardial sac can be involved in many disease processes. Certain inflammatory diseases can produce a "pericardial effusion" in which significant amounts of inflammatory fluids are accumulated in the pericardial sac. As a result, the heart becomes compressed and ineffective. A chronically inflamed and thickened pericardium may actually calcify and seriously hamper cardiac efficiency. Noninflammatory pericardial effusions commonly occur in congestive heart failure.

Bleeding into the pericardial sac or "hemopericardium" is commonly associated with penetrating heart wounds or perforation of a weakened heart muscle following myocardial infarction. Arterial bleeding into the tough, fibrous and non-extensible pericardial sac leads to compression of the encased heart and the roots of the great vessels associated with the heart. This potentially lethal condition is known as "cardiac tamponade."

In patients with pneumothorax, air under pressure may dissect along connective tissue lines into the pericardial sac, producing a "pneumopericardium." This condition is particularly serious in newborns. Pneumopericardium can be demonstrated radiographically.

On a congenital basis, the pericardium may be partially or totally absent.

Removal of Heart

Removal of the Heart. The eight great vessels must be severed, but the posterior wall of the pericardial sac should be left intact (*Atlas*, 1.61). Again, identify the transverse pericardial sinus. Mark it by placing a pencil or probe through it. Then cut across the **ascending aorta** and the

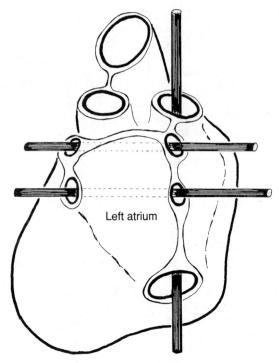

Figure 1.23. Posterior aspect of heart in anatomical position. *Horizontal rods* pass through left atrium. *Vertical rod* passes through right atrium.

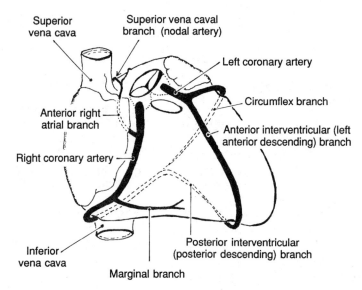

Figure 1.24. Coronary arteries.

pulmonary trunk. Next, cut the **inferior vena cava** as low as possible within the pericardial sac. Then transect the **superior vena cava** about 1 cm superior to its junction with the right atrium. Lift the heart anteriorly and superior by its apex. Then, cut across the **four pulmonary veins** where they bound the oblique sinus. Careful! Cut the pulmonary veins very close to the pericardial sac, or you will injure the left atrium. Now, the heart is held in place merely by the two layers of pericardium that separate the oblique from the transverse sinus. Incise these two layers and remove the heart. Examine the excised heart and identify the transverse pericardial sinus, curving posterior to the enclosed stems of the aorta and pulmonary trunk (*Atlas*, 1.67). Next, examine the posterior aspect of the pericardial sac. The field of dissection should compare with *Atlas*, 1.61.

Note: For instructive purposes, the heart can be conveniently placed back into the pericardial sac. This should be done whenever clarification of anatomical orientation and position is required (e.g., *anterior* or *posterior* papillary muscle; *plane* of base of heart, or *plane* of interventricular septum). Hold the isolated heart in your hand. Look at its posterior aspect (*Atlas*, 1.60B), and identify key structures. Hold it in its anatomical position in reference to your own chest. Use the roots of the pulmonary veins and of the venae cavae as reference structures. Pass two pencils or probes through the openings of the pulmonary veins in the left atrium, as indicated in Figure 1.23. Pass one probe from the superior vena cava through the right atrium into the inferior vena cava (Fig. 1.23). In the anatomical position, the probes through the venae cavae are in a vertical position, whereas the probes through the pulmonary veins are horizontally oriented.

Heart

Identify the **coronary or atrioventricular groove** (*Atlas*, 1.48A and B), a groove that runs obliquely around the heart, separating atria from ventricles. At right angles to the coronary sulcus are the **anterior and posterior interventricular grooves**. These grooves separate the ventricles from one another and, therefore, denote the position of the interventricular septum (see Fig. 1.28). The sulci contain blood vessels.

Cardiac Vessels. When dissecting the vessels, it will be necessary to remove piecemeal the epicardium and fat. Remove only enough fat to visualize the course of the vessels. Do not remove the cardiac veins as you clean the arteries. Using blunt forceps, begin with the two **coronary arteries** that originate from the **ascending aorta**. Before dissection, it is most helpful to identify the lumen of each coronary artery in the following manner: look into the aorta and identify the three aortic valvules (*Atlas*, 1.67). Find the orifice of the left coronary artery just superior to the left aortic valvule. Insert a probe into the coronary orifice. Palpate the tip of the probe between the left auricle and the pulmonary trunk. Similarly, insert a probe into the opening of the right coronary artery just superior to the right aortic valvule. Palpate the tip of the probe just to the left (anatomical position!) of the right auricle. On leaving the ascending aorta, the two coronary arteries pass anteriorly, one on each side of the root of the pulmonary trunk (Fig. 1.24; *Atlas*, 1.51).

Follow the **left coronary artery**. Between the left auricle and the pulmonary trunk, it divides into an **anterior interventricular branch** and a **circumflex branch**. The anterior interventricular branch follows the anterior interventricular groove (sulcus) to or beyond the apex. Clinicians refer to this vessel often as the *LAD*, meaning *left anterior descending* (Fig. 1.24). The circumflex branch follows the

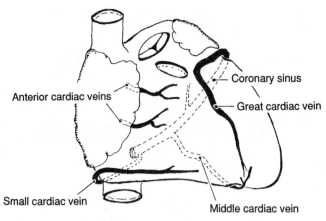

Figure 1.25. Cardiac veins.

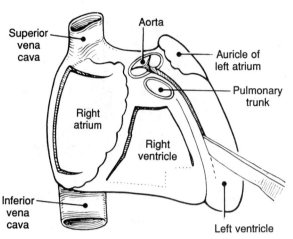

Figure 1.26. Incisions for opening right atrium and both ventricles.

coronary groove (sulcus) around the left border to the posterior surface of the heart.

Now, trace the **right coronary artery** (Fig. 1.24; *Atlas,* 1.51). It follows the coronary groove to the right border and then onto the diaphragmatic surface of the heart. Usually, it reaches the posterior interventricular groove (sulcus) in which it descends toward the apex as the **posterior interventricular branch** (posterior descending; *PDA*). At the right border of the heart, identify the usually large **marginal branch**. Follow it along the acute margin to the apex. Identify the functionally important **anterior right atrial branch** of the right coronary artery (Fig. 1.24). This branch arises close to the origin of the right coronary artery and ascends along the anteromedial wall of the right atrium. To appreciate its course, you may have to mobilize and reflect slightly the right auricle.

Locate a small but important branch of the anterior right atrial artery. Find this branch to the left and posterior to the entrance of the superior vena cava into the right atrium. This is the **superior vena caval branch**, also known as **nodal artery or sinus node artery** (Fig. 1.24). It supplies the important sinuatrial (S-A) node, which is the "pacemaker" of the heart and determines the heart rate. Occlusion of the nodal artery will lead to failure of the sinus node (sinus arrest; sinus block; cardiac arrhythmia). The nodal artery can be demonstrated radiographically with selective coronary arteriography.

Expect to find variations of the arteries and their branching patterns. These are common (*Atlas,* 1.54). In about two-thirds of the cases, the right coronary artery is dominant, i.e. posteriorly it crosses to the left side to supply the left ventricular wall and ventricular septum. The left coronary artery, in addition to supplying all of the left ventricle and ventricular septum, may send branches posteriorly to the right ventricular wall (left coronary artery dominance, about 15%). In about one-fifth of the cases, the coronary arterial pattern is balanced. The fields of distribution of the coronary arteries can be demonstrated radiographically with selective coronary arteriography (*Atlas,* 1.53). The ascending aorta and its related structures (cusps of aortic valve; coronary arteries; aortic arch) can be visualized radiographically by injecting contrast material into the root of the ascending aorta (aortic root angiogram; see Atlas, 1.52).

Cardiac Veins (Fig. 1.25; *Atlas,* 1.55). Most veins of the heart are tributaries of the **coronary sinus**. The coronary sinus is a sizable venous channel that lies in the posterior part of the coronary sulcus. The coronary sinus is about 2 to 2.5 cm in length. It empties into the right atrium. There are numerous tributaries of the coronary sinus. Identify the following two important **tributaries:**

1. **Great cardiac vein**. It begins at the apex and ascends in the anterior interventricular groove. In the coronary groove, it turns to the left and is continuous with the coronary sinus.
2. **Middle cardiac vein**. It ascends in the posterior interventricular groove and ends in the coronary sinus.

One or two **anterior cardiac veins** run from the anterior aspect of the right ventricle across the coronary sulcus to open directly into the right atrium.

Right Atrium.   Open the right atrium in the following manner (Fig. 1.26). Make a short cut through the tip of the right auricle. Next, cut with scissors through the atrial wall from the initial incision toward the inferior vena cava. Then, cut horizontally superior to the inferior vena cava, almost to the coronary groove. Turn the flap of the atrial wall, and open the right atrium widely. Remove blood clots, and wash area thoroughly with cold water. Observe the following features (Fig. 1.27; *Atlas,* 1.63A).

1. A smooth posterior atrial wall (*Note:* "posterior" in reference to the anatomical position of the heart);
2. A rough anterior atrial wall; it has comb-like parallel ridges, the **pectinate muscles**;
3. Posterior and anterior walls are separated by a vertical ridge, the **crista terminalis**;
4. The smooth posterior part receives the following veins: **superior vena cava, inferior vena cava, and coronary sinus;**
5. Remnant of the **valve of the inferior vena cava** (nonfunctional).
6. **Valve of coronary sinus;** it guards the opening of the coronary sinus that empties into the right atrium be-

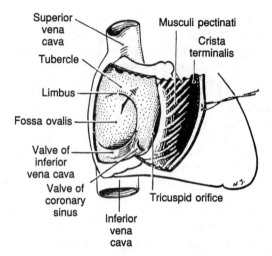

Figure 1.27. Interior of right atrium.

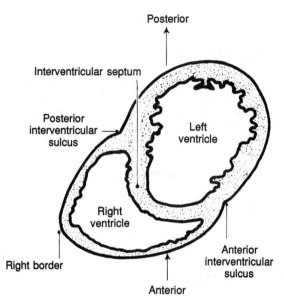

Figure 1.28. Horizontal section through right and left ventricles. *Arrows* indicate sagittal plane.

tween the opening of the inferior vena cava and the atrioventricular orifice;

7. The large **atrioventricular or tricuspid orifice**, leading forward to the right ventricle;

8. **Fossa ovalis**, an oval depression of the interatrial wall; it is the remnant of the fetal foramen ovale. In regard to the fetal circulation, it is significant that the blood flow from the inferior cava is directed toward the fossa ovalis, while blood from the superior part of the body via the superior vena cava is directed toward the tricuspid orifice (*Atlas*, 1.63**B**).

Parts of the important specialized **conduction (or conducting) system** of the heart are topographically related to the right atrium. These structures are too small to be visible in gross dissection. However, in view of their functional importance, familiarize yourself with their approximate locations. Point a probe to the vicinity of two important parts of the conduction system (*Atlas*, 1.69):

1. **Sinuatrial node** (S-A node). It lies in the crista terminalis at the junction between right atrium and superior vena cava. It is supplied by the nodal artery.

2. **Atrioventricular node** (A-V node). It lies in the lower part of the interatrial septum, near the coronary sinus opening.

Right Ventricle. Open the right ventricle in the following manner (Fig. 1.26): Pass a blunt instrument or your little finger into the pulmonary trunk (artery). Determine the level of the pulmonary valves. Make a short transverse incision into the right ventricular wall inferior to the level of the pulmonary valves. Insert your finger through the opening, and guide the scissors for the following cuts: 1 cm away from and parallel to the coronary groove toward the inferior border of the heart. Next, cautiously from the left end of the initial transverse incision, about 2 cm from and parallel to the anterior interventricular groove, toward the inferior border of the heart. Turn the flap of right ventricular wall, and open the chamber widely. Remove blood

clots; however, use considerable care in removing clotted blood to avoid damaging the delicate chordae tendineae. Rinse the right ventricle thoroughly with cold water. Observe the following features (*Atlas*, 1.64):

1. The right ventricle is crescentic on transverse section (Fig. 1.28). The interventricular septum is convex toward this chamber since the pressure is higher on the arterial than on the venous side.

2. The **right atrioventricular orifice**, situated dorsally, is large enough to admit the tips of three (average-sized) fingers.

3. The right atrioventricular orifice is guarded by **three cusps**, hence the name **tricuspid valve**. The cusps are continuous with one another at their bases. Toward the edges, they are disposed as *anterior, septal*, and *posterior*. Small secondary cusps may be present and may obscure the general arrangement.

4. The **chordae tendineae**, tendinous strands that pass from the margins and ventricular surfaces of the cusps into the apices of papillary muscles (the strands are arranged like the cords of a parachute.)

5. **Papillary muscles**. The *anterior* papillary muscle is the largest and most prominent. Its chordae tendineae are attached to the anterior and posterior cusps. The other papillary muscles are much smaller and irregular in disposition. They are designated: *posterior* and *septal*. The septal papillary muscles are very small and multiple. Each papillary muscle controls the adjacent sides of cusps (*Atlas*, 1.64**B**).

6. The interior wall of the right ventricle is roughened by muscular ridges and bridges. These are known as the **trabeculae carneae** (L. *trabs*, wooden beam; *carneus*, fleshy).

7. **Septomarginal trabecula (moderator band)**, stretching from the interventricular septum to the base of the anterior papillary muscle.

8. The **orifice of the pulmonary trunk** (pulmonary orifice). The cone-shaped portion of the chamber inferior to the orifice is the **conus arteriosus or infundibulum**. Within the right ventricle, the blood takes a U-shaped course in passing from the orifice of entrance to the orifice of exit.
9. The **valve of the pulmonary trunk** (pulmonary valve) consists of three semilunar valvules of cusps: an *anterior*, a *right*, and a *left* (*Atlas*, 1.68).

Left Atrium. Open this chamber by means of an inverted U-shaped incision through the posterior wall. Leave the openings of the pulmonary veins intact. Turn the flap inferiorly. Remove blood clots, and wash thoroughly with cold water. Observe the following features:

1. The entrances of the **four pulmonary veins** into the right and left sides of the atrium (compare *Atlas*, 1.48B).
2. The opening of the tubular left auricle.
3. The site of closure of the **foramen ovale**, situated anteriorly and to the right (anatomical position of heart!), and usually defined by a curved ridge.
4. The **left atrioventricular or mitral orifice** opening through the inferior half of the anterior wall into the left ventricle.
5. The atrial wall is smooth, except for small pectinate muscles in the left auricle.
6. Compare the thickness of the right and left atrial walls. The wall of the left atrium is distinctly thicker than that of the right atrium.

Left Ventricle. Open the left ventricle in the following manner (Fig. 1.26): Make a cut 1 cm to the left of and parallel to the anterior interventricular groove. The cut is through a wall about 1 to 1.5 cm in thickness. It should extend from the inferior border of the heart to the root of the aorta. Guide the cut with a finger passed through the left atrioventricular orifice into the left ventricle. Extend the incision along the entire length of the ascending aorta. Carefully cut exactly between the right and left coronary cusps of the aortic valve. During the prescribed cut, the circumflex artery and the great cardiac vein must be severed. Now, open the left ventricle and the length of the ascending aorta widely. Remove blood clots; however, use considerable care in removing clotted blood to avoid damaging the delicate chordae tendineae. Rinse the left ventricle thoroughly with cold water. Observe the following features (*Atlas*, 1.65):

1. The ventricular cavity is cone-shaped in outline and circular on cross section (compare Fig. 1.28).
2. The muscular wall is about 1 to 1.5 cm in thickness, but much thinner at the apex. In the normal (not necessarily in the diseased) heart, the left ventricular wall is about three times as thick as the right one.
3. The **left atrioventricular or mitral orifice.**

4. The **left atrioventricular valve (bicuspid or mitral valve)**, consisting of an *anterior* and a *posterior* cusp. The larger anterior cusp intervenes between the atrioventricular and aortic orifices.
5. **Chordae tendineae**, attached to two papillary muscles, *anterior* and *posterior*.
6. **Trabeculae carneae.**
7. **Aortic valve**, composed of three semilunar cusps: *right coronary*, *left coronary*, and *posterior or noncoronary cusp*. Observe the **nodule**, a small fibrous thickening at the middle of the free margin of each cusp (*Atlas*, 1.66). Probe the orifices of the **two coronary arteries** and study their relation to the two coronary valvules (*Atlas*, 1.68).
8. The thick and extensive **muscular part of the interventricular septum.**
9. The **membranous part of the interventricular septum**, about the size of a fingernail. It is situated just inferior to the attached margins of the right coronary and noncoronary cusps of the aortic valve. Palpate this thin, smooth, and fibrous structure between your index fingers, one in each ventricle.

The thin **membranous interventricular septum** adjoins the atrial septum. During development, the membranous interventricular septum closes last. It may be the site of a congenital defect, the membranous "ventricular septal defect" (VSD). This defect is the most common cardiac defect. It is often seen in combination with other cardiac anomalies.

Once more, review the important **conducting system** of the heart (*Atlas*, 1.69). Realize that the A-V bundle passes from the AV node to the membranous part of the interventricular septum. Subsequently, it divides into **right and left bundle branches** on either side of the muscular part of the interventricular septum. The right bundle branch connects via the septomarginal trabecula to the anterior papillary muscle. Damage to the conducting system results in various forms of cardiac arrhythmias. The dissection of the conducting system is extremely difficult.

Posterior Mediastinum

Posterior Mediastinum. Review the definition of the term "posterior mediastinum" (*P* in Fig. 1.21; *Atlas*, 1.22A). Note that it is that portion of the mediastinum anterior to the bodies of the inferior eight thoracic vertebrae and posterior to and also inferior to the pericardium. Thus, it is logical to approach the structures in the posterior mediastinum through the already opened pericardial sac: remove the posterior wall of the pericardial sac in the area of the oblique sinus (*Atlas*, 1.62). Now, the posterior relations of the heart can be examined. Most anteriorly and slightly to the right is the **esophagus**.

Temporarily, place the heart back into the opened pericardial sac. Examine its topographic relations to the esophagus. Understand why the posterior border of the heart can be best evaluated radiographically when the esophagus is filled with radiopaque material. The esophagus lies immediately posterior to the left atrium and part of the left ventricle. An enlargement of these chambers will indent the barium-filled esophagus and displace it posteriorly.

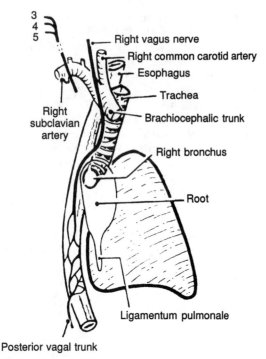

Figure 1.29. Right vagus nerve and its relation to trachea and esophagus.

> Certain heart murmurs in the left atrial area (regurgitant murmurs in mitral valve insufficiency) can be excellently recorded with the aid of a small microphone channelled into the esophagus posterior to the heart.

In the region of the posterior mediastinum, study and clean the **esophagus**, a collapsed muscular tube (*Atlas*, 1.62). Give special attention to the **two vagal nerves** and their relations to the esophagus. Identify and clean the **right vagus** posterior to the root of the right lung (Fig. 1.29; *Atlas*, 1.43). Follow the nerve to the esophagus. Identify the **left vagus** as it crosses the left side of the aortic arch. Use a probe and bluntly dissect the area where the left vagus crosses the arch. Confirm that the concavity of the arch is connected to the left pulmonary artery by a stout, obliquely set cord. This is the **ligamentum arteriosum**. Find and clean an important branch of the left vagus, the **left recurrent laryngeal nerve**, as it courses immediately posterior to the ligamentum arteriosum. Next, trace the left vagus posterior to the root of the left lung, and follow it to the esophagus (*Atlas*, 1.44). Note that the vagal fibers separate and spread out on the esophagus as the **esophageal plexus** (Fig. 1.29; *Atlas*, 1.43). Close to the diaphragm, the bundles of the esophageal plexus combine to form the two **vagal trunks**, an *anterior* and a *posterior* one. Due to the rotation of the gut during development, the bundles from the left vagus swing around to the anterior surface of the esophagus. The bundles from the right vagus come to lie dorsal to the esophagus Identify the vagal trunks as they pass through the diaphragm together with the esophagus.

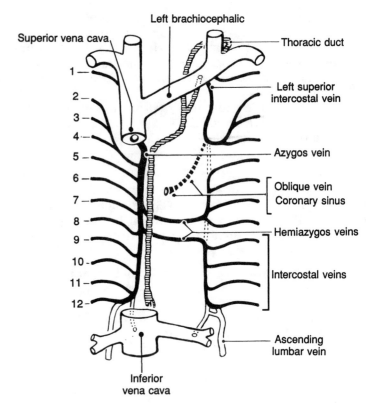

Figure 1.30. Diagram of azygos system of veins. Axiom: In order to arrive in the right or venous side of the heart, blood from the left side of the body must cross the median plane.

Pull the esophagus to the left and expose the **azygos vein.** From its arch, follow it caudally to the diaphragm (*Atlas*, 1.43, 1.83). Study a diagram of the azygos system of veins (Fig. 1.30; *Atlas*, 1.86, 1.87). Note that the intercostal veins on the right side are tributaries to the azygos vein. Observe the cross channels (irregular) bringing blood from the left side via the hemiazygos veins. Variations of the azygos system are very common. Study an azygogram (*Atlas*, 1.84).

Thoracic Duct (*Atlas*, 1.81, 1.83). This is a thin-walled, pale, and easily torn structure found between the azygos vein and the descending aorta. Carefully free this fragile structure from the surrounding fatty areolar tissue. Commonly, the duct may be plexiform in the posterior mediastinum; i.e. you may find a network of several small ducts instead of one large thoracic duct. Observe that the thoracic duct traverses the diaphragm together with the descending aorta (*Atlas* 1.78).

Identify the **descending aorta.** Clean it from the surrounding fatty areolar tissue. Look for its small variable branches to the esophagus and trachea (*Atlas*, 1.80). Identify several of its paired **posterior intercostal branches** (*Atlas*, 1.79). In addition, note at least one of the several **bronchial arteries** as they arise from the descending aorta.

Note: The sympathetic trunks lie posterior to each lung and *not* between the mediastinal pleurae (*Atlas*, 1.43, 1.44). Therefore, the sympathetic trunks are *not* contained in any subdivision of the mediastinum. However, some of its branches, the splanchnic nerves, turn medially and anteriorly and thus become part of the posterior mediastinum. Once more, identify the bilateral **splanchnic nerves** (*Atlas*, 1.83). With a probe, isolate the relatively thick **greater splanchnic nerve**. Note that it receives fibers from the 5th through the 10th thoracic sympathetic ganglia. Next, identify the much smaller **lesser splanchnic nerve** just lateral to the greater splanchnic nerve. The lesser splanchnic nerve is formed by fibers from the 10th and 11th thoracic sympathetic ganglia. Follow both nerves inferiorly. Note that they pierce the crus of the diaphragm. Their course in the abdomen will be explored later. As a variation, the splanchnic nerves are sometimes fused.

Review the classic anterior, middle, and posterior mediastinal subdivisions (*Atlas*, 1.22A). Study a transverse section through the heart and lungs (*Atlas*, 1.22B), and identify the mediastinal subdivisions in this section (*Atlas*, 1.22C). Correlate *Atlas*, 1.26 with a corresponding sagittal magnetic resonance image (MRI) of the chest (*Atlas*, 1.27). In addition, study and identify important anatomical structures in coronal transverse magnetic resonance images of the thorax (*Atlas*, 1.42).

Superior Mediastinum

Review the **boundaries of the superior mediastinum** (S in Fig. 1.21; *Atlas*, 1.22A).

1. Superiorly: superior aperture of thorax (i.e., superior entrance into thorax bounded by manubrium, 1st thoracic vertebra and the two 1st ribs; *Atlas*, 1.8).
2. Posteriorly: thoracic vertebrae 1 through 4.
3. Anteriorly: manubrium of sternum.
4. Laterally: mediastinal pleurae of the two lungs.
5. Inferiorly: a plane from sternal angle to intervertebral disc T4-T5; this plane is just superior to the limit of the pericardium.

The structures in the superior mediastinum can be better seen and explored if the manubrium of the sternum is either retracted or removed. If in doubt, check with your instructor.

Identify the **thymus** (*Atlas*, 1.70). In the adult cadaver, it is represented by a (functionally inactive) fatty mass that lies immediately posterior to the manubrium in the anterior portion of the superior mediastinum. Do not overlook the thymus just because it resembles fat. Observe that the arteries supplying the thymus are (in part) derived from the internal thoracic arteries. In the newborn, the thymus is a broad, lobulated, active structure that can be readily visualized on a routine chest radiograph. In the infant and child, the thymus is a prominent, active organ of glandular texture. After puberty, the organ undergoes involution, and it may be scarcely recognizable in old age.

Remove the thymus but do not damage the left brachiocephalic vein that lies posterior to it (*Atlas*, 1.70, 1.72). Now, clean the great veins (*Atlas*, 1.72). Halfway along the right margin of the manubrium, the **two brachiocephalic veins** (innominate veins) meet to form the **superior vena**

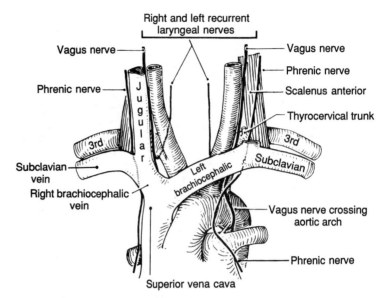

Figure 1.31. Great veins, arteries and related nerves.

cava. On the right side, identify again the **azygos vein.** It arches over the root of the lung to empty into the superior vena cava (*Atlas*, 1.43, 1.86). Cut the superior vena cava just superior to the entrance of the azygos vein. Reflect the great veins in order to expose the **arch of the aorta** and the great arteries arising from it (Fig. 1.31; *Atlas*, 1.57). These vessels can be demonstrated radiographically (*Atlas*, 1.56). Thus, abnormalities within these arteries as well as variations in the origins of the branches of the aortic arch can be detected (*Atlas*, 1.58). In addition, abnormalities of the aortic arch itself can be visualized (*Atlas*, 1.59).

Clean the aortic arch and the three great arteries arising from it (*Atlas*, 1.72, 1.78).

1. **Brachiocephalic trunk** (innominate artery), arising from the summit of the aortic arch.
2. **Left common carotid artery.**
3. **Left subclavian artery.** It lies immediately posterior to the left common carotid artery. Both arteries ascend almost vertically. Be aware of important variations in the origins of arterial branches from the aortic arch (*Atlas*, 1.58).

The **aortic arch**, by definition, begins and ends at the same level: this is the sternal angle anteriorly, and the intervertebral disc T4-T5 posteriorly. Observe that the aorta arches over the left bronchus and then becomes the descending aorta. Further caudally, the esophagus is interposed between it and the pericardial sac (*Atlas*, 1.62). Verify that the aortic arch passes from anterior to posterior. Therefore, by necessity, the aortic arch is crossed by two nerves that descend vertically. These are the **left phrenic nerve** and the **left vagus** (*Atlas*, 1.72).

At the level of the **aortic arch** (*Atlas*, 1.74B), review all pertinent topographic relations. Study a suitable transverse section (*Atlas*, 1.74C) and relate your findings to a corresponding MRI (*Atlas*, 1.74A).

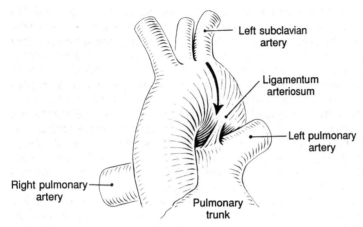

Figure 1.32. Ligamentum arteriosum (obliterated ductus arteriosus).

Left Phrenic Nerve (Fig. 1.31; *Atlas*, 1.44, 1.72). It descends from the neck, enters the thorax between the subclavian artery and subclavian vein, and reaches the aortic arch. After crossing the arch, it lies approximately 1 cm anterior to the root of the lung. Subsequently, it lies on the left side of the pericardial sac. Restore its position, and review the course of the nerve to the diaphragm.

Left Vagus (*Atlas*, 1.44, 1.72, 1.76). It descends from the neck along the posterolateral side of the left common carotid artery. Find it in the angular interval between the left common carotid and subclavian arteries. Trace it across the left side of the aortic arch. Since it is on its way to the esophagus, it passes posterior to the root of the left lung; i.e., posterior to bronchus, pulmonary artery, and pulmonary veins (see Fig. 1.33). If not already done during the dissection of the posterior mediastinum, use a probe and dissect bluntly the area where the vagus crosses the aortic arch. Confirm that the concavity of the arch is connected to the left pulmonary artery by a stout, obliquely set cord. This is the **ligamentum arteriosum**, the remnant of the ductus arteriosus (Fig. 1.32; *Atlas*, 1.75). Find and clean the **left recurrent laryngeal nerve**. It is an important branch of the left vagus. Locate it immediately posterior to the ligamentum arteriosum. Follow it for a short distance superiorly. Later, the nerve will be followed to its termination in the larynx.

> The aortic arch is also crossed by two slender **cardiac nerves** (*Atlas*, 1.72, 1.75), which may now be difficult to find. Often, these nerves are mistaken for connective tissue strings or fascia. They arise in the neck from the sympathetic trunk and from the vagus. They pass to the superficial cardiac plexus situated just to the right of the ligamentum arteriosum.

Identify the **right phrenic nerve.** Review the positions and relationships of the **right vagus** nerve (Fig. 1.33; *Atlas*, 1.43, 1.72, 1.75). Note that this nerve takes a course

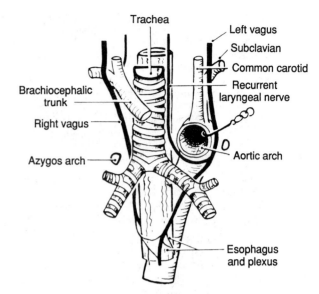

Figure 1.33. Right and left vagus, their recurrent laryngeal nerve branches, and their relations to trachea and esophagus.

along the right side of the trachea and toward the posterior aspect of the root of the lung. Some branches arise from the vagus and cross the trachea anteriorly (*Atlas*, 1.75); these are cardiac branches on their way to the deep cardiac plexus.

> The right recurrent laryngeal nerve, which cannot be demonstrated at this time, loops around the right subclavian artery (*Atlas*, 1.72, 1.73). Since this vessel lies too high to be part of the superior mediastinum, the right recurrent laryngeal nerve is not part of it either. In contrast, the left recurrent laryngeal nerve with its close relation to the aortic arch traverses the superior mediastinum. Thus, in cases of mediastinal tumors, the left recurrent laryngeal nerve is likely to be compromised, resulting in paralysis of the left vocal cord (with associated hoarseness).

If not already done, detach the ascending portion of the aorta from the pericardial sac. Reflect the aortic arch to the left (let your partner hold it, or use a pin to hold it in the reflected position). Once again, identify the ligamentum arteriosum and the left recurrent laryngeal nerve. Observe and clean a number of fine branches from both vagi and sympathetic trunks as they course toward an area between the aortic arch and the bifurcation of the trachea (*Atlas*, 1.75). This is the site of the **deep cardiac plexus** that is much more extensive than the superficial cardiac plexus. Review the nerve supply of the thoracic contents (*Atlas*, 1.41, 1.82).

Observe the **tracheobronchial lymph nodes** on both sides of the trachea and in the vicinity of its bifurcation (*Atlas*, 1.75, 1.78). This mass of pigmented nodes fills the angle within the fork of the trachea and intervenes between the right pulmonary artery and esophagus. Be familiar with the passageways through which the nodes are drained (*Atlas*, 1.81).

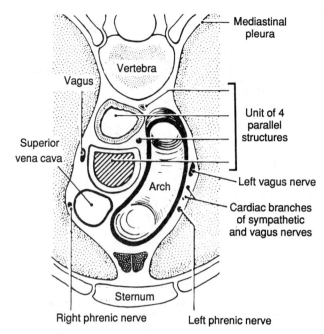

Figure 1.34. Transverse section through superior mediastinum at level of aortic arch (viewed superiorly).

Identify and study the **bifurcation of the trachea** (Fig. 1.33; *Atlas*, 1.76, 1.78). Palpate the anterior and posterior surface of the trachea near its bifurcation. Review the four major structures topographically related to the bifurcation of the trachea (*Atlas*, 1.77): these are sequentially from deep to superficial: lymph nodes at the tracheal bifurcation; pulmonary arteries; ascending aorta and arch of aorta; brachiocephalic veins forming the superior vena cava. Next, identify individual **tracheal rings.** Verify that these "rings" are imperfect: Only the anterior two-thirds of the circumference consists of cartilage. Posteriorly, the tracheal tube is completed by a musculofibrous membrane. With sturdy scissors, incise the right main bronchus. Carry the incision to the tracheal bifurcation. Identify the **carina.** It is a ridge on the inside of the tracheal bifurcation.

During bronchoscopy, the **carina** serves as an important landmark. It stands between the superior ends of the right and left main bronchi.

Foreign bodies (paper clips, small metal objects, etc.) are usually aspirated into the right main bronchus. Understand why: (a) the right main bronchus is more vertical, shorter, and wider than the left one (*Atlas*, 1.76); (b) the carina is usually positioned slightly to the left of the median plane.

Superior to the level of the aortic arch (*Atlas*, 1.71**B**) there are four parallel vertically running structures: **esophagus, trachea, left recurrent laryngeal nerve, and thoracic duct.** Study these relations in the cadaver and in suitable transverse sections (*Atlas*, 1.71**A** and **C**). Observe the **esophagus** anterior to the vertebral column and projecting slightly to the left of the trachea. The **trachea** is immediately anterior to the esophagus. In the angle between esophagus and trachea, the **left recurrent laryngeal nerve** ascends to the larynx. The **thoracic duct** is small, thinwalled and easily torn. Make an attempt to find the thoracic duct superior to the level of the aortic arch. With a blunt probe, search in the area posterior to the left subclavian artery where it ascends subpleurally on the side of the esophagus (*Atlas*, 1.71**C**, 1.76). Do not waste appreciable time. The structure will be examined again during dissection of the neck.

Review the superior vena cava and its tributaries (*Atlas*, 1.86, 1.87). Compression (obstruction) of this large vessel leads to a characteristic aggregate of signs and symptoms known as the **superior vena cava syndrome.** Obstruction of the superior vena cava most often is caused by malignant disease of the chest such as bronchogenic carcinoma. In most cases, tumors of the right lung are responsible for compression of this right-sided vessel. Blood from the upper limbs, head, and neck cannot freely drain to the heart; it must find its way to the heart via collateral venous drainage. As a result, the upper torso, head and neck show evidence of increased blood volume, such as grossly distended veins and capillary leakage.

Realize that the superior mediastinum is only an arbitrary subdivision. Many vital structures on their way to or from the neck pass through this space. Therefore, this region should be reviewed again during dissection of the neck.

Keep all dissected structures moist with preservative fluid to avoid deterioration. Return the thoracic viscera (heart, lungs) into the chest cavity for convenient storage. In addition, retain the removed anterior chest wall for future review of surface relationships. Ask your instructor if additional procedures should be followed before you end the dissection of the thorax.

CHAPTER 2

THE ABDOMEN

Anterior Abdominal Wall

General Remarks

The contents of the abdominal cavity are protected in front and on the flanks by a wall made up of several layers. These layers are (*Atlas*, 2.16A):

1. Skin
2. Superficial fascia:
   a. fatty layer (of Camper)
   b. membranous layer (of Scarpa)
Three flat muscles:
3. External oblique
4. Internal oblique three flat muscles
5. Transversus
6. Fascia transversalis
7. Extraperitoneal fatty areolar tissue
8. Peritoneum

On each side of the midline, extending down the length of the anterior abdominal wall, the three flat muscles are reinforced by a longitudinal strap-like muscle. This muscle, the **rectus abdominis**, is enclosed in a sheath produced by the aponeuroses of the three flat muscles (*Atlas*, 2.5A).

The ventral rami of the lower six thoracic nerves enter and supply the abdominal wall (*Atlas*, 2.7). Note that T10 supplies the skin around the umbilicus. Three nerves (T7, T8, T9) supply the region superior to the umbilicus; and three nerves (T11, T12, L1) supply the region inferior to the umbilicus.

In the male, the **testes** are housed in a special outpouching of the anterior abdominal wall, the **scrotum**. The scrotum consists of skin and superficial fascia that is void of fat. Each testis is connected to intrapelvic structures via the **ductus deferens**. The duct and its associated vessels and nerves constitute the major components of the **spermatic cord**. This cord traverses the abdominal wall through an obliquely set canal, the **inguinal canal**. The inguinal canal is of great clinical importance, since loops of intestine may herniate through it. Therefore, this region of the anterior abdominal wall should be studied with particular attention.

In the female, the inguinal canal is relatively small. It contains the **round ligament of the uterus**, a tape-like structure corresponding in position to the spermatic cord of the male. Compare male with female cadavers. If you dissect a female cadaver, substitute in the text "round ligament" for "spermatic cord."

Important Landmarks

Palpate the following (Fig. 2.1; *Atlas*, 2.1A):

1. **Xiphisternal junction**, at the inferior end of the body of the sternum;
2. **Costal margin**, consisting of the upturned ends of cartilages 7 to 10;
3. **Pubic symphysis**, marking the lowest limit of the anterior abdominal wall in the median plane;
4. **Pubic crest**, extending laterally from the symphysis;
5. **Pubic tubercle**, at the lateral end of the pubic crest;
6. **Inguinal ligament**, stretching from the pubic tubercle to the anterior superior iliac spine;
7. **Anterior superior iliac spine**, at the anterior end of the iliac crest;
8. **Tubercle of the crest**, at the most lateral point of the crest.

Before you begin . . .

The three flat muscles (external oblique, internal oblique, transversus) will be studied, particularly in the important inguinal region. The composition and contents of the rectus sheath will be explored. Finally, the anterior abdominal wall will be reflected so that:

1. Full access to the contents of the abdominopelvic cavity is ensured.

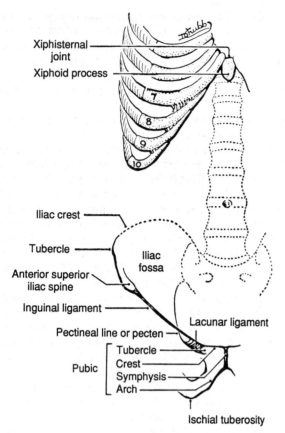

Figure 2.1. Landmarks and boundaries of the anterior abdominal wall.

2. Most components of the abdominal wall can be repositioned for future studies. These studies include a review of the inguinal canal and of the various layers of the abdominal wall.

Skin Incisions

Place the cadaver into the supine position (face up). Put a block transversely beneath the lumbar region of the back. This procedure stretches the anterior abdominal wall. Make the following skin incisions according to Figure 2.2:

1. Make a midline skin incision from the xiphisternal junction to the symphysis pubis, encircling the umbilicus (C to E).
2. If not already done, make a transverse incision from the superior end of the vertical incision laterally until stopped by the table (C to D).
3. From the inferior end of the vertical incision cut along the pubic crest. Below the course of the inguinal ligament, extend the incision to the anterior superior iliac spine and along the iliac crest (E to F).
4. Reflect the skin of the abdomen laterally.

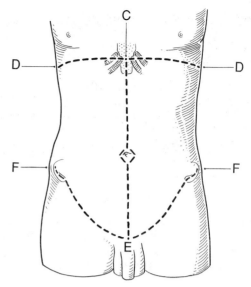

Figure 2.2. Skin incisions.

Dissection of Anterior Abdominal Wall and Inguinal Canal

The **superficial fascia (Camper's fascia)** may contain various amounts of fat. In this fascia observe the superficial epigastric vein. It passes inferiorly from near the umbilicus toward the inguinal region (*Atlas*, 2.5).

> The right and left superficial epigastric veins are of potential clinical importance: The veins and their anastomoses with the lateral thoracic veins constitute important collateral venous channels to the upper part of the body. These collateral channels are utilized and engorged in patients whose venous blood cannot freely return to the heart (obstruction of the inferior vena cava or of the portal vein). Under these pathological conditions, the superficial veins in the abdominal wall, especially around the umbilicus, become greatly dilated and tortuous. This phenomenon, known as *caput medusae*, is of important diagnostic value.

The **membranous, deep layer of the superficial fascia (Scarpa's fascia)** lies superficial to the aponeurosis of the external oblique (Fig. 2.3). It is mainly composed of fibrous tissue. It is unique in that it is continuous with the superficial perineal fascia (Colles' fascia) and dartos fascia which surround the shaft of the penis and the scrotal sac. In the lower abdominal wall, Scarpa's fascia is separated from the underlying aponeurosis of the external oblique only by the deep investing fascia of the external oblique (all muscles have an investing fascia). Sometimes it is difficult to separate the deep investing fascia of the external oblique from Scarpa's fascia. This fascial arrangement must be understood in order to appreciate certain clinical conditions in which Scarpa's fascia and the aponeurosis of the external oblique are forcefully separated and a potential space is created between the two; see clinical comments

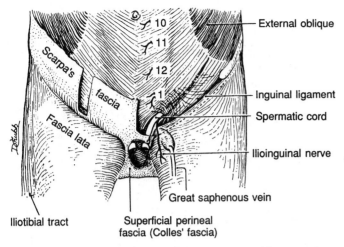

Labels on figure: External oblique, Inguinal ligament, Spermatic cord, Ilioinguinal nerve, Great saphenous vein, Superficial perineal fascia (Colles' fascia), Iliotibial tract, Fascia lata, Scarpa's fascia, 10, 11, 12, 1

Figure 2.3. Scarpa's and Colles' fasciae, external oblique, and superficial inguinal ring (penis and scrotum cut away).

(screened material). Explore Scarpa's fascia. It is best distinguished from the underlying aponeurosis at a point approximately 3 cm superior to the iliac crest in the anterior axillary line. At this point, incise Scarpa's fascia without cutting into the fleshy fibers of the external oblique. Make sure that the proper plane between Scarpa's fascia and muscular aponeurosis has been reached. Then, continue the incision medially to the midline, about 4 cm superior to the superior end of the pubic symphysis. Inferiorly, **Scarpa's fascia** ends by being attached to the **fascia lata** (i.e., deep fascia of the thigh) along a line 2 cm below the inguinal ligament. Verify this important fact by inserting your index finger between Scarpa's fascia and the aponeurosis of the external oblique. With gentle sweeping movements of the finger, verify and demonstrate that the finger is prevented from descending into the thigh. In contrast, you will be able to push your finger into the scrotal sac and toward the perineum (Fig. 2.3).

> The clinician must be aware of the fascial arrangements of the external genitalia and of the lower abdominal wall. If the penile urethra is injured (perineal injuries in car accidents; falling astride onto sharp objects such as fence poles, etc.), urine may escape from the urethra into the scrotum. From there it may readily spread superiorly into the lower abdominal wall between Scarpa's fascia and the aponeurosis of the external oblique (Fig. 2.3). The clinical picture of this urinary extravasation may be dramatic with extensive, red edematous swelling of the scrotum, penis and lower abdominal wall. Of course, urinary extravasation into the thigh does *not* occur. This clinical picture can only be understood properly if one is mindful of the previously mentioned fascial arrangements.

Cutaneous Nerves (*Atlas*, 2.5A, 2.6). Do not injure the underlying aponeurosis of the external oblique. Incise the superficial fascia 5 cm from the midline. Make this incision from the xiphoid process to the symphysis pubis. With the finger or the handle of a scalpel, detach the fascia medially for about 2.5 cm. Now, palpate the **anterior cutaneous nerves**. These nerves are in series with those in the

thoracic region. The anterior cutaneous nerves of the abdomen are terminal twigs of the ventral rami (T7 to L1). About 4 cm superior to the pubic crest, look for the **anterior cutaneous branch of the iliohypogastric nerve** (L1), the lowest branch of that nerve on the anterior abdominal wall (*Atlas*, 2.6). Review the distribution of a spinal nerve (*Atlas*, 1.20).

The fleshy fibers of the **external oblique** originate superior to the costal margin (*Atlas*, 2.7). Observe the fleshy digitations of the external oblique from each of the lower eight ribs (the upper four interdigitate with serratus anterior, the lower four with the latissimus dorsi). Between the digitations, observe the **lateral cutaneous nerves** (T7 to T12). Each nerve divides into a small posterior branch and a large anterior branch. The **posterior branches** turn posteriorly over the latissimus dorsi. The anterior branches descend, in the superficial fascia, in line with the fibers of the external oblique (*Atlas*, 2.7). Trace at least one **anterior branch** anteriorly to the abdominal wall.

Remove all remains of the superficial fascia. Clean the surface of the **external oblique**. Clearly distinguish between muscular and aponeurotic portion. Observe the curved line of union between these two portions (*Atlas*, 2.5, 2.7). Notice the **linea alba** (*Atlas*, 2.6). It is a whitish groove in the midline of the abdominal wall, formed by interlacing fibers from the right and left sides. About halfway between the xiphoid process and the pubic symphysis, the linea alba is interrupted by the umbilicus.

Inguinal Canal. The inguinal region is of considerable clinical importance because inguinal hernias may occur here, particularly in males. Dissection of the inguinal region and its canal is difficult and often frustrating. Understand that the **inguinal canal** is an **obliquely set tunnel** that traverses the anterior abdominal wall. This tunnel runs parallel to and just superior to the medial half of the inguinal ligament. It is 3 to 5 cm in length. It extends between the **superficial inguinal ring** (an opening in the aponeurosis of the external oblique) and the **deep (internal) inguinal ring** (an opening in the transversalis fascia). During its course between these openings, the inguinal canal passes through the arched aponeurotic and muscular layers of the anterior abdominal wall formed by the three flat muscles (Fig. 2.4): external oblique (aponeurotic), internal oblique and transversus abdominis (muscular). Thus, the inguinal canal can be likened to an arcade of three arches formed by the three flat abdominal muscles (Fig. 2.5). The arches formed by the internal oblique and transversus abdominis are often fused and cannot be completely separated. In the male, the inguinal canal is traversed by the spermatic cord. In the female, the inguinal canal is less well defined; it contains the round ligament of the uterus.

In preparation for the anticipated dissection, study a schema of the inguinal canal (*Atlas*, 2.16A). Realize that the spermatic cord traverses obliquely the various layers of the anterior abdominal wall, specifically the three flat muscles. Also note that various abdominal layers make contributions to the spermatic cord as so-called "coverings" (for example, the external oblique, and frequently also the transversus abdominis, contribute to the cremaster muscle).

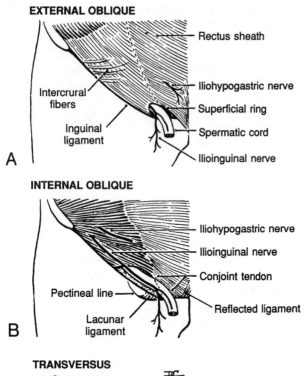

EXTERNAL OBLIQUE

- Rectus sheath
- Iliohypogastric nerve
- Superficial ring
- Spermatic cord
- Ilioinguinal nerve

Intercrural fibers

Inguinal ligament

A

INTERNAL OBLIQUE

- Iliohypogastric nerve
- Ilioinguinal nerve
- Conjoint tendon
- Reflected ligament

Pectineal line

Lacunar ligament

B

TRANSVERSUS

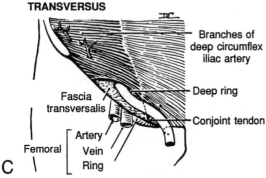

- Branches of deep circumflex iliac artery
- Deep ring
- Conjoint tendon

Fascia transversalis

Femoral { Artery / Vein / Ring

C

Figure 2.4. Contributions of the three flat abdominal muscles to the inguinal canal.

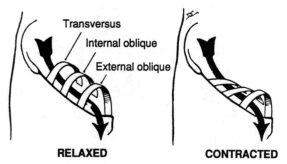

Transversus
Internal oblique
External oblique

RELAXED   **CONTRACTED**

Figure 2.5. The inguinal canal resembles an arcade of three arches traversed by the spermatic cord.

Dissecting instructions are provided for male cadavers. Dissection will proceed from superficial to deep. Each section of the canal (*superficial inguinal ring and aponeurosis of external oblique; internal oblique; transversus abdominis; deep inguinal ring and transversalis fascia*) will be clearly identified. If possible, review suitable prosections or museum specimens before commencing with your own dissection.

Superficial Inguinal Ring and Aponeurosis of External Oblique. The aponeurosis of the external oblique forms the first and most superficial arch traversed by the spermatic cord (Fig. 2.5). Carefully clean the aponeurosis of the external oblique in the inguinal region. Identify the following structures (*Atlas*, 2.8):

1. **Superficial inguinal ring.** It is, of course, subcutaneous. Delineate the arch-like, triangular aperture in the aponeurosis for the passage of the spermatic cord in the male (or for the passage of the round ligament in the female). The base of this triangular aperture is formed by the pubic crest; its sides are the medial and lateral crura.
2. **Lateral (inferior) crus.** It is formed by the portion of the aponeurosis attaching to the pubic tubercle via the inguinal ligament. The spermatic cord rests on the inferior part of the lateral crus.
3. **Medial (superior) crus** (*Atlas*, 2.8). It is that portion of the aponeurosis that diverges to attach to the pubic bone and crest medial to the pubic tubercle.
4. **Intercrural fibers.** Lateral to the apex of the triangular gap. They prevent the crura from spreading apart (*Atlas*, 2.8).
5. **Inguinal ligament** or Poupart's ligament (*Atlas*, 2.8). It forms the free inferior border of the aponeurosis of the external oblique. Notice and palpate its attachment to the anterior superior iliac spine and to the pubic tubercle. The **lacunar ligament** (which cannot be inspected at this time) consists of fibers that are reflected from the medial end of the inguinal ligament to the pecten pubis.

Identify but do not disturb the **spermatic cord** (round ligament in the female) as it traverses the superficial inguinal ring (*Atlas*, 2.5). Note the **ilioinguinal nerve** that emerges from the ring lateral to the spermatic cord. This nerve sends sensory twigs to the external genitalia and the medial aspect of the thigh. Do not destroy the proximal portion of the nerve (it will be used as a guiding structure for finding the plane between the internal oblique and the transversus abdominis). Clean the space between the spermatic cord and the fundiform ligament of the penis. Remove fat and small external pudendal vessels contained in this space (*Atlas*, 2.5). Before proceeding to the next deeper arch formed by the internal oblique (Fig. 2.5), the aponeurosis of the external oblique in the inguinal region must be reflected. Proceed as follows: With a pair of scissors, split the fleshy fibers of the external oblique for approximately 10 cm. Start the incision about 5 cm superior to the iliac crest and proceed medially in the direction of the muscle fibers. Insert two fingers into the incision, and separate the fibers of the external oblique from the fascia of the underlying internal oblique. Notice that the fibers of the internal oblique take a different direction (*Atlas*, 2.6). Enlarge the incision. Free the posterior (deep) surface of the external oblique as far as possible with your hand. Me-

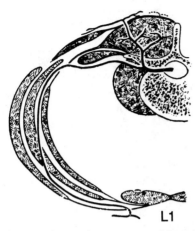

Figure 2.6. Course of ventral nerve ramus L1 in abdominal wall.

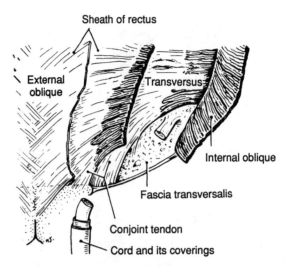

Figure 2.7. Conjoint tendon and fascia transversalis.

dially, the fingers cannot proceed beyond the rectus sheath which is partially formed by the aponeurosis of the external oblique. Extend the incision medially in the direction of the aponeurotic fibers of the external oblique. Cut as far as 2.5 cm superior to the superficial inguinal ring. The next objective is to reflect the external oblique and expose the internal oblique.

Internal Oblique (*Atlas*, 2.10, 2.12). This is the second and next deeper arch of the arcade (Fig. 2.5). To demonstrate this muscle and its contribution to the inguinal canal, it will be necessary to find the plane between the **external oblique** and the underlying **internal oblique.** Proceed as follows:

1. Keep your hand as a guide in the plane between the two oblique muscles.
2. Cut the external oblique: From the iliac crest superiorly, curving medially about 5 cm in front of the digitations of the serratus anterior, to a point corresponding approximately to the 5th costal cartilage.
3. Reflect the inferior part of the divided external oblique inferiorly.
4. Reflect the larger superior part of the muscle medially until stopped by the rectus sheath. Now, the anterior surface of the internal oblique is exposed (*Atlas*, 2.6).
5. Examine the inferior portion of the internal oblique as it forms the second arch of the arcade (Fig. 2.5). Use a probe and create a small gap between this arch and the traversing spermatic cord. Lateral to the spermatic cord, notice small muscle slips connecting the internal oblique with the spermatic cord. This is the muscular contribution of the internal oblique to the cremaster muscle. Verify that the fibers of the internal oblique become aponeurotic as they approach their insertion into the pubic crest and the pecten pubis just medial to the inguinal canal. At that point, the tendinous fibers of the internal oblique join the tendinous fibers of the transversus abdominis; this *joint tendon* is appropriately known as the **conjoint tendon** (*Atlas*, 2.12, 2.13). Identify it.

Transversus Abdominis (*Atlas*, 2.12). This is the third and deepest arch of the arcade (Fig. 2.5). As pointed out earlier, the musculotendinous arches formed by the internal oblique and transversus abdominis are often fused and cannot be completely separated.

Check with your instructor to determine if you should attempt to separate internal oblique from transversus abdominis. If in the affirmative, proceed as follows: Clean the anterior surface of the internal oblique and demonstrate the course of its muscle fibers. Do not injure the **ilioinguinal nerve.** Clean this nerve and follow it proximally to the point where it traverses the internal oblique (*Atlas*, 2.5). Now, use the nerve as a guiding structure to determine the plane between the internal oblique and the underlying transversus abdominis. The ilioinguinal nerve, a branch of L1, runs in the space between the two innermost muscles (Fig. 2.6). With a pair of scissors, split the internal oblique along its fiber course where it is traversed by the ilioinguinal nerve (about 2 to 3 cm above the inferior border of the muscle). Insert your finger into the plane between the internal oblique and the transversus abdominis. Push the finger inferiorly and separate the inferior borders of the two muscles. Difficulties will be encountered if the two muscles are fused inferolaterally.

At any rate, the tendinous portions of the internal oblique and the transversus abdominis are always fused medial to the inguinal canal where they insert, as the **conjoint tendon**, into the pubic crest and pecten pubis (Fig. 2.7; *Atlas*, 2.12, 2.14). Verify this fact in the cadaver.

Deep Inguinal Ring and Transversalis Fascia. Hold the free inferior margin of the transversus abdominis (or the margin of the fused internal oblique and the transversus) anteriorly and superiorly. Sweep the handle of the scalpel or a probe between it and the underlying **fascia transversalis** (Fig. 2.7; *Atlas*, 2.15, 2.16A). This fascia is the internal investing layer which lines the entire abdominal wall. Notice that it is somewhat transparent. Through it you can see some yellowish extraperitoneal fat and areolar tissue. The next deeper layer is the peritoneum which cannot be seen at this time. Roll the spermatic cord laterally and observe the **inferior epigastric vessels** shining through

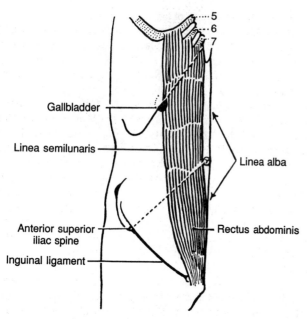

Figure 2.8.   Rectus abdominis.

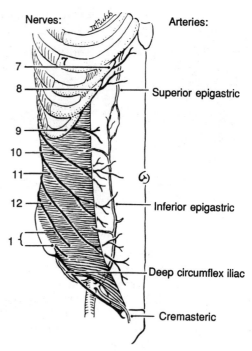

Figure 2.9.   Nerves and arteries within the rectus sheath.

the fascia transversalis (*Atlas*, 2.12, 2.14). Just lateral to these inferior epigastric vessels is the **internal opening of the inguinal canal, the deep inguinal ring.** Push a probe medially along the spermatic cord toward the deep inguinal ring. This orifice will be examined again later from its inner aspect during dissection of pelvic structures.

Review the inguinal canal and its walls. Gently push a probe through the superficial inguinal ring parallel to the spermatic cord. Hold the probe in place while examining the inner aspect of the abdominal wall. Find the probe pushing against the **deep inguinal ring.** The length of the obliquely set inguinal canal is about 3 to 5 cm. Verify this. **Review the walls of the inguinal canal** (Fig. 2.4, 2.5; *Atlas*, 2.8, 2.10 through 2.13):

1. *Anterior:* Mainly the aponeurosis of the external oblique;
2. *Inferior* (floor): Inguinal ligament and lacunar ligament, i.e., fibers of the medial end of the inguinal ligament that are rolled under the spermatic cord and attach to the pubic pecten;
3. *Superior* (roof): Arches of the internal oblique and the transversus abdominis;
4. *Posterior:* Fascia transversalis, reinforced medially by the conjoint tendon.

The inguinal canal is like an arcade of three arches traversed by the spermatic cord (Fig. 2.5). During standing, coughing, or vigorous straining, the abdominal muscles contract. The arched fleshy fibers of the internal oblique and transversus cause the roof of the canal to become lower and taut. The action is essentially that of a half-sphincter.

An enlarged or congenitally patent inguinal canal is a potential channel through which abdominal viscera may protrude. The protruding viscera are contained in a hernial sac, which is an outpouching of the peritoneal membrane. Hernias through the ingui-

nal canal are called **indirect hernias.** Indirect inguinal hernias are located *lateral* to the inferior epigastric vessels (*Atlas*, 2.16B).

Great and prolonged increase in intra-abdominal pressure may eventually produce an outward bulging of a sac whose walls are composed of peritoneum, extraperitoneal fat, and fascia transversalis. If this sac (hernial sac) protrudes *medial* to the inferior epigastric vessels, the condition of a **direct inguinal hernia** exists (*Atlas*, 2.16C).

Realize that there are other potentially weak areas through which hernias can occur. Refer to *Atlas*, 2.9 to study the sites of a femoral hernia and an obturator hernia. In comparison with the inguinal hernias, the femoral and obturator hernias are relatively rare.

The elicitation of the **cremasteric reflex** is part of every routine physical examination in the male patient. When the skin on the inner side of the thigh is scratched, the testicle on the same side is drawn upward. The afferent fibers of this reflex are carried in the genital branch of the genitofemoral nerve (*Atlas*, 5.7). Sensory (afferent) fibers of this nerve supply the skin of the scrotum and the adjacent thigh. Motor fibers of this nerve supply the cremaster muscle (efferent reflex arc). Centrally in the spinal cord, the reflex involves segments L1 and L2.

Rectus Abdominis (Fig. 2.8; *Atlas*, 2.5A). Reposition the cut halves of the external oblique. Outline the approximate location of the **rectus abdominis.** Note that the muscle is three times as wide cranially as it is caudally. The fleshy fibers of the rectus are inserted into the cartilages of ribs 5 to 7. Inferiorly, the muscle arises from the symphysis and body of the pubis. On the anterior surface of the inferior part of the rectus abdominis you may find a small triangular muscle, the pyramidalis. It is functionally unimportant. Now, open the **rectus sheath** vertically to display its contents:

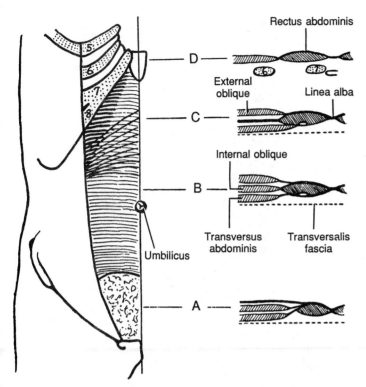

Figure 2.10. Posterior wall of rectus sheath (*left*), and transverse sections of rectus sheath at four different levels (*A, B, C,* and *D*).

1. Below the umbilicus, keep the vertical incision about 12 mm from the midline.
2. Superior to the umbilicus, make the vertical incision about 25 mm from the midline.
3. Observe that the rectus sheath is firmly attached to the rectus muscle at the three **tendinous insertions.** Sever these connections with a scalpel.
4. Carefully mobilize the rectus muscle with your hands, but do not remove it. Note that the anterior branches of six spinal nerves (T7 to T12) pierce the rectus sheath laterally. These nerves enter and supply the muscle (Fig. 2.9, *Atlas,* 2.6).
5. In its middle, divide the rectus muscle transversely. Carefully reflect the two halves superiorly and inferiorly, respectively.
6. On the posterior (deep) surface of the inferior half, observe the large **inferior epigastric vessels.**
7. On the posterior (deep) surface of the superior half, note the smaller **superior epigastric vessels.**

The superior and inferior epigastric arteries and veins anastomose (Fig. 2.9, *Atlas,* 2.6). If the venous blood from the inferior part of the body cannot return freely to the heart (obstruction of inferior vena cava), the anastomosing inferior and superior epigastric veins provide an important collateral venous channel to the superior part of the body. Conversely, collateral arterial circulation via the superior and inferior epigastric arteries provides channels for arterial blood flow to the lower part of the body if the aorta is occluded (e.g., in coarctation of aorta).

Study the **rectus sheath** (Fig. 2.10, *Atlas,* 2.4). Examine the **posterior layer or wall** of the sheath. Identify the **arcuate line,** midway between the symphysis pubis and the umbilicus (*Atlas,* 2.6). At the level of the arcuate line, the inferior epigastric vessels enter the rectus sheath. Verify this.

The aponeuroses of the three flat abdominal muscles contribute to the formation of the **rectus sheath.** Below the arcuate line, all aponeurotic layers pass ventral to the rectus (Fig. 2.10A); only the transversalis fascia remains dorsal to the muscle. Above the level of the arcuate line, the aponeurosis of the internal oblique splits: Together with the aponeurosis of the transversus it forms the posterior layer; together with the aponeurosis of the external oblique, it forms the anterior layer of the rectus sheath (Fig. 2.10B and C). At the level of the xiphoid process, only the aponeurosis of the external oblique contributes to the rectus sheath (Fig. 2.10D).

Inferior to the arcuate line, remove the **transversalis fascia.** Remove the **extraperitoneal fat** and areolar tissue, and thus expose the **peritoneum.** Do not incise this membrane.

The **linea alba** (*Atlas,* 2.10) is formed by decussating fibers of the aponeuroses of the right and left flat abdominal muscles (external oblique; internal oblique; transversus). Superior to the umbilicus, the linea alba is a band, about 2 cm wide (Fig. 2.8). Inferior to the umbilicus, it is a thin line since the two recti muscles come into contact with each other. The linea alba is a raphe or decussation, and therefore it is extensile.

The next objective is to reflect the anterior abdominal wall in such a manner that:

1. Full access to the contents of the abdominopelvic cavity is ensured.
2. Most components of the abdominal wall can be repositioned for future studies.

Proceed in the following manner: Detach the fleshy fibers of the rectus from ribs 5 to 7, and sever the superior epigastric artery close to the muscle. Make a vertical incision through the linea alba, keeping on the left side about 1 cm from the midline (to preserve the obliterated umbilical vein). Make a 3-cm long vertical incision just left of the xiphoid process. Be careful not to injure the contents of the abdominal cavity. Place the index finger of one hand through the incision into the abdominal cavity. With your finger, pull the anterior abdominal wall anteriorly, thereby creating a gap between abdominal wall and abdominal contents. Now, it is safe to extend the vertical incision inferiorly. Cut around the umbilicus on the left side so that it remains attached to the right side of the abdominal wall. Below the umbilicus, continue the incision on the left, about 5 mm from the midline and as close as possible to the left rectus sheath (to preserve the obliterated urachus). Continue the incision to the symphysis pubis.

Subsequently, place one hand into the left side of the abdominal cavity to separate abdominal wall from abdominal contents. With the scalpel in the other hand, detach the left abdominal wall from the rib cage. Starting at the xiphoid process, follow the inferior border of rib 10; then carry the cut to the left iliac crest. Reflect the left side of the anterior abdominal wall inferiorly.

Before reflecting the right side of the abdominal wall, establish the following facts:

1. The **falciform ligament** spans the space between the anterior abdominal wall and liver (*Atlas*, 2.22, 2.23).
2. Contained in the inferior free margin of the falciform ligament is the **ligamentum teres**. This is the obliterated umbilical vein that, in the fetus, carried blood from the umbilical cord to the liver.

Make sure that your dissecting partners have seen these two structures. Now, detach the falciform ligament from the anterior abdominal wall and sever the ligamentum teres. Subsequently, reflect the right side of the anterior abdominal wall in the same manner as the left side.

Review the various layers of the **abdominal wall**. At the rib cage, observe the attachments of the three severed, flat abdominal muscles:

1. The origin of the **external oblique** from the *external* surface of the lower ribs;
2. The insertion of the **internal oblique** into the *inferior* surface of the lower ribs;
3. The origin of the **transversus abdominis** from the *inner* surfaces of the lower ribs.

Look at the peritoneal aspect of the umbilical region (*Atlas*, 2.23). The obliterated remains of fetal structures radiate from the umbilical region. They are:

1. The obliterated umbilical vein or **ligamentum teres** of the liver (already seen);
2. The obliterated allantoic duct (urachus) or **median umbilical ligament**, in the midline ascending from the apex of the bladder;
3. The obliterated umbilical artery or **medial umbilical ligament**, one on each side.

Scrotum, Spermatic Cord, and Testis

Exposure of Spermatic Cord and Testis. Free the cord from the surrounding fat. Push your index finger into the scrotal sac so that the finger intervenes between testis medially and scrotal wall laterally. With the finger in this position, make an incision halfway down the scrotum, through the skin, dartos, and superficial fascia. Free the testis and cord from the surrounding areolar tissue and shell it out of the scrotum. Snip the band of tissue that anchors the inferior pole of the testis to the scrotum. This is the **gubernaculum testis.**

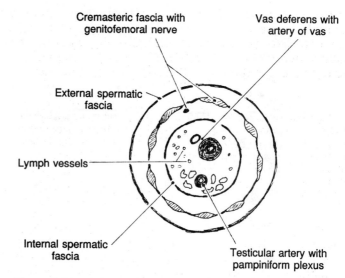

Figure 2.11. Schematic transverse section through spermatic cord.

Observe that the **scrotal sac** is divided into two pouches by a median septum. Verify that the superficial fascia of the scrotum is void of fat. It contains a layer of involuntary muscle fibers, the **dartos**, which controls the surface area of the scrotum.

Coverings of the Cord (*Atlas*, 2.16A, 2.19B). Carefully incise the tubular coverings of the cord longitudinally:

1. **External spermatic fascia,** the thin outermost covering;
2. **Cremasteric fascia,** the middle covering; it is areolar and contains loops of cremaster muscle;
3. **Internal spermatic fascia,** the filmy innermost covering of the spermatic cord.

Constituents of the Cord. The **ductus (vas) deferens** is easily identified. It is located in the posterior portion of the cord, and it is hard and cord-like in consistency. Free it for 5 to 8 cm. Look for the small **deferent artery** that clings to it. Free a larger artery, the **testicular artery,** which runs with the **pampiniform plexus of veins.** Trace the ductus deferens up to the deep inguinal ring and note that it hooks around the lateral side of the inferior epigastric vessels. Be aware of, but do not search for other components of the cord: *lymph vessels* that drain the testis (not the scrotum); *autonomic nerve fibers* running with the testicular artery and the ductus deferens. Review once more the constituents of the spermatic cord and their derivation (*Atlas*, 2.16A). Study and understand a transverse section through the spermatic cord (Fig. 2.11).

Testis (*Atlas*, 2.17, 2.19). Carefully remove any superficial areolar tissue that may adhere to the **tunica vaginalis testis.** The tunica vaginalis is a closed serous sac of peritoneal origin. During development, the testis and epididymis invaginated into the posterior wall of this sac. Demonstrate the extent of the sac by injecting air or water into it (use syringe and fine needle). Observe that the (artificially distended) cavity covers the anterior, medial, and lateral surfaces of the testis (but not its posterior surface).

> Under pathological conditions, the potential space of tunica vaginalis testis may be enlarged and distended by blood (hematocele) or serous fluid (hydrocele). A hydrocele can eventually become as large as or larger than a fist. Taking into account the topographic relations of tunica vaginalis and testis, understand that in hydrocele the testis can only be palpated *posterior* to the swelling; i.e., where the testis is *not* covered with tunica vaginalis.

Incise the tunica vaginalis testis and inspect the interior of the serous sac. On the lateral side, identify the **sinus** of the epididymis that separates the testis from the **body of the epididymis** (*Atlas*, 2.19A). The visceral layer of the sac covers the testis and the head of the epididymis. Carefully incise the sac at its reflection from the testis.

Trace the vas deferens to the tail of the **epididymis** (*Atlas*, 2.19C). Here, the vas is thin-walled and easily torn. Unravel part of the epididymis. The epididymis consists of a single convoluted duct of considerable length. With a probe, free some of the 15 to 20 fine **efferent ductules** between the superior pole of the testis and the head of the epididymis. From the cord, trace blood vessels to the testis (*Atlas*, 2.19D).

Longitudinally, incise the anterior aspect of the testis from its superior to its inferior pole (*Atlas*, 2.17). Notice the thickness of its fibrous capsule, the **tunica albuginea.** Look for fibrous strands that divide the interior of the testis into numerous lobules. Tease some of these lobules apart, and note the fine thread-like **seminiferous tubules.**

The **lymphatic drainage of the scrotal sac and its contents** is of clinical importance. Realize that lymphatics from the penis and also from the scrotum (an outpouching of the abdominal wall) drain to nodes that receive lymph vessels from the lower abdominal wall and lower limb: the superficial inguinal nodes (*Atlas*, 2.18). In contrast, lymphatics from the right and left testes drain into deeply positioned right and left lateral nodes, respectively. Subsequently, these lateral nodes empty into the preaortic lymph nodes (*Atlas*, 2.18). Thus, inflammation of the penis or the scrotal sac will most likely be associated with enlargement of the superficial inguinal nodes. Testicular tumors, spreading along lymph vessels, will involve lateral and preaortic nodes. These latter nodes cannot be palpated on physical examination. However, they can be evaluated with a CT or MRI scan (*Atlas*, 2.112).

Abdominopelvic Cavity

General Remarks

The **peritoneum** is a thin, translucent, serous membrane. To understand its complexities, certain fundamental facts must be appreciated:

1. It lines the walls of the abdominal cavity.
2. It forms a completely closed sac or cavity, except in the female where the funnel-shaped infundibulum of each uterine tube opens into it.
3. Immediately outside of it is an extraperitoneal (subperitoneal) fatty layer. In this layer, the organs and their vessels develop and lie.
4. "Retroperitoneal" organs remain behind (retro) the sac and are merely covered in front with peritoneum. In general, this applies to the urinary system.
5. An organ which invaginates the sac is invested in peritoneum. The outer investment is the **serous coat** of the organ. In general, this applies to the gastrointestinal system.
6. The mobility of an organ depends to a great extent on its peritoneal covering.
7. Two layers of peritoneum are attached to each of the two curvatures of the stomach. They are the two **omenta.** The **lesser omentum** is attached to the *lesser* curvature of the stomach, and the **greater omentum** is attached to the *greater* curvature.
8. **Mesenteries** are two layers of peritoneum that "sling" the intestine from the posterior abdominal wall. Vessels and nerves travel to and from the intestine between the two layers.
9. All other double layers and folds of peritoneum are called **peritoneal ligaments.**
10. **Folds or plicae** may be produced by blood vessels and ducts lifting the peritoneum off the body wall.
11. Everywhere within the peritoneal cavity, peritoneum is in contact with peritoneum. The cavity is merely a potential space containing a small amount of lubricating serous fluid. Thus, intra-abdominal organs can move upon each other without significant friction.

> Under certain pathological conditions, the potential space of the peritoneal cavity may be distended into an actual space containing up to several liters of fluid. This accumulation of serous fluid in the peritoneal cavity is known as ascites. Also, other substances (e.g., blood from a ruptured spleen, bile from a ruptured bile duct, fecal matter from ruptured intestine) may accumulate in the abdominal cavity.

Inspection of Abdominal Cavity and Contents

Work will be much more pleasant if you clean the entire surface of the peritoneal cavity with a damp sponge. Always keep the cavity and its contents moist with mold-deterrent preservative fluid.

Inspect. Do not dissect at this time. Study the dispositions of various organs and of the peritoneum. You may encounter pathological conditions (e.g., cancer; enlarged liver or spleen; etc.). As a result of old inflammatory processes, *adhesions* (strands of fibrous tissue) may exist between the opposing surfaces of peritoneal membranes. These adhesions must be broken down with your fingers.

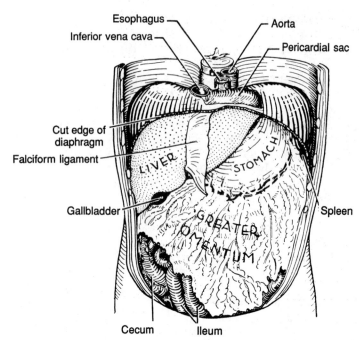

Esophagus — — Aorta

Inferior vena cava — — Pericardial sac

Cut edge of diaphragm

Falciform ligament —

Gallbladder —   — Spleen

Cecum   Ileum

Figure 2.12. Abdominal contents including gallbladder and spleen. Cut edge of diaphragm.

Identify, merely identify the following structures (Fig. 2.12; *Atlas*, 2.2A, 2.21A):

1. **Diaphragm,** forming the roof of the abdomen.
2. **Liver,** divided into a **right** and a **left lobe** by the **falciform ligament.** This ligament connects the liver to the diaphragm and to the anterior abdominal wall in the median plane. Place your opened hand into the potential space between diaphragm and right lobe of liver.
3. **Gallbladder;** it projects to the lateral margin of the right rectus abdominis (Fig. 2.8). It is attached to the visceral (inferior) surface of liver. It reaches beyond the sharp inferior border of the liver.
4. **Stomach or gaster** (*Atlas*, 2.2A, 2.25); it may be dilated and conspicuous or contracted and less evident. It is connected to the liver by the lesser omentum. Identify the greater curvature. Verify that the greater omentum is attached to it.
5. **Greater omentum** (Fig. 2.12); it is attached to the caudal border of the greater curvature of the stomach. Spread out this structure to appreciate its size and extent. It covers anteriorly the transverse colon and extends inferiorly to cover portions of the small intestine. Expect to find considerable variations in size and thickness. In emaciated cadavers, it may be very thin; in obese cadavers, the greater omentum contains a considerable amount of fat and, therefore, it may be of remarkable thickness and weight. Observe these variations in different cadavers. Be aware that the greater omentum has mobility and can wrap itself around inflamed areas to wall them off and prevent spread of infection. In that way, adhesions are created. These must be broken down, using your fingers or blunt dissection.

6. **Spleen or lien** (Figs. 2.12, 2.13; *Atlas*, 2.2A and **B**); it lies posterior to the stomach in contact with the diaphragm. It is connected to the left part of the greater curvature of the stomach by two layers of peritoneum, the **gastrolienal (gastrosplenic) ligament** (*Atlas*, 2.27).

   Now, reflect the greater omentum cranially over the costal margin and thereby uncover the following structures:

7. **Small intestine** (*Atlas*, 2.2A, 2.21A); the mobile coils of the jejunum and ileum are visible (combined length approximately 6 m). The small intestine terminates by emptying into the cecum, a large blind pouch of the large intestine (Fig. 2.13).
8. **Large intestine** (Fig. 2.13; *Atlas*, 2.2A, 2.71); the large intestine frames the small intestine on three sides:
   a. On the right side, the **cecum** and the **ascending colon.**
   b. Superiorly, the **transverse colon.**
   c. On the left side, the **descending colon** and the **sigmoid colon.**

In the abdomen, follow the **alimentary canal (GI tract)** from its beginning to its end. Realize that certain parts of the GI tract are not immediately accessible (e.g., duodenum) and, therefore, cannot be demonstrated at this time. Study the names and general dispositions of the parts of the GI tract from proximal to distal ends (*Atlas*, 2.2).

Correlate your gross anatomical observations with a suitable magnetic resonance image (*Atlas*, 2.75C).

Identify the **stomach.** The exit from the stomach is the **pylorus.** Observe the right concave border of the stomach. This is the **lesser curvature.** The lesser curvature and the first 3 cm of the duodenum are the attachment sites for the **lesser omentum,** which continues to the liver (*Atlas*, 2.2A, 2.25). The lesser omentum is divisible into two parts: The **hepatogastric** and the **hepatoduodenal ligaments** (Fig. 2.14). The **greater curvature** of the stomach is long and convex. Attached to it is the **greater omentum.** The two important parts of the greater omentum are its **gastrocolic** (from stomach to colon) and **gastrosplenic** (from stomach to spleen) **portions** (Fig. 2.14; *Atlas*, 2.26, 2.27).

Next, **inspect the small intestine.** There are three parts: **Duodenum, jejunum,** and **ileum.**

The **duodenum** (*Atlas*, 2.2A) immediately succeeds the pyloric portion of the stomach. Its first inch is mobile and was noted in association with the hepatoduodenal ligament (Fig. 2.14). The remainder of the duodenum is inaccessible at the present time. Realize that it is C-shaped and molded around the head of the pancreas. The duodenum is attached to the structures ventral to the posterior abdominal wall. Find its termination, the **duodenojejunal junction:** Pull the mobile small intestine to the right side, then follow the jejunum proximally as far as possible. Find the point where the immobile duodenum ends and the mobile jejunum begins. This is the duodenojejunal junction (Fig. 2.13; *Atlas*, 2.2A, 2.76).

Immediately succeeding the duodenum is the mobile part of the small intestine. It consists of **jejunum** (proxi-

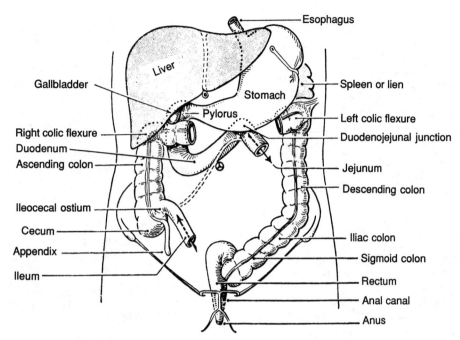

Figure 2.13. Various parts of the digestive tract, and disposition of organs.

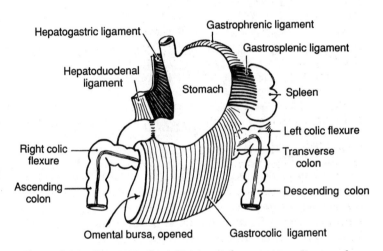

Figure 2.14. Diagram of subdivisions of greater omentum and lesser omentum, and various peritoneal ligaments.

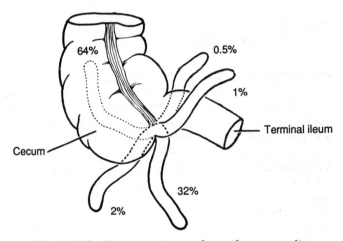

Figure 2.15. Various positions of vermiform appendix.

mal 2/5) and **ileum** (distal 3/5). The ileum empties into the **cecum** at the **ileocecal orifice or junction**. Note that the distance between the duodenojejunal junction and ileocecal junction is about 15 to 20 cm in the adult. Yet, the total length of small intestine accommodated between these two points is about 20 ft (or 6 m). Find out how this is possible. Verify that the **root of the mesentery** of the mobile part of the small intestine stretches diagonally across the posterior wall from the duodenojejunal to the ileocecal junction (Fig. 2.13; *Atlas*, 2.76, 2.82). This root is only 15 to 20 cm long. However, the **intestinal border of the mesentery** is elaborately ruffled to accommodate the substantial length of jejunum and ileum. The small intestine is so convoluted and mobile that you can pass many feet of it through your hands without knowing whether you are

proceeding to its duodenal end or its cecal end. However, by placing a hand on each side of the mesentery and drawing the fingers anteriorly from root to intestinal border, the convolutions are locally untwisted and the direction of the gut becomes obvious.

Next, turn your attention to the **large intestine** (*Atlas*, 2.2A). It consists of **cecum** with attached **appendix, colon** (ascending; transverse, descending; sigmoid), **rectum,** and **anal canal**. Observe the following features:

1. **Cecum** (L. *caecus*, blind); extends inferiorly beyond the ileocecal junction into the right iliac fossa. The length of its mesentery, i.e., the degree of its mobility, varies considerably.
2. **Vermiform appendix** (L. *vermis*, worm; *forma*, shape; *appendere*, to hang on); opens into the cecum infe-

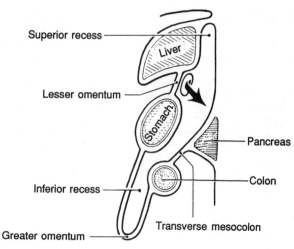

Figure 2.16. Transverse colon and its mesentery. Walls of the omental bursa (lesser sac). The *arrow* passes through the omental (epiploic) foramen.

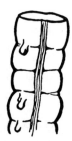

Figure 2.17. Segment of colon showing appendices epiploicae, haustra, and one of the three teniae.

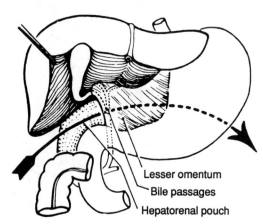

Figure 2.18. Entrance into omental bursa through omental (epiploic) foramen. The *broken line* of the *arrow* passes through the omental bursa and posterior to the stomach.

rior to the ileocecal orifice (Fig. 2.13; *Atlas*, 2.2A, 2.72); may occupy any position consistent with its length; most commonly found retrocecal, i.e., posterior to the cecum (Fig. 2.15; *Atlas*, 2.73); its mesentery is a triangular fold of peritoneum, the mesoappendix (*Atlas*, 2.74).

3. **Ascending colon** (Gr. *kolon*, large intestine; hollow); has no mesentery; therefore, it is attached to the posterior abdominal wall; ascends to the liver where it makes a right-angle bend. This is the **right colic flexure or hepatic flexure** (Fig. 2.13).

4. **Transverse colon**; extends transversely from **right colic flexure** to **left colic flexure or splenic flexure.** The left colic flexure is attached to the diaphragm by the **phrenicocolic ligament,** which also forms a shelf to support the spleen (*Atlas*, 2.62). The left colic flexure is at a more superior level and a more posterior plane than the right colic flexure. Between the two flexures, the transverse colon is freely movable. Its mesentery, the **transverse mesocolon,** is connected to the inferior border of the pancreas (Fig. 2.16). Also adherent to the transverse colon is the **greater omentum** (Fig. 2.16). The portion of the greater omentum between stomach and transverse colon is called the gastrocolic ligament (Fig. 2.14).

5. **Descending colon;** descends from the sharply curved left colic flexure to the pelvic brim. It is of smaller caliber than the ascending colon. Its posterior surface is attached to the posterior abdominal wall.

6. **Sigmoid colon** (resembling the Greek letter *sigma*); it has a long mesentery and, therefore, considerable freedom of movement. Identify the point where the mesentery, the **sigmoid mesocolon,** ends. Here, the sigmoid colon is continuous with the rectum (*Atlas*, 2.2A, 3.9).

7. **Rectum** (L. *rectus*, straight). The rectum is only partially covered with peritoneum (*Atlas*, 3.8, 3.17). Its relation to other pelvic structures will be studied later.

8. The outer longitudinal muscular coat of the large intestine is concentrated into three narrow bands, the **teniae coli.** The three teniae begin at the appendix (*Atlas*, 2.71, 2.74). The **anterior tenia** is easily visible in gross specimens.

9. Since the teniae are shorter than the other layers of the colon, they cause the formation of characteristic sacculations called **haustra** (plural: *haustra*; singular: *haustrum*; Fig. 2.17; *Atlas*, 2.71, 2.72). Appreciate a view of the haustra in a double-contrast radiograph of the large intestine (*Atlas*, 2.75).

10. **Appendices epiploicae** are small bags of fat which hang from the colon throughout its length (Fig. 2.17; *Atlas*, 2.71).

11. Study radiographs of the large intestine (*Atlas*, 2.75). Identify the rectum and the various portions of the colon. Realize that the contrast material (barium) is infused into the large intestine via the rectum (barium enema). Note that the contrast material normally does not enter the small intestine. This fact is due to a normally competent ileocecal valve.

Now, return the greater omentum to its original position. Study the upper abdominal viscera and their disposition in the abdominal cavity:

Liver or Hepar (Gr. *hepar*, liver). It is the largest organ in the male and non-pregnant female, weighing 1.2 to 1.6 kg. Note that its **right lobe** is about six times as large as

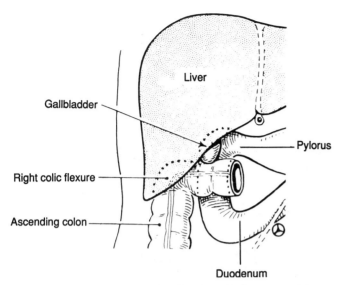

Figure 2.19. Interrelations of gallbladder, duodenum, and transverse colon (anterior view).

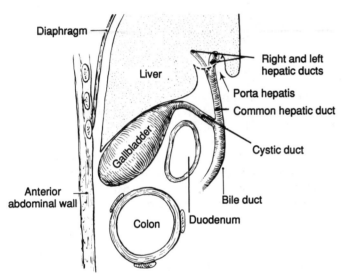

Figure 2.20. Interrelations of gallbladder, duodenum, and transverse colon (paramedian section through gallbladder).

the **left**. Observe the two surfaces of the liver, the **diaphragmatic surface** and the **visceral surface**:

1. **Diaphragmatic surface**; in contact with the diaphragm; very extensive, convex, and smooth (*Atlas*, 2.22).
2. **Visceral surface**; in contact with viscera (stomach, duodenum, colon, right kidney); concave and irregular, facing inferiorly, to the left, and posteriorly. Pull the sharp inferior margin of the liver anteriorly, expose the visceral surface (Fig. 2.18; *Atlas*, 2.36, 2.38), and observe two important structures:
   a. The **gallbladder**; study its four contact relations: liver, duodenum, colon, and anterior abdominal wall (Figs. 2.19 and 2.20; *Atlas*, 2.51).

These relations are of clinical importance. An inflamed gallbladder can become adherent to the intestinal tract, notably to the duodenum and/or the transverse colon with which the gallbladder is in close contact (Figs. 2.19 and 2.20; *Atlas*, 2.51). Subsequently, a fistula between gallbladder and GI tract (cholecystoenteric fistula) may develop through which bile or gallstones can enter the GI tract. For example, a large single gallstone could perforate into the duodenum and pass through the jejunum and ileum all the way to the ileocecal valve. If it cannot pass through this narrow valve, bowel obstruction (gallstone ileus) will result, with disastrous consequences. Conversely, air or gas from the GI tract can enter the gallbladder through a cholecystoenteric fistula. This air can be visualized radiographically; it is an important diagnostic sign.

Realize that the size of the gallbladder varies from patient to patient (subject to subject). Gallbladders can be very small or very large. This is a variation of normal. Study radiographs of the biliary passages and the gallbladder (*Atlas*, 2.42, 2.44). Be aware of considerable variations.

b. The **porta hepatis** (*Atlas*, 2.36, 2.38, 2.39B, 2.40). The porta hepatis is the "doorway" to the liver. Identify it by looking for a 5 cm transverse fissure through which vessels, ducts, and nerves enter and exit.

Once again, identify the **lesser omentum** as it stretches from the lesser curvature of the stomach and from the initial portion of the duodenum to the visceral surface of the liver (Fig. 2.18; *Atlas*, 2.25A and B). Focus your attention on the right free margin of the lesser omentum, the **hepatoduodenal ligament**. Between the two peritoneal layers of this ligament are the structures that pass to the porta hepatis: **Hepatic artery, portal vein, bile passages**, autonomic nerves, and lymphatics. Stand on the right side of the cadaver. With the hand palm up, place your index finger behind (dorsal to) the hepatoduodenal ligament in the direction of the *arrow* shown in Figure 2.18. Your finger will pass through the **omental foramen** (epiploic foramen; foramen of Winslow) into the **omental bursa or lesser sac** (*Atlas*, 2.25 through 2.27). Anterior to your finger is the hepatoduodenal ligament with its important contents.

Omental Bursa and Peritoneal Reflections

The **exploration of the omental bursa** (lesser sac) will be easier if **its anterior wall, the lesser omentum**, is partially removed: Break through the filmy membrane that stretches between the lesser curvature of the stomach and liver. Leave the hepatoduodenal ligament and its contents undisturbed. Place your hand into the widely opened lesser sac and study its extent.

1. Push your finger horizontally toward the far left. Here, the **peritoneal attachments of the spleen** are the boundaries of the lesser sac (Fig. 2.21; *Atlas*, 2.27).
2. Direct your fingers inferiorly (Fig. 2.16; *Atlas*, 2.26). They will pass posterior to the stomach and, at the same time, anterior to the pancreas and transverse

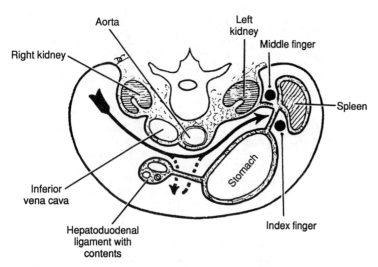

Figure 2.21. Horizontal extent of omental bursa (lesser sac). Fingers are positioned to palpate the "pedicle" of the spleen.

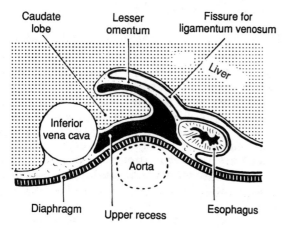

Figure 2.22. Boundaries of superior recess of omental bursa (transverse section; inferior view).

mesocolon. Then, the fingers will pass toward the **inferior recess** that lies between the two double layers of the gastrocolic ligament. Normally, these two double layers fuse during fetal development; as a result, the inferior recess is obliterated. Understand that the greater omentum is composed of four layers of peritoneum. If the greater omentum is incised between the transverse colon and the stomach, surgical access can be gained to the omental bursa (lesser sac). This procedure is employed in surgical approaches to the pancreas.

3. Pass your middle finger superiorly in the median plane between the liver and the posterior aspect of diaphragm (Fig. 2.16; *Atlas*, 2.26). Your finger is now in the **superior recess** of the omental bursa. Palpate the structures bordering this cul-de-sac (Fig. 2.22): Posterior to your finger is the diaphragm; anteriorly, the caudate lobe of the liver; to the left, the abdominal portion of the esophagus; to the right, the large inferior vena cava.

Next **examine the peritoneal attachments of the spleen** (Fig. 2.21; *Atlas*, 2.27). Stand on the right side of

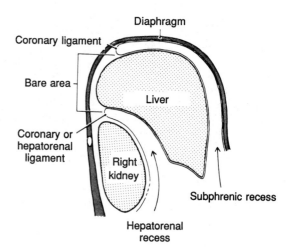

Figure 2.23. Paramedian section through diaphragm, liver, and right kidney. Subphrenic recess and hepatorenal recess or pouch (of Morison).

the cadaver and push your right hand between diaphragm and spleen until the spleen lies scooped in the palm. Pass your middle finger dorsal to the spleen until stopped by the **splenorenal ligament** that stretches from spleen to kidney. Now, place your left fingers into the lesser sac and palpate the intervening splenorenal ligament. Next, leave your left hand in the omental bursa, place the right index finger between greater curvature of stomach and spleen, and palpate the intervening **gastrosplenic ligament** (Fig. 2.21 or *Atlas*, 2.27). Understand that these two ligaments, splenorenal and gastrosplenic, suspend the spleen between the kidney and the stomach. They form a **pedicle** (stalk) that transmits blood vessels to and from the hilus of the spleen. From your observations and from the diagram in Figure 2.21 it should be obvious that:

1. The splenorenal and gastrosplenic ligaments are double layers of peritoneum.
2. Their inner layers are composed of peritoneum of the omental bursa (lesser sac).
3. Their outer layers are composed of peritoneum of the peritoneal cavity (greater sac).
4. Both ligaments form the left boundary of the omental bursa.
5. The spleen itself is covered with peritoneum of the greater sac.

Now examine the **peritoneal attachments of the liver** (Fig. 2.23; *Atlas*, 2.37). Provide better access to the hepatic region by cutting the right costal cartilages 6 and 7 near the xiphisternal junction and by partially incising the diaphragm.

Once again, identify the **falciform ligament of the liver** (*Atlas*, 2.22). Place your right hand between the diaphragm and the left lobe of the liver; simultaneously, place your left hand between the diaphragm and the larger right hepatic lobe. Verify that:

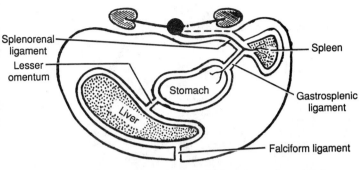

Figure 2.24. Peritoneal investment of liver, stomach, and spleen, and related peritoneal ligaments: falciform ligament; lesser omentum; gastrosplenic ligament; splenorenal ligament.

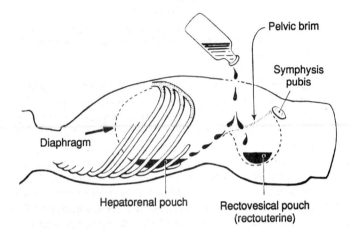

Figure 2.25. Most dorsal parts of the peritoneal cavity. Fluids may collect in the recesses (pouches) when the subject lies recumbent.

1. The hands cannot meet because of the intervening falciform ligament (compare Fig. 2.24).
2. The hands can be pushed dorsally for a considerable distance between the diaphragm and the diaphragmatic surface of the liver until stopped by the reflections of the peritoneum from the liver onto the diaphragm (Fig. 2.23).

These peritoneal reflections from the liver onto the diaphragm leave an irregular triangular area of the liver without peritoneal covering. Therefore, this uncovered area is called the **bare area** of the liver (Fig. 2.23; *Atlas*, 2.36). *Atlas*, 2.37 shows the area of the diaphragm which is in contact with the bare area of the liver. The peritoneal reflections around the bare area are called the **coronary ligament** (Fig. 2.23; *Atlas*, 2.34, 2.37). The peritoneal fold attaching the left tip of the left hepatic lobe to the diaphragm is the **left triangular ligament** (*Atlas*, 2.34, 2.36). Palpate it. The cranial reflection of the coronary ligament is continuous with the falciform ligament. The caudal part of the coronary ligament is reflected onto the diaphragm and the right kidney; therefore, it is alternatively called the **hepatorenal ligament** (Fig. 2.23).

Inferior to the hepatorenal ligament is a potential peritoneal space, the **hepatorenal pouch or recess** (of Mori-

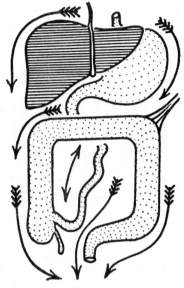

Figure 2.26. Gutters in the peritoneal cavity.

son). This pouch is bounded by the liver, the right kidney, the colon, and the duodenum. It is surgically important. It lies at the lowest point of the peritoneal cavity when the subject is recumbent (Fig. 2.25).

Peritoneal Gutters (Fig. 2.26). The mesentery of the mobile small intestine, the ascending colon, and the descending colon are attached to the posterior abdominal wall in a characteristic fashion. As a result, **four gutters** exist that can conveniently conduct materials (ascites, inflammatory material, blood, bile, etc.) from one point of the peritoneal cavity to another. Identify in the cadaver (Fig. 2.26):

1. The **right lateral (paracolic) gutter,** to the right of the ascending colon; it may conduct fluid from the omental bursa via the hepatorenal pouch into the pelvis.
2. The **left lateral (paracolic) gutter** to the left of the descending colon; it is closed cranially by the phrenicocolic ligament (*Atlas*, 2.62).
3. The **gutter to the right of the mesentery;** it is closed cranially and caudally.
4. The **gutter to the left of the mesentery;** it opens widely into the pelvis.

The **paracolic gutters** are of considerable clinical importance. They provide the pathways for flow of ascites and for the spread of intraperitoneal infections. Infectious material in the abdomen can be transported along these gutters into the pelvis; conversely, infections arising in the pelvis may extend superiorly. In a similar fashion, the paracolic gutters can provide pathways for the spread of tumor deposits (seeded metastases). Any medical student who considers the normal and pathological anatomy of the abdomen vital to his or her career should read the fascinating book *Dynamic Radiology of the Abdomen*, 3rd Edition, by M. A. Meyers, (Springer-Verlag, 1988). The book contains numerous, well labeled color plates of transverse sections through the abdominal cavity. Normal anatomic relationships and variants are presented.

Before you begin . . .

Do *not* dissect at this time. Just understand that the following steps and procedures are planned: The vessels and ducts connecting the porta hepatis with other abdominal structures will be demonstrated. Next, the branches of the three unpaired abdominal arteries (celiac; superior mesenteric; inferior mesenteric) will be followed to their fields of supply. Similarly, the venous drainage of the GI tract into the portal venous system will be studied. Subsequently, the entire GI tract will be removed as a unit together with its three unpaired organs (liver; pancreas; spleen). This en bloc extirpation offers several advantages:

1. No essential structures will be destroyed. The unity of the GI tract will be maintained.
2. The removed GI tract can be placed on a separate table or tray for convenient and more accessible examination. The student will be able to study the GI tract repeatedly and in detail, even while fellow students are engaged in the dissection of other areas.
3. Once placed on a table or tray, the student will have the challenging task to lay out the viscera in their *characteristic anatomical configuration*. This exercise alone is a valuable and impressive learning experience.
4. It should be noted that the knowledge gained from this en bloc extirpation and examination will prepare the student well for subsequent pathology and autopsy exposure. Pathologists routinely remove organ systems en bloc. Often, the viscera of the neck and thorax are removed as a block together with the upper part of the GI system (stomach, duodenum, liver, pancreas, and spleen) while the bulk of the small and large gut is separated at the duodenojejunal junction (at the suspensory muscle of the duodenum, also known as the ligament of Treitz) and remains in the abdomen for practical reasons. However, complete en bloc extirpations are also employed in pathology. We have opted for complete removal of the GI tract in order to maintain continuity of the GI tract and in order to expose the posterior abdominal wall and to facilitate access into the pelvis.
5. If so desired, the entire GI tract can be placed back into the abdominal cavity, and topographic relations with other structures can be reestablished.
6. Not every gross anatomy instructor favors en bloc extirpation of the GI tract. Please, consult with your instructor before you proceed with the actual dissection within the abdominal cavity.

Bile Passages, Celiac Trunk, and Portal Vein

The following dissection requires time, patience, and adequate preparation on your part. Insert your finger into the omental (epiploic) foramen. Anterior to your finger lies the remaining free edge of the lesser omentum, the **hepatoduodenal ligament,** with its **contents: bile passages, hepatic artery, portal vein, autonomic nerves, and**

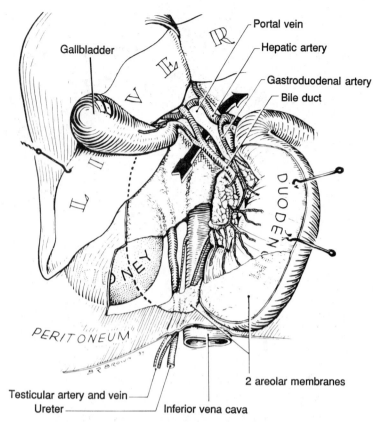

Figure 2.27. Structures contained in hepatoduodenal ligament. Omental (epiploic) foramen marked by *arrow.*

lymphatics. Replace the finger with a roll of white paper. Then, remove the peritoneum from the right free edge of the lesser omentum until the **bile duct** is exposed (Fig. 2.27; *Atlas*, 2.50). The bile duct has the caliber of a pencil. It is thin-walled and usually empty and collapsed. By careful dissection, establish that the bile duct is connected to the gallbladder via the **cystic duct** (*Atlas*, 2.38, 2.66). Then, follow the bile passages toward the liver and identify the **common hepatic duct,** and the rather short right and left hepatic ducts. Be mindful of the possible variations of the cystic and hepatic ducts (Atlas, 2.43). Study radiographs of the biliary passages (*Atlas*, 2.42, 2.44).

Note that the structures in the hepatoduodenal ligament are surrounded and accompanied by a substantial network of **autonomic nerve fibers** that originate from the celiac ganglia (around the root of the celiac artery). To simplify the field of dissection, you may discard these nerves. Look for at least one of several **hepatic lymph nodes** located around the bile duct and the portal vein (*Atlas*, 2.106B). Focus your attention on the bile passages and blood vessels. Carefully free the **hepatic artery proper,** which lies on the left side of the bile duct (Fig. 2.27; *Atlas*, 2.38, 2.50). Proceed with intelligence. Be aware of the ramifications of the **common hepatic artery** and of its origin from the **celiac trunk** (Fig. 2.28; *Atlas*, 2.32, 2.33). Follow the common hepatic artery back to the celiac trunk, a very short, unpaired vessel that originates directly from the abdominal aorta immediately caudal to the diaphragm (*Atlas*, 2.102). At the superior border of the first portion of

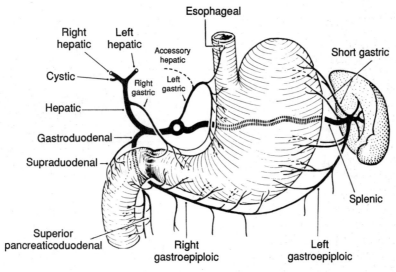

Figure 2.28. Celiac trunk (artery) and its branches.

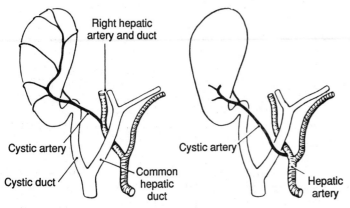

Figure 2.29. Where to look for the cystic artery.

arteries may also originate separately from the celiac trunk. There may be *accessory* right or left hepatic arteries; these are vessels that are additional to those arteries originating according to the usual standard pattern. Surgeons must be aware of these variations. The blood supply of the liver may be seriously disturbed (liver necrosis) following unintended ligation of arteries solely supplying certain parts of the liver. For example, during gastrectomy (surgical removal of the stomach) a "replaced" left hepatic artery (originating from the left gastric artery) could be unintentionally ligated, thus endangering the entire blood supply to the left lobe of the liver.

Study a celiac arteriogram (*Atlas*, 2.31), and compare it with a diagram of branches of the celiac trunk (*Atlas*, 2.32). Note that the contrast material has reached the liver via the hepatic arteries. The splenic artery is characteristically tortuous.

the duodenum, the **common hepatic artery** divides into the **gastroduodenal artery** and the **hepatic artery proper.** Dissect the hepatic artery and its branches (Fig. 2.28; *Atlas*, 2.40):

1. **Right gastric artery,** to the lesser curvature of the stomach;
2. **Left hepatic artery,** to the left lobe of the liver;
3. **Right hepatic artery,** to the right lobe of the liver;
4. **Cystic artery** (Fig. 2.29), a slender branch, usually arising from the right hepatic artery.

Anatomical dissectors and surgeons alike must be aware of common variations in the hepatic and cystic arterial supply. If the arterial distribution in the cadaver does not conform with the usual pattern (Figs. 2.28 and 2.29; *Atlas*, 2.38) consider alternate possibilities (*Atlas*, 2.41, 2.48, 2.49A and **B**). Variations in the origin and course of the hepatic artery are common (40%). In about 12% of the cases, the right hepatic artery is aberrant or "replaced" and arises as a separate vessel from the superior mesenteric artery. The left hepatic artery may be "replaced", i.e., it may take origin from the left gastric artery (*Atlas*, 2.48). The right and left hepatic

Next, dissect the two other branches of the celiac trunk:

1. The large **splenic artery** (Fig. 2.28; *Atlas*, 2.65A and **B**); follow it for 2 to 3 cm along the superior border of the pancreas. Do not dissect it further at this time.
2. The **left gastric artery** (Fig. 2.28; *Atlas*, 2.33); follow it to the lesser curvature of the stomach. Observe that it anastomoses with the **right gastric artery** to form an arterial arch along the lesser curvature.

Along the greater curvature of the stomach, examine the **right and left gastroepiploic arteries** that often form an arterial arch. Clean the **right gastroepiploic artery** and follow it behind the first part of the duodenum where it arises from the gastroduodenal artery. Next, carefully clean the **left gastroepiploic artery,** and follow it through the fatty greater omentum toward the spleen. Leave the gastroepiploic arteries attached to the greater curvature of the stomach, but sever the greater omentum (gastrocolic ligament) just inferior to these arteries. The greater omentum is still attached to the transverse colon. Understand why the detachment of the gastrocolic ligament from the stomach provides a wide access to the omental bursa (Fig.

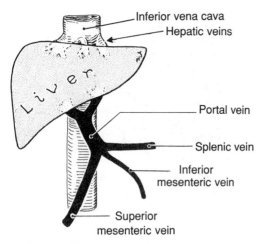

Figure 2.30. Portal vein and its tributaries.

2.16), particularly if the stomach is pulled superiorly. Observe that the pancreas is readily accessible. Let your partner pull the spleen anteriorly while you are tracing the left gastroepiploic artery to the hilus of the spleen and to the splenic artery (Fig. 2.28; *Atlas*, 2.33). Next, complete the dissection of the **splenic artery.** Observe that it contributes branches to the body and tail of the pancreas (*Atlas*, 2.65). Look for short gastric branches from the splenic artery to the fundus of the stomach (Fig. 2.28; *Atlas*, 2.33).

Carefully mobilize the tail and then the body of the pancreas. Note that the **splenic vein** lies inferior to the splenic artery (*Atlas*, 2.60, 2.62, 2.64). Follow the splenic vein to the **portal vein** (*Atlas*, 2.53). Observe that the **superior mesenteric vein** is the largest tributary of the portal vein. The **inferior mesenteric vein** may empty into either the splenic vein or the superior mesenteric vein, or it may join the portal vein at the junction of the splenic and superior mesenteric veins (Fig. 2.30). Look for the **gastric veins** that carry blood from the esophagus and the lesser curvature of the stomach to the portal vein. Review the portal system of veins (Fig. 2.30; *Atlas*, 2.53, 2.54).

> **Portal hypertension** (i.e., portal venous pressure above 20 cm H₂0) may result from suprahepatic causes (e.g., heart failure), intrahepatic causes (e.g., cirrhosis), or infrahepatic causes (e.g., portal vein thrombosis; tumor compression of portal vein). As a consequence of portal venous hypertension, the portal venous blood cannot freely drain, the esophageal and gastric veins become engorged, dilated, and eventually varicose. Rupture and extensive bleeding from these **esophageogastric varices** is an alarming and serious complication of portal venous hypertension. An understanding of the anatomy of the portal venous system is a prerequisite for intelligent diagnosis and treatment. Esophageal varices can be demonstrated radiographically (*Atlas*, 2.55).

Superior and Inferior Mesenteric Vessels

The **superior mesenteric artery (SMA)** is an unpaired vessel that arises from the abdominal aorta about 1 cm caudal to the celiac trunk. It has about the same diameter

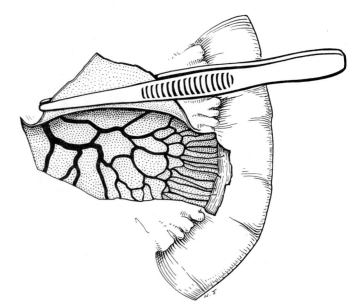

Figure 2.31. Exposure of blood vessels contained in the mesentery.

as the celiac trunk (*Atlas*, 2.98, 2.102). The objective is to **demonstrate the extensive field supply** of the superior mesenteric artery: Duodenum, except its superior portion; jejunum and ileum; cecum and appendix; ascending colon; approximately one-half of the transverse colon (*Atlas*, 2.78). Reflect tail and body of the pancreas to the right, then carefully free the origin and initial portion of the superior mesenteric artery. Note the dense nervous network surrounding the vessel. This is the **superior mesenteric plexus of nerves.** Remove it to the extent necessary. Follow the artery to the point where it crosses anterior to the inferior part of the duodenum (*Atlas*, 2.65A and **C**). Do not damage branches to the pancreas and duodenum. The **superior mesenteric vein** lies immediately to the right of the artery. It drains the same area supplied by the artery.

Next, follow the superior mesenteric vessels to the various parts of the small and large intestine. Use the following approach: lift the transverse colon, with the attached greater omentum, superiorly over the chest margin and retain it there. Draw the small intestine to the left, and have your partner stretch the mesentery taut. Palpate the superior mesenteric vessels just to the right of the duodenojejunal junction. Then, using scissors or two pairs of blunt forceps, expose the vessels between the two layers of the mesentery (Fig. 2.31). Now, identify and follow the branches of the superior mesenteric artery. Realize that these branches are named according to the structures that they supply:

1. **Intestinal arteries,** 15 to 18 arteries to jejunum and ileum; arteries unite to form loops or arches from which straight terminal branches arise. These are the **vasa recta** that pass alternately to opposite sides of the jejunum and ileum (Figs. 2.31, 2.32, and 2.33). The vasa recta do not anastomose within the mesentery; thus, "windows" appear between the vessels (Fig. 2.32). In the ileum, the arterial loops and arches become more

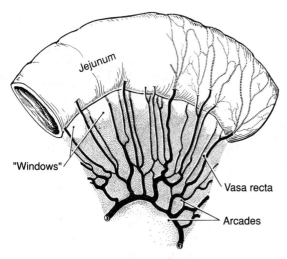

Figure 2.32. Arteries of the jejunum.

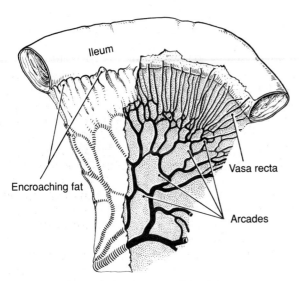

Figure 2.33. Arteries of the ileum.

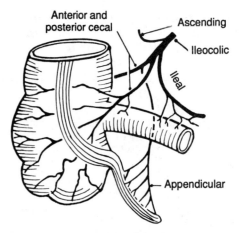

Figure 2.34. Branches of the ileocolic artery.

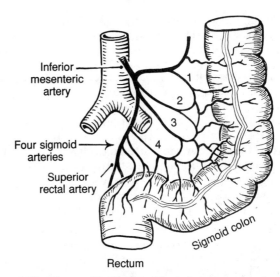

Figure 2.35. Sigmoid branches of the inferior mesenteric artery.

complex, and the vasa recta become progressively shorter (Fig. 2.33). Demonstrate a few arterial arches and vasa recta in the jejunum and ileum. Study a superior mesenteric arteriogram (*Atlas*, 2.79, 2.81).

2. **Ileocolic artery** (Fig. 2.34; *Atlas*, 2.78); passes to the right iliac fossa; supplies cecum and appendix (appendicular artery); anastomoses with ileal branches and with the right colic artery.

3. **Right colic artery** (*Atlas*, 2.78); arises from either the superior mesenteric or the ileocolic artery; supplies ascending colon; anastomoses with neighboring arteries.

4. **Middle colic artery** (*Atlas*, 2.78); supplies the right half of the transverse colon; anastomoses with neighboring arteries.

The tributaries of the **superior mesenteric vein** correspond to the branches of the superior mesenteric artery. Identify the superior mesenteric vein and trace it to the **portal vein** (*Atlas*, 2.53, 2.64A).

The mesentery contains a large aggregate of **lymph nodes** (numbering between 100 and 200). In most cases, these nodes are small. However, if there was prior inflammatory or malignant bowel disease, some of the nodes can be of substantial size. Make an attempt to identify nodes along the branches (tributaries) of the superior mesenteric vessels. Eventually, larger lymphatic branches lead into the **superior mesenteric nodes** that are located near the point of origin of the superior mesenteric artery from the abdominal aorta (*Atlas*, 2.105, 2.106).

The **inferior mesenteric artery (IMA)** is an unpaired vessel that arises from the abdominal aorta, about 3 cm cranial to the aortic bifurcation. The inferior mesenteric artery is much smaller than the superior mesenteric artery (*Atlas*, 2.98, 2.102). The objective is to **demonstrate the field of supply** of this artery: left half of transverse colon; descending colon; sigmoid colon; the greater part of the rectum (*Atlas*, 2.82). First palpate and then dissect the origin of the inferior mesenteric artery. It is surrounded by the inferior mesenteric plexus of nerves. Trace the artery toward the large intestine, and identify its branches:

1. **Left colic artery** (*Atlas*, 2.82); runs toward the left colic flexure; supplies the descending colon and the left half of the transverse colon; anastomoses with the middle colic artery.
2. **Sigmoid arteries** (Fig. 2.35; *Atlas*, 2.82); usually four branches that form arches.
3. **Superior rectal artery** (Fig. 2.35); supplies the proximal part of the rectum; divides into a right and a left branch that descend on either side of the rectum (*Atlas*, 3.14). Study an inferior mesenteric arteriogram (*Atlas*, 2.83).

The branches of the superior and inferior mesenteric arteries form a series of anastomosing loops along the colon. The result is a continuous **marginal artery** (of Drummond) situated along the wall of the large gut (Fig. 2.36). There are areas where the anastomoses are insufficiently developed, and hence there is less effective collateral circulation (+ in Fig. 2.36). This fact is of clinical importance in cases of mesenteric artery occlusion (thrombosis; embolism).

The tributaries of the **inferior mesenteric vein** correspond to the branches of the inferior mesenteric artery. Identify the inferior mesenteric vein and trace it to the **portal vein** (*Atlas*, 2.53, 2.54). The inferior mesenteric vessels are accompanied by lymph vessels and **lymph nodes** that drain into the **inferior mesenteric nodes** around the root of the inferior mesenteric artery (*Atlas*, 2.106A). Identify one representative node in the mesentery. If there was prior cancer of the rectum or the sigmoid colon, the inferior mesenteric nodes are probably pathologically enlarged.

Be aware that the **superior rectal vein** originates from the rectal venous plexus (*Atlas*, 2.53, 2.54). The rectal venous plexus is also drained by the middle and inferior rectal veins that, in turn, empty into the caval system of veins. In portal venous hypertension, blood flow in the superior rectal vein may be reversed: portal blood may be carried to the rectal plexus and, from there, shunted into the caval system. The resulting increased blood flow and pressure in the rectal venous plexus leads to the development of hemorrhoids. Thus, in case of hemorrhoids, the physician must always evaluate the condition of the portal venous system.

The portal venous system has no valves. This fact explains why the blood flow in the portal system can be easily reversed.

Removal of the GI Tract

Next, remove the entire GI tract together with its three unpaired organs (liver; pancreas; spleen). Proceed with this en bloc extirpation in the following manner:

1. Tie two strings about 2.5 cm apart tightly around the **rectum.** Cut the rectum between the two strings to prevent escape of its contents.
2. Cut the **inferior mesenteric artery** close to the abdominal aorta. Leave a 1-cm stump attached to the

aorta for future reference of this vessel. At the same time, you will also cut through autonomic nerve fibers originating in the inferior celiac ganglion.

3. Cut through the V-shaped **mesentery of the sigmoid colon** (*Atlas*, 2.76). Keep to its lateral side in order *not* to damage the inferior mesenteric vessels or the left ureter.
4. With your fingers, detach the **descending colon** from the posterior abdominal wall. At the left colic flexure, cut through the **phrenicocolic ligament** (*Atlas*, 2.61, 2.62). The phrenicocolic ligament provides a shelf for the spleen. Thus, after sectioning the ligament, the **spleen** is sufficiently mobilized.
5. Detach the **ascending colon** from the posterior abdominal wall. Keep to its lateral side in order *not* to damage the vessels supplying the colon.
6. Pull the transverse colon with the attached greater omentum caudally, and expose the **origin of the superior mesenteric artery.** Sever this vessel close to the abdominal aorta. In doing so, you will also cut through autonomic nerve fibers arising from the superior mesenteric ganglion. If the right hepatic artery arises from the superior mesenteric artery (12%), be sure to include it in this section.
7. Sever the **celiac trunk** at its origin from the aorta. Make sure to include all its branches. By necessity, you will also cut through autonomic nerve fibers originating from the celiac ganglia.
8. Tie a string around the **esophagus** close to the diaphragm. If the thorax has already been dissected, tie the string around the esophagus within the thorax just superior to the diaphragm. Cut the esophagus and the vagal nerves superior to the string (to avoid escape of gastric contents). Using blunt dissection, free the distal portion of the esophagus from the esophageal hiatus of the diaphragm (*Atlas*, 2.100, 2.101) and pull it into the abdominal cavity. (If the thorax has not been dissected as yet, cut the tied esophagus just inferior to the diaphragm). Free the **stomach** completely so that it is only attached to the duodenum and blood vessels. Cut vagal branches to the celiac plexus of nerves.
9. The **duodenojejunal junction or flexure** is held in place by a fibromuscular band, the **suspensory muscle of the duodenum** (ligament of Treitz). This structure passes from the posterior aspect of the ascending part of the duodenum and the duodenojejunal flexure to the right crus of the diaphragm. Palpate this supporting structure and sever it close to the duodenojejunal junction. With your fingers, detach the **duodenum** and **pancreas** from the posterior abdominal wall. Do *not* damage the bile passages or vessels of the pancreaticoduodenal region.
10. Identify the **inferior vena cava** as it approaches the dorsal surface of the liver (*Atlas*, 2.50). Lift the liver anteriorly and superiorly, and follow the inferior cava to the point where it is attached to the dorsal surface of the liver. At this level, cut through this large vessel as close to the liver as possible (*Atlas*, 2.36).

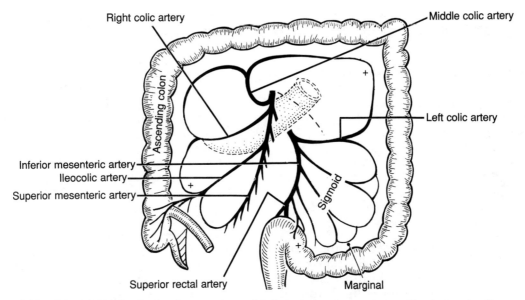

Figure 2.36. Arterial supply of colon by superior and inferior mesenteric arteries. The + denotes three weak points in the marginal anastomoses.

11. The last organ to be mobilized is the **liver:** incise the **falciform ligament** between the diaphragm and the diaphragmatic surface of the liver. Cut the **left triangular ligament** and then the anterior portion of the **coronary ligament** (Fig. 2.23). Forcibly pull the liver inferiorly with one hand and **cut the inferior vena cava** at the point where it pierces the diaphragm (*Atlas*, 2.100). Cut along the remaining portion of the coronary ligament. Again, observe the hepatorenal ligament as you cut through it (Fig. 2.23).

12. Finally, **remove the detached GI tract together with the liver, the pancreas, and the spleen.** Carefully lift the organs out of the abdominal cavity. Avoid tearing the fragile inferior mesenteric vein; thus, support the weight of the sigmoid colon and the descending colon with one hand. Place the organs on a tray or table, and arrange them in their *characteristic anatomical configuration* (*Atlas*, 2.2A). This is an instructive exercise that will contribute greatly to your understanding of the disposition of the GI tract and its three unpaired organs (liver; pancreas; spleen). Now, the various organs, their interconnections, and their blood vessels can be conveniently examined in greater detail.

Detailed Examination of GI Tract and Its Unpaired Organs

Identify the main **tributaries of the portal vein** (splenic; superior mesenteric; inferior mesenteric; *Atlas*, 2.53). Clean these vessels and the portal vein. Make a special effort to trace **esophageal and gastric veins** to the portal vein. Does your cadaver specimen have esophageogastric varices?

Clean the **celiac trunk.** Observe strands of **autonomic nerve fibers** accompanying the celiac trunk and its

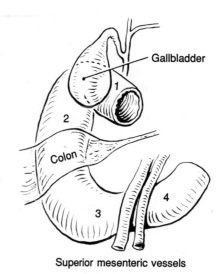

Figure 2.37. Three structures that are related anteriorly to the four parts (*1, 2, 3, 4*) of the duodenum: gallbladder, transverse colon, and superior mesenteric vessels.

branches. These fibers are derived from the celiac plexus of nerves. Review (*Atlas*, 2.32, 2.65) and then clean all **branches of the celiac trunk: splenic, left gastric, hepatic.** Follow the gastroduodenal artery and note a branch that supplies the posterior aspect of the pancreas and duodenum (posterior superior pancreaticoduodenal artery; *Atlas*, 2.65B). Realize that the splenic artery sends branches to the body and tail of the pancreas (*Atlas*, 2.65). Look for **lymph nodes** along the course of the splenic artery. These nodes receive lymphatic drainage from the tail of the pancreas and from the spleen, hence the term **pancreaticosplenic nodes** (*Atlas*, 2.105).

Pick up the severed end of the superior mesenteric artery. Clean and follow its branches to the head of the pancreas and the three distal portions of the duodenum. Re-

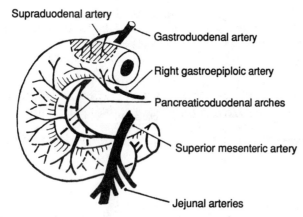

Figure 2.38. Blood supply of duodenum.

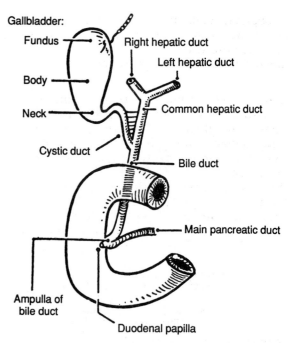

Figure 2.39. Bile passages (anterior view).

view the relations of the duodenum, pancreas, and superior mesenteric vessels (Fig. 2.37; *Atlas*, 2.64, 2.86): the four portions of the duodenum are molded around the head of the pancreas. Near the junction of its third and fourth portions, the duodenum is crossed ventrally by the superior mesenteric vessels. Verify this fact. Review the blood supply to the duodenum and pancreas (Fig. 2.38; *Atlas*, 2.65). If present as a variation, identify and follow the right hepatic artery from the superior mesenteric artery to the porta hepatis.

Review the **bile passages** (Fig. 2.39 or *Atlas*, 2.66). Turn the duodenum and pancreas slightly as to make their posterior surfaces accessible. Follow the **bile duct** to a groove on the posterior surface of the head of the pancreas (*Atlas*, 2.64B). With probe and scissors, carefully free the duct from surrounding pancreatic tissue. Follow it to the point where it passes obliquely through the wall of the descending (second) portion of the duodenum. The opening into the duodenum is the **major duodenal papilla** (of Vater). Take great care *not* to destroy the **main pancreatic duct** that (usually) joins the terminal portion of the bile duct (Fig. 2.39). Notice that the wall of the common terminal portion of both ducts is thickened. This is due to a smooth sphincter muscle, the **sphincter of Oddi.** Follow the main pancreatic duct for 5 cm into the substance of the pancreas. Note numerous small ducts which drain into the main duct. In addition, an accessory duct may open separately into the duodenum (*Atlas*, 2.66). Open the duodenum by a 5 cm incision just opposite the entrance of the bile duct. Observe the **major duodenal papilla** and the **hood-like plica** that covers it (*Atlas*, 2.67).If an accessory pancreatic duct is present, there may be a minor duodenal papilla about 2 cm superior to the major papilla. Be aware of the variability of pancreatic ducts (*Atlas*, 2.70).

The bile passages and the pancreatic ducts can be demonstrated radiographically. This can be accomplished by *endoscopic retrograde cholangiography and pancreatography (ERCP).* A fiberoptic endoscope is passed through the patient's mouth, esophagus, and stomach into the second portion of the duodenum. Under visual control, the major duodenal papilla (of Vater) is cannulated, and a radiopaque dye is injected in a retrograde fashion (i.e., in the opposite direction of the usual flow of fluids). In this manner, the pancreatic and biliary systems can be evaluated radiographically. Correlate your gross anatomical knowledge of these systems with a suitable image obtained with ERCP (*Atlas*, 2.68).

Examine the **bile duct** throughout its entire length. Does your cadaver specimen have a gallbladder? Is there evidence that a cholecystectomy had been performed prior to death? If the gallbladder is present, follow the **cystic duct** to the **gallbladder.** With probe and forceps, carefully remove part of the fundus of the gallbladder from its bed. Notice numerous small veins that plunge directly from the gallbladder into the liver (a magnifying glass is helpful). These small veins are of surgical importance. Immediately after cholecystectomy (removal of the gallbladder), the surgeon must overcome the problem of blood oozing from the gallbladder bed. Incise the gallbladder and examine its contents (bile; are there gallstones?). Observe the characteristic honeycombed mucosa of the gallbladder. Be aware of the variations (*Atlas*, 2.43, 2.45, 2.46).

Next, examine the **liver.** Note that its sharp inferior border separates the visceral from the diaphragmatic surface. On the posterior aspect, observe the triangular, granulated **bare area.** Here, the liver was attached to the diaphragm (Fig. 2.23; *Atlas*, 2.37). Around the bare area, note the peritoneal reflections of the **coronary ligament.**

Observe the **four lobes of the liver**: *right, left, quadrate,* and *caudate* (Figs. 2.40 and 2.41; *Atlas*, 2.39). Note the H-shaped deep fissures and wide sulci defining the four lobes (Fig. 2.41):

1. **Right sagittal fossa**; posteriorly forming a groove for the inferior vena cava (IVC), and inferiorly forming the shallow bed for the gallbladder.

2. **Left sagittal fissure;** accommodates the ligamentum venosum posteriorly, and the round ligament (ligamentum teres) inferiorly.
3. **Transverse fissure, the porta hepatis.**

Review all structures passing through the porta hepatis. Examine the small segment of **inferior vena cava** (IVC) that is attached to its groove. Note that the two or three large **hepatic veins** drain directly into it. Be fully aware of the difference between portal vein and hepatic veins (*Atlas*, 2.54).

Realize that the liver has a substantial lymphatic drainage. At the porta hepatis, there are several lymph vessels that drain into **hepatic lymph nodes** (*Atlas*, 2.106B). Make an attempt to find a representative node (usually not larger than a small bean) around the bile duct and portal vein. From there, the lymphatics drain into the **celiac nodes** around the root of the celiac artery.

Section part of the liver (*Atlas*, 2.56). Observe:

1. Branches of portal vein, hepatic artery, and bile ducts (stained green) lying together and being surrounded by the perivascular fibrous capsule.
2. Hepatic veins, unaccompanied (lying alone) and having no capsule.

Clinical Observations. The liver is subject to many pathological changes, and some of these are likely to be encountered in the gross anatomical laboratory. The liver may be smooth and considerably enlarged. This happens most often in passive liver congestion due to cardiac insufficiency (cardiac liver). In contrast, the liver may appear small and show a regular formation of small nodules throughout. Such a finding is most likely a case of liver cirrhosis (frequently the result of alcoholism). Metastatic (secondary) tumors are often encountered. These vary widely in appearance. You may find numerous small white nodules bulging over the surface, or you may find an occasional single large node.

Be aware of the fact that the liver can be subdivided into segments, similar to those in the lung (*Atlas*, 2.58, 2.59). Each segment contains its own branch of the hepatic artery, bile duct, and portal vein. This segmentation is of surgical relevance since parts of a diseased liver can be removed segmentally without indiscriminately interrupting the functionally important triad of hepatic artery, bile duct, and portal vein.

The patency of portal triads and particularly of hepatic veins can be readily assessed with an ultrasound scan (*Atlas*, 2.57).

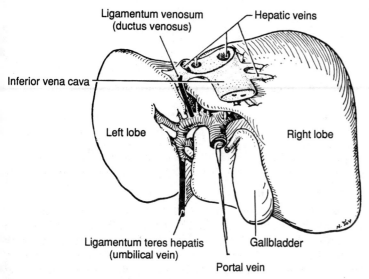

Figure 2.40. Visceral and dorsal surfaces of liver (posterior view). Portal vein and inferior vena cava.

Spleen (*Atlas*, 2.62, 2.63). Sizes and weights vary considerably. Observe:

1. **Hilus;** for entrance and exit of splenic vessels;

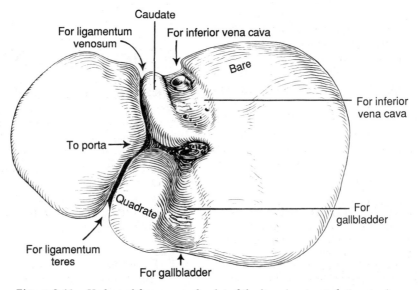

Figure 2.41. H-shaped fissures and sulci of the liver (posteroinferior view).

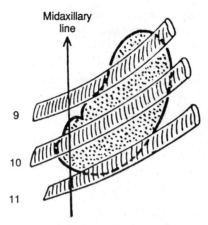

Figure 2.42. Spleen in relation to ribs.

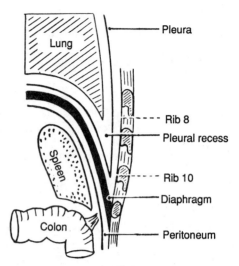

Figure 2.43. Topographic relations of spleen. Coronal section in midaxillary line.

2. **Borders;** anterior and superior borders are sharp and often notched; posterior and inferior borders are rounded;
3. **Visceral surface;** divided according to contact areas with other viscera: gastric, renal, pancreatic, and colic;
4. **Diaphragmatic surface;** convex and smooth.

Place your hand into the (now empty) left hypochondriac region, where the spleen was located. Realize the topographical relationship of spleen to ribs 9, 10, and 11 (Fig. 2.42). Push a probe horizontally through the 9th intercostal space, about 2 to 3 cm posterior to the midaxillary line. Realize that the instrument passes through the pleural cavity and through the diaphragm into the abdominal cavity and then into the spleen (Fig. 2.43; *Atlas*, 2.61). These topographical relations are of great importance in evaluating stab wounds and injuries associated with displaced rib fractures.

The anterior notched border of the spleen can often be visualized on plain radiographic films. Verify the close relationship between spleen and colon. The anterior notched border of the spleen can occasionally produce a characteristic scalloping of the colonic surface near the left (splenic) flexure. A pathologically enlarged spleen may indent the fundus or the greater curvature of the stomach. This fact is useful in diagnostic radiology.

In about 10 to 20% of cases, one or more small "accessory spleens" may exist. They are usually located in the splenic hilus or along the splenic vessels. Does the cadaver you are working on have an accessory spleen?

Interior Organ Inspection. The interior of representative portions of the GI tract should be inspected. Study prosected specimens and specially prepared museum specimens. If these are not available, use the removed GI tract of the cadaver and observe the following:

1. **Stomach** (*Atlas*, 2.28B); longitudinal ridges along the lesser curvature; pyloric sphincter and orifice (*Atlas*, 2.28C). Study radiographs of the upper gastrointestinal (GI) system (*Atlas*, 2.29, 2.30).

2. **Duodenum** (*Atlas*, 2.67); major and minor duodenal papillae (seen before); pronounced plicae circulares.
3. **Jejunum** (*Atlas*, 2.77A); tall, closely packed plicae circulares.
4. **Ileum** (*Atlas*, 2.77B and C); few plicae circulares in upper part; absence of plicae in lower part; look for a Meckel's diverticulum, found in 2% of all cases (*Atlas*, 2.72).
5. **Ileocecal region** (*Atlas*, 2.72); open the cecum. Clean the region with sponge and water. Study the ileocecal orifice and the orifice of the vermiform appendix. Section the appendix and examine its interior surface.
6. **Colon** (*Atlas*, 2.72, 2.77D); haustra (sacculations); the crescentic fold between the haustra are called the plicae semilunares. Correlate your gross anatomical observations with a suitable radiograph (*Atlas*, 2.75).

Store the detached GI tract with its three unpaired organs in a plastic bag for future reference. Make sure the specimen is well moistened with preservative fluid.

Posterior Abdominal Viscera

General Remarks and Orientation

Work will be more pleasant if you sponge the posterior abdominal region and pouches. It is impossible to dissect nerves and vessels in a pool of liquefied fat. Always keep the specimen moist with mold-deterrent preservative fluid.

Palpate the kidneys and the suprarenal (adrenal) glands. The suprarenal glands are friable and very easily torn. Note that the suprarenal glands are closely related to the cranial poles of the kidneys. Only a film of fatty tissue intervenes between kidney and suprarenal gland. Once again, identify the abdominal aorta and its bifurcation. To the right of the aorta observe the inferior vena cava (IVC).

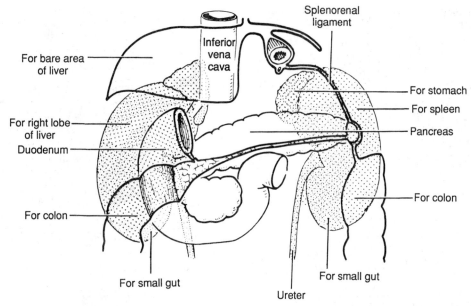

Figure 2.44. Anterior relations of kidneys and suprarenal glands.

Before continuing with the dissection, review the posterior abdominal viscera and their ventral relations (Fig. 2.44; *Atlas*, 2.84A).

Point your finger to the caudal part of the **right kidney.** Here, it was in contact with the right colic flexure. About three-fourths of the ventral surface is still covered with parietal peritoneum. Here, the right kidney was in contact with the visceral surface of the liver (hepatorenal recess; compare Fig. 2.23). Place your finger on the medial border of the right kidney. Here, it was in contact with the descending portion of the duodenum. Examine the **left kidney.** At about the middle of its ventral surface, it was in contact with the tail of the pancreas (Fig. 2.44). Caudal to this pancreatic area is a region that was in contact with the left colic flexure.

Before you begin . . .

The parietal peritoneal covering of the posterior abdominal wall will be removed. This procedure will completely expose the abdominal aorta and its branches and the inferior vena cava and its tributaries. The kidneys will be shelled out of their fatty capsules. Next, their vessels and excretory ducts (ureters) will be studied. After ventral reflection of the kidneys and removal of the fatty renal capsule, the posterior abdominal wall will be accessible. Its muscles will be studied. Then, the lumbar plexus of nerves will be examined. Finally, the roof of the abdominal cavity, the diaphragm, will be studied.

Testicular and Ovarian Vessels

Testicular and Ovarian Arteries and Veins (*Atlas*, 2.85). *Note:* The testicular (male) and ovarian (female) vessels are small and easily damaged or lost; the corresponding veins

are usually much larger. Observe these vessels shining through the parietal peritoneal covering.

In the **male cadaver,** note that the testicular vessels cross the ureter (*Atlas*, 2.85, 3.18, 3.29). The ureter must *not* be damaged during dissection. Pick up the testicular vessels at the deep inguinal ring. Free them and follow them superiorly. Observe (*Atlas*, 2.85):

1. The **left testicular vein** drains into the **left renal vein.**
2. The **right testicular vein** drains directly into the **IVC.**
3. The **right** and **left testicular arteries** originate directly from the aorta, inferior to the origin of the renal arteries.

In the **female cadaver,** dissect the corresponding **ovarian vessels** (*Atlas*, 3.45). They cross the external iliac vessels very close to the ureter.

Kidneys and Suprarenal Glands

Kidneys (L. *renes*, kidneys). The kidney is embedded in a substantial mass of fat, the **perirenal fat or adipose (fatty) capsule.** Observe that little fatty tissue lies in front of the kidney. Most of the fat lies lateral and posterior to the organ (*Atlas*, 2.108). The **renal fascia** encloses both the kidney and its fatty capsule. Verify that the kidneys are *not* rigidly fixed to the posterior abdominal wall. In fact, in the living subject, they move slightly up and down during respiration.

With your fingers, shell out the kidneys from the renal fascia and fatty capsule. The superior pole is separated from the suprarenal gland by a thin layer of fat. Carefully pass your fingers between kidney and suprarenal gland and separate the two organs. Note the characteristic bean shape of the kidney (*Atlas*, 2.87).

The approximate measurements of an adult kidney are: length, 11 to 12 cm; breadth, 5 to 8 cm; thickness, 3 to 4 cm. The weight of each kidney varies from 120 to 170 g. In one out of 400 cases, you may find a "horseshoe" kidney. This is an anomaly (*Atlas*, 2.97D).

Left Kidney (*Atlas*, 2.85). Dissect the **left renal vein** from IVC to the hilus of the left kidney. Observe and dissect venous tributaries: **left testicular or ovarian vein** (already seen), and **venous channels from the left suprarenal gland**. In order to have full access to the renal artery, the left renal vein must be severed close to the IVC and reflected toward the left. Now, find the **left renal artery**. Follow this large vessel to the renal hilus. Usually, the artery divides into two branches before it enters the kidney. Accessory renal arteries are common. Observe fine branches to the ureter and to the suprarenal gland. The renal arteries are accompanied by autonomic nerve fibers (*Atlas*, 2.104). Identify strands of autonomic nerves surrounding the left renal artery.

Left Renal Pelvis and Ureter. Reflect the left kidney anteriorly and toward the right. At the most posterior part of the hilus, identify the **renal pelvis** and its inferior continuation, the **ureter**. Follow and dissect the ureter. Observe:

1. **Abdominal part of ureter** (*Atlas*, 2.85); crosses the psoas major muscle; runs obliquely posterior to the testicular (ovarian) vessels. Verify that the superior portion of the right ureter runs lateral to the IVC.
2. **Pelvic part of ureter**; dissect it for a short distance along the wall of the pelvic cavity. Its junction with the urinary bladder will be seen later.

Right Kidney. Dissect the relatively short right renal vein from IVC to the hilus of the right kidney (*Atlas*, 2.85). Since the left renal vein was severed earlier, the IVC can easily be reflected inferiorly and slightly to the right. This procedure will expose the **right renal artery** (or arteries). Identify the **renal pelvis**, and follow the **ureter** caudally. Observe the relations between right ureter, right testicular (ovarian) vessels, and psoas muscle. (If the right ureter passes posterior to the IVC, it is called "retrocaval ureter" (*Atlas*, 2.97C). This condition may interfere with proper drainage of urine from the right kidney).

Next, reflect the kidneys and remove the substantial fatty renal capsule and the renal fascia by forcibly pulling it off the posterior abdominal wall. Clean the posterior abdominal wall, and sponge the entire area clean. Identify the following muscles (Fig. 2.45; *Atlas*, 2.85): **Transversus abdominis, quadratus lumborum, iliacus,** and **psoas major**. Also, identify the floating **12th rib** and the **diaphragm**. Now, study the topographic relations between kidneys and the posterior abdominal wall. Verify that the dorsal surface of each kidney is in contact with the diaphragm, psoas major, quadratus lumborum, and the posterior tendinous portion of the transversus abdominis. The superior pole of the right kidney lies at the level of the 12th rib. The left kidney is positioned somewhat higher; its superior pole lies at the level of the 11th rib (Fig. 2.45).

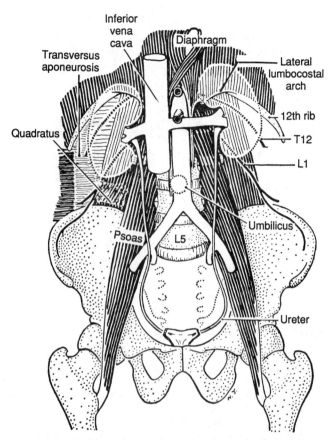

Figure 2.45. Posterior relations of the kidneys.

The liver is responsible for "pushing" the right kidney down (and the right lung up).

The traditional surgical approach to the kidney is the lumbar renal or retroperitoneal approach. Lumbar nephrectomy (extirpation of kidney via the retroperitoneal lumbar route) is indicated when contamination of the peritoneal cavity is likely (inflammatory renal disease, calculi). The lumbar approach to the kidney (*Atlas*, 2.107 through 2.110) is an optional exercise described in Appendix I. The transabdominal approach to the kidney is mainly employed for surgery of the renal vessels and kidney transplants.

The arterial distribution in the kidney is of surgical importance. Usually, the renal artery divides into an anterior and posterior branch. These branches supply the anterior and posterior halves of the kidney, respectively (*Atlas*, 2.95, 2.96). There are no anastomoses. Thus, there are no large vessels in the longitudinal plane of the kidney. Hence, surgical procedures along this plane (nephrotomy) offer the advantage of minimal hemorrhage. Study a corrosion cast of a segmental artery (*Atlas*, 2.92). Correlate the renal arterial distribution with a renal arteriogram (*Atlas*, 2.93).

Kidney on Section (Fig. 2.46; *Atlas*, 2.89). Do *not* sever the kidneys from their vessels or ureters. Divide the left kidney into anterior and posterior halves by splitting it longitudinally along its convex, lateral border. Identify and observe:

1. **Fibrous capsule,** which can be easily stripped off;

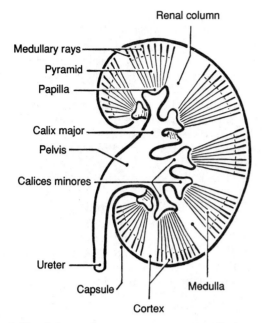

Medullary rays
Pyramid
Papilla
Calix major
Pelvis
Calices minores
Ureter
Capsule
Cortex
Medulla
Renal column

Figure 2.46. Schema of macroscopic structure of kidney on longitudinal section.

2. **Renal cortex;** the outer one-third; of granulated appearance (microanatomy: consists of glomeruli and convoluted tubules);
3. **Renal medulla,** consists of:
   a. **Renal pyramids** (microanatomy: loops of Henle; collecting ducts join a central tube which opens at a renal papilla);
   b. **Renal columns** (microanatomy: interlobular arteries and veins);
4. **Renal papillae;** in groups of two or three, projecting into small cups, the calyces minores;
5. **Calyces minores,** unite to form two or three **calyces majores;** the major calyces unite to form the **renal pelvis,** which leads to the **ureter.**

> As a clinical correlation, study the renal collecting structures in a pyelogram (*Atlas*, 2.90). Normally, the renal pelvis is found at the level of the spinous process L1. Be aware of variations (*Atlas*, 2.97A through E).

Suprarenal (Adrenal) Glands (*Atlas*, 2.85). These glands deteriorate rapidly after death. Depending on the quality of body embalmment, they may or may not be well preserved. The right and left adrenal glands differ in gross morphology and their topographic relationships. Verify that the right adrenal gland is roughly triangular in shape, has only a loose attachment to the superior pole of the right kidney, and lies just posterior to the inferior vena cava. Observe that the left adrenal gland is semilunar in shape and is closely adjacent to the superior and medial border of the left kidney (occasionally extending to the level of the renal hilus). Realize that numerous arteries supply the suprarenal glands (*Atlas*, 2.98). These vessels are derived from the aorta, renal artery, and inferior phrenic ar-

tery. The venous blood is emptied either into the renal vein or inferior vena cava. The suprarenals receive numerous sympathetic nerve fibers. Section one gland, and distinguish between cortex and medulla.

> Realize that kidneys and adrenal glands have a separate embryonic origin. Therefore, the development and position of the adrenal glands is usually unaffected by renal abnormalities or anomalous renal positions. The adrenal glands develop in their normal position just lateral to the celiac trunk.
> The adrenal glands can usually be well demonstrated and morphologically evaluated by computed tomography (CT).

Review the abdominal aorta and its branches. Identify (*Atlas*, 2.98):

1. **Branches to the GI tract and its three unpaired organs** (celiac; superior mesenteric; inferior mesenteric);
2. **Branches to the three paired organs** (suprarenal; renal; testicular or ovarian);
3. **Branches to walls** of the abdominal cavity (phrenic; lumbar); realize that there are four paired **lumbar arteries** that are responsible for the segmental blood supply of the lumbar region. Identify at least one representative lumbar vessel. Trace it as closely as possible to its origin from the dorsal aspect of the abdominal aorta. Notice that the lumbar arteries disappear in the depth of muscles positioned on either side of the vertebral column (*Atlas*, 2.98).
4. **Bifurcation of abdominal aorta,** at the level of L4. The umbilicus projects just superior to the bifurcation (Fig. 2.45 or *Atlas*, 2.1D).
5. **Common iliac arteries,** which divide into internal and external iliac arteries (*Atlas*, 2.1C).

Review the **inferior vena cava (IVC)** and its tributaries (*Atlas*, 2.99). Recapitulate the **portacaval system** (*Atlas*, 2.54).

Posterior Abdominal Wall

Once again, identify the muscles of the posterior abdominal wall (*Atlas*, 2.103):

1. **Psoas major;** arises from lumbar vertebrae (sides; intervertebral discs; transverse processes); ventral to the psoas major, the long flat tendon of the psoas minor can be observed.
2. **Iliacus;** occupies the extensive iliac fossa; iliacus and psoas form a functional unit; thus, they are referred to as **iliopsoas.** The iliopsoas is the most powerful flexor of the thigh.
3. **Quadratus lumborum;** thick, rhomboidal muscular sheet, running from iliac crest to lumbar transverse

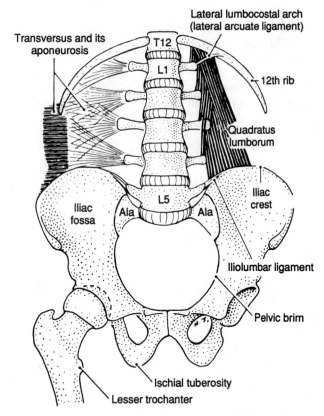

Figure 2.47. Muscles of posterior abdominal wall (excluding the psoas major muscle).

processes and rib 12; flexes vertebral column (Fig. 2.47; *Atlas*, 2.1**B**).

4. **Transversus abdominis** (Fig. 2.47); running horizontally posterior to the oblique borders of the quadratus lumborum.

Nerves of the Posterior Abdominal Wall (*Atlas*, 2.103). These are ventral rami of T12 to L5 that are derived from the lumbar nerve plexus. Carefully remove the fascia from the posterior abdominal muscles to expose the nerves. Expect to find variations. The usual pattern is as follows:

1. **Subcostal nerve** (T12); about 1 cm caudal to rib 12.
2. **Iliohypogastric** and **ilioinguinal nerves** (L1); descending steeply in front of the quadratus lumborum. Frequently, the two nerves arise from a common trunk and do not separate until they reach the transversus abdominis muscle. Positively identify the ilioinguinal nerve. Identify it again at the anterior abdominal wall. Trace it back from the superficial inguinal ring (*Atlas*, 2.5) to the plane between internal oblique and transversus abdominis (*Atlas*, 2.10, 2.12). Establish its continuity at the posterior abdominal wall. *Note:* Variations of these two nerves are common. Occasionally, the ilioinguinal nerve is absent.
3. **Genitofemoral nerve** (*Atlas*, 2.103); piercing the anterior surface of the psoas. It supplies a small portion of

skin inferior and medial to the inguinal ligament as well as the cremaster muscle.

4. **Lateral cutaneous nerve of thigh** (*Atlas*, 2.103); it passes deep to the inguinal ligament near the anterior superior iliac spine. This nerve supplies the lateral aspect of the thigh with sensory fibers.
5. **Femoral nerve** (L2, L3, L4). Large nerve lying in the angle between psoas and iliacus, and then deep to the inguinal ligament; provides motor and sensory contributions to the anterior and medial thigh.
6. **Obturator nerve** (L2, L3, L4); at the medial border of the psoas. Find the nerve in the following manner:
   a. Identify the obturator foramen in the skeleton. Palpate the obturator groove from inside the pelvis.
   b. Now, palpate the obturator groove from inside the pelvis in the cadaver. This is precisely the point where the obturator nerve passes from the pelvis into the thigh (*Atlas*, 3.34, 3.38, 3.40). Free the nerve with a probe, and follow it superiorly to the medial border of the psoas.
7. **Lumbosacral trunk** (*Atlas*, 2.103, 3.33, 3.34, 3.35). This large trunk consists of ventral rami of part of L4 and all of L5. The trunk runs caudally to the sacral plexus. The large and flat lumbosacral trunk is tightly applied to the ala of the sacrum. It is difficult to see with the psoas muscle in place.
8. **Sympathetic trunk** (*Atlas*, 2.103, 2.104, 3.33, 3.34). Trace the continuity of the sympathetic trunk from the thoracic cavity to the abdominal cavity. Look for rami communicantes passing from ganglia to lumbar nerves. **Review the autonomic nerve supply of the abdomen** (*Atlas*, 2.104).

The origin of the nerves of the posterior abdominal wall (paragraphs 1–7 above) from the lumbar plexus can only be studied after careful removal of the psoas major muscle. Since the nerves traverse the muscle at different depths, it is necessary to remove the psoas in a piecemeal fashion. Ask your instructor if the psoas muscle should be removed on both sides. Usually it is sufficient to demonstrate the lumbar plexus on one side only. Using fingers and forceps, peel up the muscle and remove it gradually bit by bit. Study the **lumbar plexus**. Identify the **lumbosacral trunk** (*Atlas*, 2.103, 3.33).

Diaphragm

Diaphragm (*Atlas*, 2.100, 2.103). The diaphragm forms the roof of the abdominal cavity. Strip parietal peritoneum and areolar tissue off its fleshy fibers.
   Identify:

1. **Sternal part;**
2. **Costal part;** from the inferior six ribs; interdigitating with transversus abdominis;
3. **Lumbar part;**
   a. **Right crus;** just lateral to the esophageal hiatus, look for a muscle slip running in an inferomedial di-

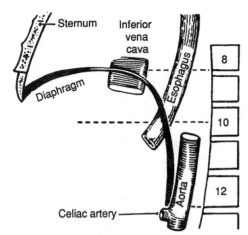

Figure 2.48. Diaphragm at levels of T8 through T12: The more superior the vertebral level, the more anterior is the opening in the diaphragm.

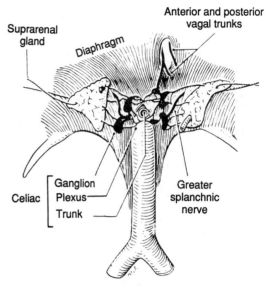

Figure 2.49. Celiac plexus and ganglia located on each side of the celiac trunk at vertebral level T12/L1.

rection. This is the remaining portion of the suspensory muscle of the duodenum (ligament of Treitz) that supports the duodenojejunal flexure.

b. **Left crus;**
c. Fleshy fibers from the **arcuate ligaments** (lumbocostal arches);
4. **Medial arcuate ligament;** a tendinous arch providing a gap for the psoas muscle;
5. **Lateral arcuate ligament;** across the superior portion of the quadratus lumborum;
6. **Central tendon.**

Study the three large openings in the diaphragm (Fig. 2.48; *Atlas*, 2.100, 2.101). Readily identify the two openings from which the traversing structures have been removed: **vena cava foramen** and **esophageal hiatus.** The aorta (still in place) traverses the **aortic hiatus.** Note that this hiatus is formed by the union of the medial tendinous margins of the two crura, known as the median arcuate ligament. Identify the thoracic vertebral levels at which the openings in the diaphragm occur (Fig. 2.48; *Atlas*, 2.101). *Observe:* The higher the vertebral level, the more ventral is the hiatus (opening) in the diaphragm.

The **greater splanchnic nerves** traverse the crura (*Atlas*, 2.104). To find them, proceed in the following manner: in the thorax, identify the greater splanchnic nerve on one side. Follow it to the diaphragm. Parallel to the nerve, push a probe through the diaphragm. Pick up the probe and splanchnic nerve at the abdominal aspect of the crura (*Atlas*, 2.104). Note that the main portion of the splanchnic nerve runs toward the celiac ganglion (Fig. 2.49; *Atlas*, 2.104). Review the autonomic nerve supply of the abdomen.

Transverse Sections Through Abdomen. Integrate gross anatomical studies of the abdomen with transverse sectional anatomy. Use actual transverse sectional slices or plastic-embedded sliced specimens if available. Knowledge of transverse sectional anatomy is of considerable importance in view of the wide clinical use of computerized tomography (CT) and/or magnetic resonance images (MRI) for diagnostic purposes. Refer to *Atlas*, 2.112, and study abdominal transverse sections at three important levels: at the level of the liver and spleen, at the level of the renal vessels, and at the level of the inferior poles of the kidneys. Study the corresponding magnetic resonance images and appreciate the fact that significant structural information can be obtained in the living person with this technology. The physician must be able to analyze these transverse sectional images and to distinguish normal from abnormal. Remember that it is clinical convention to view transverse CT and MRI sections from inferior; thus, right-sided structures (e.g., liver) appear on the left side of the printed image.

Other Sections Through Abdomen. Using the technique of ultrasound, one can obtain various sections through parts of the abdomen, particularly through soft tissues and blood vessels. Although these images appear somewhat distorted in comparison with the actual anatomical field, they nevertheless can provide most valuable diagnostic information. Refer to *Atlas*, 2.111, and appreciate examples of abdominal ultrasound images. Refer to a suitable cadaver and identify the anatomical fields displayed in the shown ultrasound images. In addition, study coronal and sagittal MRI scans of the abdomen (*Atlas*, 2.113).

CHAPTER 3

THE PELVIS AND PERINEUM

Laboratory Approach to Pelvis and Perineum

The dissection of the pelvis and perineum requires time, skill, and patience. Dissection is difficult because (1) only one or two students can work simultaneously on the spatially limited dissection field, (2) the topography of various anatomical structures is complex, and (3) there are considerable anatomical differences between male and female specimens.

Requirements and expectations for this anatomical region vary greatly from school to school. It is possible that your teaching faculty may want to make changes in the dissection sequence or approach. Please, check with your instructors.

The method presented in this chapter has been chosen because it has been used successfully in a number of schools. *Definitions, Important Landmarks* and the *Anal Region* are covered initially. Subsequently, the chapter is divided into two separate sections, taking into account the differences between male and female specimens: (1) *Male Pelvis and Perineum* and (2) *Female Pelvis and Perineum*. Students are urged to exchange information in the dissection of specimens from the opposite sex. Obviously, students will be expected to demonstrate knowledge of both male and female anatomy in the pelvic and perineal regions.

General Remarks and Definitions

The **pelvis** (L. *pelvis*, basin) is divided into the greater pelvis and lesser pelvis. By definition, the **pelvic brim** is the circumference of a plane dividing the two pelvic portions (Fig. 3.1). The **greater pelvis** (pelvis major; false pelvis) is situated superior to the pelvic brim, and is bounded on either side by the ilium. The **lesser pelvis** (pelvis minor; true pelvis) is situated caudal to the pelvic brim.

The walls of the pelvic cavity are in part lined with muscles (see Fig. 3.4; *Atlas*, 3.60**B**). No muscle crosses the pelvic brim (if muscles crossed the pelvic brim, they would interfere with childbirth by partially obstructing the pelvic inlet).

The **floor of the pelvis** is formed by muscles collectively called the **pelvic diaphragm** (Fig. 3.1). The principal organs contained in the pelvic cavity have their outlet in the median plane (Fig. 3.2). They pass through the pelvic floor and are anchored to it. The GI tract (rectum) lies posteriorly and passes through the **anal region** or "anal triangle." The urinary system lies anteriorly. The genital system takes an intermediate position. Both systems (urinary and genital) pass through the **urogenital region** or "urogenital triangle" of the pelvic floor. Together, the **anal triangle** and the **urogenital triangle** form the diamond-shaped **perineum** or perineal region (Fig. 3.3).

The **peritoneal cavity** extends into the lesser pelvis (hence the term "abdominopelvic cavity"). In the lesser pelvis, the **peritoneum** partially invests several pelvic organs, notably the rectum and bladder (see Fig. 3.16), and in the female also the uterus (see Fig. 3.28).

Pelvic Fascia (Fig. 3.4). The pelvic fascia consists of **two parts:** (1) **parietal pelvic fascia** and (2) **visceral pelvic fascia.** The intrapelvic surfaces of the muscles lining the

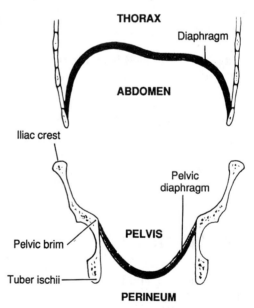

Figure 3.1. Diaphragm and pelvic diaphragm (coronal section). The perineum is the region inferior to the pelvic diaphragm.

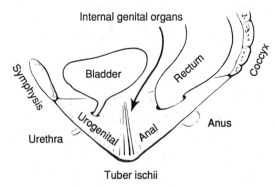

Figure 3.2. Urinary system passing through "urogenital triangle," digestive system traversing "anal triangle" of the diamond-shaped floor of the pelvis (pelvic diaphragm).

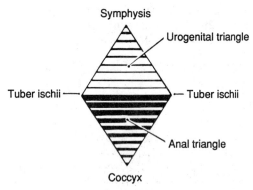

Figure 3.3. Diamond-shaped perineal region. Urogenital and anal triangles.

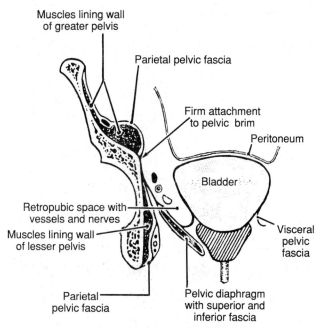

Figure 3.4. Diagram of pelvic fascia and retropubic space (male pelvis; coronal section).

walls of the pelvic cavity are covered with the **parietal pelvic fascia.** This fascia is firmly attached to the **pelvic brim** (which runs anteriorly toward the pubic symphysis). The parietal pelvic fascia is also continuous with the fascia lining both the superior and inferior surfaces of the pelvic diaphragm. The **visceral pelvic fascia** provides a fascial covering for the pelvic viscera (e.g., for the bladder; Fig. 3.4).

The space between parietal pelvic fascia and bladder, particularly posterior to the pubic region but also extending laterally, is called the **retropubic space.** This space contains extraperitoneal fat and areolar tissue, blood vessels, and nerves (Fig. 3.4).

The structures that fill the inferior aperture (outlet) of the pelvis are called the **perineum.** The perineum is a diamond-shaped area (Fig. 3.3) extending from symphysis pubis to coccyx. A transverse line between the right and left ischial tuberosities divides the perineal region into two triangular areas, the **urogenital region (triangle)** and the **anal region (triangle).**

Important Landmarks

Refer to an articulated bony pelvis, preferably one with intact ligaments. Feel free to orientate the pelvis in such a manner that its position compares with that of the cadaver under dissection. Observe the following (*Atlas*, 3.1 to 3.7):

1. The **bony pelvis** is formed by:
   a. **Right hip bone** (os coxae), anteriorly and laterally on the right.
   b. **Left hip bone** (os coxae), anteriorly and laterally on the left.
   c. **Sacrum and coccyx,** parts of the vertebral column, interposed dorsally between the two hip bones.
2. **Pelvic brim** (*Atlas*, 3.2B); surrounds the **pelvic inlet or superior aperture** of the pelvis; extends from the **promontory** of the sacrum dorsally to the **symphysis pubis** ventrally; distinguish the three parts of the pelvic brim:
   a. Anterior border of ala of sacrum (sacral part);
   b. Arcuate line (iliac part);
   c. Pecten pubis and pubic crest (pubic part).
3. In the **erect posture** (anatomical position), the anterior superior iliac spines and the upper end of the symphysis pubis occupy the same vertical plane (*Atlas*, 3.1C). In this position, the plane of the superior aperture (pelvic inlet) forms an angle of 50° to 60° with the horizontal plane. Verify this.
4. **Obturator foramen** (*Atlas*, 5.1A); this foramen is closed by the obturator membrane (*Atlas*, 3.4); superiorly, the obturator canal (for obturator nerve and vessels) traverses the membrane.
5. **Ischial tuberosity** (*Atlas*, 3.6).
6. **Ischial spine** (*Atlas*, 3.6, 5.1B).
7. **Sacrospinous and sacrotuberous ligaments** (anterior view, *Atlas*, 3.4; posterior view, *Atlas*, 3.6; medial view, *Atlas*, 3.40); the sacrospinous ligament stretches from coccyx to ischial spine. The sacrotuberous ligament stretches from sacrum to ischial tuberosity. The sacrospinous and sacrotuberous ligaments form the partial boundaries for two foramina: **lesser sciatic foramen** and **greater sciatic foramen.**

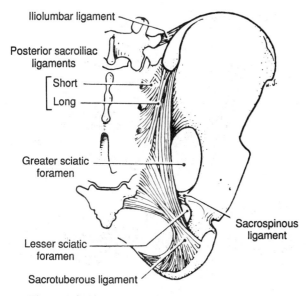

Figure 3.5. Ligaments of the pelvis (dorsal view).

Note: The term "sciatic" is interchangeable with "ischiadic" (*Nomina Anatomica*).

8. **Pubic arch** (*Atlas*, 5.1A); compare male and female pelves (*Atlas*, 3.1A, 3.2A). In the female, the pubic arch is much wider.

9. **Sacrum** (L. *sacer*, sacred); on the ventral or pelvic surface, observe (see Fig. 3.6; *Atlas*, 4.23A): **Anterior sacral foramina** for the passage of ventral nerve rami S1 to S4, and the **promontory**. On the dorsal surface observe (*Atlas*, 4.24): **Dorsal sacral foramina** for the passage of dorsal nerve rami S1 to S4. Superiorly, observe the **sacral canal** which transmits spinal nerves S1 to S5 on their way to the sacral foramina.

10. **Sacroiliac articulation;** a joint (synovial type) between the auricular surfaces of sacrum and ilium (*Atlas*, 3.1B, 3.2B); held together by anterior sacroiliac ligaments (*Atlas*, 3.4) and posterior sacroiliac ligaments (Fig. 3.5; *Atlas*, 3.6).

11. **Coccyx** (Gr. *kokkyx*, cuckoo; resembling a cuckoo's bill); three to five rudimentary vertebrae (Fig. 3.6; *Atlas*, 4.23).

12. Realize that the **hip bone** (os coxae; innominate bone) consists of three parts: Ilium, ischium, pubis. These three elements meet at the acetabulum, the cup-shaped cavity for the head of the femur. In the child, the three parts of the hip bone are not fused with each other. However, by age 16, fusion occurs.

Familiarize yourself with some measurements of the female pelvis. These measurements are of obstetrical importance. Obtain an articulated female pelvis and observe the following (*Atlas*, 3.3):

1. A line connecting the superior end of the symphysis pubis with the coccyx lies in the horizontal plane (in the anatomical position);

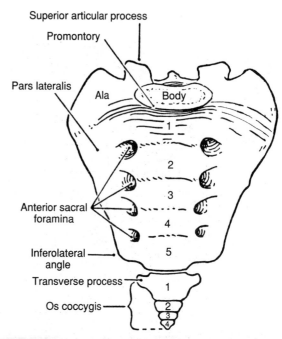

Figure 3.6. Anterior surface of sacrum and coccyx.

2. At the **superior pelvic aperture or pelvic inlet**, identify the midsagittal line connecting the superior end of the symphysis pubis with the promontory of the sacrum. This line indicates the plane of the pelvic inlet or brim. The plane of the pelvic inlet forms an angle about 60° with the horizontal plane;

3. **Transverse diameter** (13.5 cm); it is measured across the greatest width of the superior aperture.

4. A line connecting the lower end of the symphysis pubis with the tip of the coccyx is the **anteroposterior or conjugate diameter** (10.5 to 11 cm). It indicates the **pelvic outlet or the inferior pelvic aperture.** The plane of the pelvic outlet forms an angle of about 15° with the horizontal plane.

5. The transverse diameter (11 cm) of the pelvic outlet is measured between the two ischial tuberosities.

6. The pubic arch in the female is wide. The subpubic angle measures about 90° (*Atlas*, 3.2A). In the male, the subpubic angle measures only about 60° (*Atlas*, 3.1A).

Study a radiograph of the pelvis (*Atlas*, 4.22).

Anal Region (Triangle)

Before you begin . . .

Do not dissect at this time. Understand that the next objective is the study of the **anal region (triangle)** and its nerve and blood supply. This is best accomplished by placing the cadaver into the prone position. By reflecting the gluteus maximus and partially exposing the gluteal region, it will be easier to trace nerves and blood vessels to the perineal region.

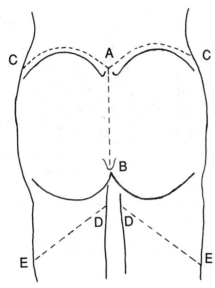

Figure 3.7. Skin incisions.

Skin Incisions. Turn the cadaver into the prone position (face down). Make skin incisions according to Figure 3.7.

1. A median vertical cut from the lower lumbar region to coccyx (*A* to *B*);
2. From point A lateralward just above the iliac crest, until stopped by the table (*A* to *C*);
3. From the medial aspect of the thigh (about 2.5 cm below the gluteal fold) to the lateral part of the thigh about 15 cm below the greater trochanter (*D* to *E*);
4. From points *B* to *D*.

To save time, remove skin and subcutaneous fat in one piece (from skin down to deep fascia enveloping both gluteus maximus and the thigh). This approach will destroy some of the cutaneous nerves of the gluteal region. Realize, however, that these cutaneous nerves do exist (*Atlas*, 5.7B). Do not cut too deeply across the posterior aspect of the thigh (*D* to *E*), otherwise the posterior cutaneous nerve of the thigh (*Atlas*, 5.7B) will be injured.

Dissection. Remove skin and subcutaneous tissue. Expose the **gluteus maximus** (*Atlas*, 5.31). Define the superior and inferior borders of this vast rhomboidal muscle. If the lower limb has already been dissected earlier, simply reflect the gluteus maximus laterally and proceed with the exploration of the anal region. Otherwise, reflect the gluteus maximus in the following manner:

1. Detach its superior portion close to the ilium.
2. With a scalpel, cut through its fibers very close to their origin from the posterior surface of the sacrum and coccyx.
3. Place your fingers under the inferior portion of the muscle. Realize that it is attached to the sacrotuberous ligament. Now, carefully detach the gluteus maximus

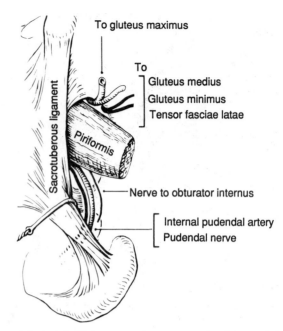

Figure 3.8. Pudendal nerve and internal pudendal vessels leaving the gluteal region through the lesser sciatic foramen.

from the sacrotuberous ligament, using a pair of scissors. Do *not* cut the ligament.

4. It is not necessary to reflect the muscle completely. Reflect the muscle laterally to the point where the inferior gluteal nerve and vessels enter it (i.e., near its "center").

Refer to an articulated bony pelvis, preferably one with its ligaments intact. Hold this orientation specimen in such a manner that its position corresponds to the region under dissection. Identify the **greater and lesser sciatic foramina.** Palpate the **ischial spine** and **ischial tuberosity.** Now, coming from the gluteal region, palpate the same structures in the cadaver. Force your finger through the greater sciatic foramen. Observe that your finger passes along with the piriformis muscle and the sciatic nerve (*Atlas*, 5.37).

Next, push your finger through the lesser sciatic foramen into the ischioanal (ischiorectal) fossa of the anal triangle. The finger runs in the same direction as the pudendal nerve and the internal pudendal vessels (Fig. 3.8; *Atlas*, 5.36). These vessels and nerve fibers supply the perineal structures (*Atlas*, 3.39).

Note: Before proceeding with the dissection of the ischioanal (ischiorectal) fossa and its contents, the anal canal should be distended and stabilized. This is best done by inserting a super-size tampon, along with its plastic insertion tube, into the anal canal. This procedure adds rigidity and stability to the anus and makes dissection of the anal triangle considerably easier.

The **ischioanal (ischiorectal) fossa** (Figs. 3.9 and 3.10; *Atlas*, 3.60B) is a large, wedge-shaped space on either side of the anus. Its surfaces are formed by the fasciae of the obturator internus and levator ani. Its base is the skin of the perineum (skin of anal triangle).

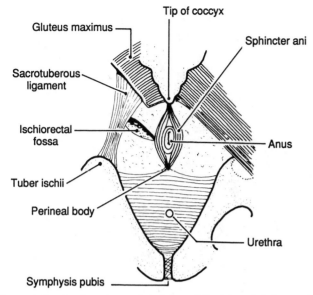

Figure 3.9. Anal region and ischioanal (ischiorectal) fossa. Cadaver in the prone position.

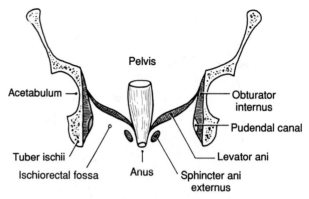

Figure 3.10. Ischioanal (ischiorectal) fossa and anus (coronal section).

The ischioanal fossa is filled with soft fat. This tissue accommodates the distended rectum. Incise the fat of the ischioanal fossa (Fig. 3.9): with the blade directed toward the anus, start the incision roughly midway between ischial tuberosity and coccyx. Insert the blade approximately 4 cm deep. As the anus is approached, gradually withdraw the scalpel. Insert your finger into the incision. Palpate the distinct strands of the **inferior rectal (hemorrhoidal) nerve and vessels.** Enlarge the opening with your finger. In a piecemeal fashion, remove the fat with a forceps. Dry the area with paper towels. Observe vessels and nerves traversing the fossa from the lateral wall toward the anus (*Atlas*, 3.61; note that the *Atlas* illustration is 180° reversed from your dissection field with the cadaver in the prone position).

Infections of the ischioanal (ischiorectal) fossa may result in the formation of an abscess. The abscess may spontaneously open into the rectum or through the skin into the perineal region. Surgeons must be aware of the fact that the right and left ischioanal fossae communicate via the deep postanal space (which lies posterior to the anus between superficial and deep external sphincter). As a result, an infection in one ischioanal fossa may eventually involve a semicircular area around the posterior aspect of the anus.

Clean the **sphincter ani externus** (*Atlas*, 3.61). It consists of three parts (*Atlas*, 3.62):

1. Subcutaneous part, delicate, encircling the anal orifice;
2. Superficial part, anchoring the anus to the perineal body ventrally and to the coccyx posteriorly;
3. Deep part, forming a wide encircling band; it is fused with the levator ani (puborectal sling). During defeca-

tion, the puborectal sling and all parts of the sphincter ani externus relax.

Temporarily remove the stabilizing tampon from the anal canal. With a gloved hand, insert your middle finger into the rectum. At the same time, place the fingers of your other hand on the sphincter ani externus within the ischioanal fossa. Appreciate the thickness of this muscle. Subsequently, insert the tampon again into the anal canal (or use a new tampon).

Clean the fascia of the **obturator internus** within the ischioanal fossa. The inferior portion of the obturator fascia is thickened. It splits to form a fibrous canal, the **pudendal canal** (*Atlas*, 3.60B, 3.61). The canal contains the **pudendal nerve** and the **internal pudendal vessels.** These structures run along the ischiopubic ramus toward the urogenital diaphragm (*Atlas*, 3.39). Carefully incise the obturator fascia along the ischiopubic ramus and just ventral to the sacrotuberous ligament. With a probe, pick up the contents of the pudendal canal (*Atlas*, 3.61). Carefully push the probe into the canal. Then, push forward along the ischiopubic ramus toward the inferior portion of the symphysis pubis. This is the course of the pudendal nerve and the internal pudendal vessels to the urogenital diaphragm and the dorsum of the penis (clitoris in the female).

MALE PELVIS AND PERINEUM

Male Urogenital Region (Triangle)

General Remarks and Orientation

The **perineum** is the area between the thighs. The perineal region is diamond-shaped and divided into two triangular areas, the **anal region** and the **urogenital region** (Fig. 3.3). The anal region has already been studied (see earlier part of this chapter). Now, the urogenital region (triangle) must be dissected. This will be done by using the

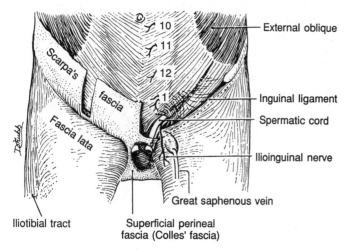

Figure 3.11. Attachments of membranous layer of superficial fascia (Colles' fascia). It is continuous with Scarpa's fascia of the lower abdominal wall (penis and scrotum cut away).

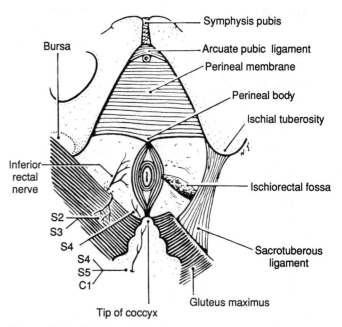

Figure 3.12. Pubic arch and urogenital diaphragm: perineal membrane (inferior fascia of urogenital diaphragm); perineal body (central tendon of perineum).

so-called *"Traditional Approach,"* which is preferred by many anatomists: The cadaver is in the supine position (face up). The thighs are widely stretched apart. The dissector sits or stands in front of the exposed perineal region (just as a urologist would). Usually, only one student can work on the region at a given time. The lighting must be excellent.

Place the cadaver in the supine position. Stretch the thighs widely apart. This can be accomplished by using either wooden boards placed between the feet or by abducting the lower limbs with the aid of ropes.

Note: The scrotum has been dissected earlier together with the structures of the anterior abdominal wall, the spermatic cord, and the testes. Review this material.

Skin Incisions. Make a midline incision. Start posterior to (below) the shaft of the penis. Split the scrotum into right and left halves. Carry the cut posteriorly to the already dissected anal triangle.

Dissection. Carefully reflect the skin flaps of the urogenital region. Note that the **superficial fascia** consists of two layers, a superficial fatty layer and a deeper membranous layer. Observe that the **fatty layer** is continuous with the dartos muscle of the scrotum anteriorly, the subcutaneous tissue surrounding the anus posteriorly, and the subcutaneous fatty layer of the medial sides of the thighs laterally. The **membranous layer** (Colles' fascia; superficial perineal fascia) is an aponeurotic structure of considerable strength. It is continuous with dartos fascia and the membranous layer of the superficial fascia (Scarpa's fascia) of the lower anterior abdominal wall (Fig. 3.11). Note that the membranous layer is firmly attached to the rami of pubis and ischium as far back as the ischial tuberosity (*Atlas*, 3.61). Posteriorly and in the median plane, the membrane blends with the perineal body at the base of the urogenital triangle.

Superficial Perineal Space. Incise the **membranous layer** of the superficial fascia (Colles' fascia) about 2 to 3 cm from the median plane. With a probe, pick up the **posterior scrotal nerves** and vessels (*Atlas*, 3.61). Insert your fingertip deep to the fascia. Your finger is now in the **superficial perineal space or pouch.** Confirm the posterior extent of the space by placing a finger of the other hand into the ischioanal fossa. Observe that the posterior portion of the membranous layer is between both fingertips. The **contents of the superficial perineal pouch** include three paired muscles and portions of the penile erectile tissue: the crura and the bulb of the penis.

Identify and clean the **three paired muscles** within the superficial perineal pouch (*Atlas*, 3.59F, 3.61):

1. **Transversus perinei superficialis** (superficial transverse perineal muscle), a slender muscle passing from ischial tuberosity to the perineal body. Note that the

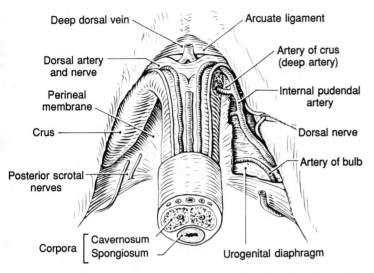

Figure 3.13. Urogenital diaphragm and penis. Deep dorsal vein of penis (cut) passing inferior to symphysis pubis.

perineal body (or central tendon) is a fibromuscular node in the median plane (Fig. 3.12). At this point, several perineal muscles converge and interlace.

2. **Ischiocavernosus**, arising from the ischial tuberosity and covering the crus of the corpus cavernosum on the same side. *Function:* alters erection, once achieved, by forcing blood from the cavernous tissue of the crus of the penis into the distal part of the corpus cavernosum penis.

3. **Bulbospongiosus;** the right and left muscles together are shaped like a feather. It arises from a median raphe and from the perineal body, and it encircles the bulb and the adjacent part of the corpus spongiosum penis. Raise the thin anterior, free border of the muscle. *Function:* The paired bulbospongiosi form a sphincter that empties part of the spongy urethra. Also, it alters erection, once achieved, by forcing blood from the spongy portion of the bulb into the distal part of the corpus spongiosum penis.

Separate the three superficial perineal muscles from each other until a small triangular area comes into view. This is part of the **inferior fascia of the urogenital (U-G) diaphragm** (*Atlas,* 3.61). To expose and view the entire inferior fascia, the following structures must be removed: the three paired perineal muscles (see paragraphs 1 to 3 listed previously), the right and left crura of the penis, and the bulb of the penis. Before reflecting these structures, dissect the penis:

Penis (L. *penis,* tail)**, Fascia, Vessels, and Nerves.** Remove the skin of the penis leaving the glans intact. The **superficial fascia** is devoid of fat. It contains superficial veins that drain to the inguinal region. Deep to the loose superficial fascia is the tight tubular investing sheath, the **deep fascia of the penis** (*Atlas,* 3.70) that holds the erectile tissue components together. Carefully incise the deep fascia between the glans and the symphysis pubis. On the dorsum of the shaft of the penis identify:

1. The unpaired **deep dorsal vein of the penis** (Fig. 3.13); follow the vein where it passes just inferior to the symphysis pubis. Most of the blood from the penis drains through this vein into the prostatic venous plexus.
2. The paired **dorsal arteries of the penis,** branches of the internal pudendal arteries (Fig. 3.13, *Atlas,* 3.69, 3.70).
3. The paired **dorsal nerves of the penis,** branches of the pudendal nerves (Fig. 3.13; *Atlas,* 3.39, 3.70).

Now, the **three superficial perineal muscles** will be removed. Use the **perineal body** (or central tendon) as a reference point (Fig. 3.12; *Atlas,* 3.61). First, remove the slender **transversus perinei superficialis,** thereby fully exposing the posterior extent of the **superficial perineal space or pouch.** Next, split the **bulbospongiosus muscle** at its raphe (*Atlas,* 3.61) and remove it, thereby exposing the **bulb of the penis** (*Atlas,* 3.62, 3.72, 3.74). Subsequently, clear away the **ischiocavernosus muscle** on both sides, thereby exposing the right and left **crura of the penis.** Study the components of the erectile tissues of the penis (*Atlas,* 3.72, 3.74). The **glans penis** is the distal expansion of the corpus spongiosum. The glans (L., *glans,* acorn) is pierced by the spongy urethra.

Spongy Urethra or Penile Urethra. Realize that the *entire* male urethra consists of three portions: prostatic, membranous, and spongy (see Fig. 3.15). At this point, only the **spongy (penile) portion** of the urethra will be examined. As the name implies, the spongy urethra runs within the corpus spongiosum penis. Examine the **external urethral orifice** near the tip of the glans penis. Push a probe into it. The next objective is to open the entire penile urethra in a longitudinal direction: push a probe into the navicular fossa of the glans (*Atlas,* 3.71). With a sharp scalpel, cut longitudinally through the ventral (inferior) part of the glans until stopped by the probe. Push the probe deeper (more proximal) into the spongy urethra. Continue to split it until reaching the bulb of the corpus spongiosum. Here the urethra bends at almost a right angle and passes through the urogenital diaphragm (see Fig. 3.15). Examine the mucous membrane of the spongy urethra. Note the orifices of tiny mucous glands (*Atlas,* 3.71).

Next, mobilize the penis by cutting the **suspensory ligament of the penis,** a triangular band attached anteriorly to the symphysis pubis (Fig. 3.14; *Atlas,* 3.66). Observe the **deep dorsal vein of the penis** passing inferior to the pubic arch into the pelvis (*Atlas,* 3.68, 3.69). Cut the vein. Now, free the crura. Next, pull gently on the bulb and, using a sharp blade, detach it from the inferior surface of the U-G diaphragm. In doing so, you are cutting through blood vessels to the penis (see below) and through the **urethra** at the junction of the spongy portion and the distal portion of the membranous urethra (Fig. 3.15; *Atlas,* 3.72, 3.73). Realize that the short membranous portion of the urethra lies within the urogenital diaphragm. It will be examined later.

Detach the **penis** entirely by cutting through the right and left dorsal nerves and dorsal arteries of the penis near the symphysis pubis. Make two **transverse sections** through the glans penis (*Atlas,* 3.67A): Make a more distal cross section at the level of the navicular fossa of the spongy

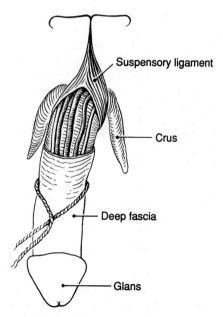

Figure 3.14. Suspensory ligament of penis: a triangular band attached anterior to the symphysis pubis.

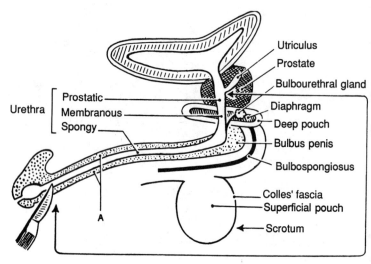

Figure 3.15. Diagram of male urethra.

urethra (section *C*). Note the erectile tissue surrounding the urethra. Make another more proximal cross section through the glans penis (section *B*). Study and understand the anatomical relations of **corona of glans, corpus cavernosum, and corpus spongiosum**. Once more, verify that the spongy urethra is contained within the corpus spongiosum. Next, make another transverse section through the proximal part of the penis near its bulb (*Atlas*, 3.68, 3.69). Observe the dark red cavernous structure of the erectile tissue of the corpus spongiosum and the two corpora cavernosa. Within the corpus cavernosum, identify the bilateral **deep artery of the penis** that supplies the necessary blood to the erectile tissue. Realize that these arteries and also the artery to the bulb (i.e., to the corpus spongiosum) are **branches of the internal pudendal artery.** This artery runs within the pudendal canal toward the symphysis pubis. Its branches include: artery to the bulb, deep artery of penis, and dorsal artery of penis (*Atlas*, 3.69). Store the detached penis in a plastic bag for future reference.

Examine the exposed **inferior fascia of the urogenital diaphragm** (Fig. 3.12; *Atlas*, 3.59D, 3.69). Positively identify the sectioned urethra. Push a probe into the short **membranous portion of the urethra** which traverses the urogenital triangle close to the symphysis pubis.

Deep Perineal Space. Incise the inferior fascia of the U-G diaphragm and remove it. You have now opened the **deep perineal space or pouch** (*Atlas*, 3.59C). The contents of this space are:

1. **Membranous urethra.** It traverses the deep perineal pouch and extends from the inferior fascia inferiorly to the superior fascia of the U-G diaphragm superiorly. This part of the urethra is superlative in being the shortest (1 to 2 cm), the thinnest, the narrowest, and the least dilatable.

2. **Sphincter urethrae.** This important striated muscle surrounds the membranous urethra. When the muscle contracts, it compresses the urethra and stops the flow of urine.

3. **Transverse perinei profundus** (deep transverse perineal muscle). This paired muscle originates at the pubic arch and meets the opposite muscle in a tendinous median raphe. The muscle and its raphe are attached to the perineal body.

4. Other smaller structures include the **artery to the bulb,** the paired **bulbourethral glands** (Cowper's glands), and **branches of the pudendal nerve,** which supplies all muscles of the urogenital region.

Spread apart the muscle fibers of the deep perineal space and expose a small portion of the **superior fascia of the U-G diaphragm** (*Atlas*, 3.59B). Realize that the **prostate gland** rests on the pelvic aspect of this superior fascia (Fig. 3.15; *Atlas*, 3.8). In addition, the superior fascia is related to the levator ani (*Atlas*, 3.20), particularly its anterior portion, the **pubococcygeus** or "puborectal sling."

Review the various layers of the perineum in the male (*Atlas*, 3.59, left column). Build up from deep to superficial (**A** through **F**).

Have all students of your group seen and studied the structures of the male urogenital triangle? If so, you may remove wooden boards and/or ropes used to spread the lower limbs apart. Now, return to the pelvic region.

Peritoneum in the Male Pelvis

Examine the **peritoneum** in the male pelvis (Fig. 3.16, *Atlas*, 3.9). The peritoneum passes from the anterior abdominal wall (1) to the level of the pubic bone (2) on to the superior surface of the urinary bladder (3). Next, it passes approximately 2 cm inferiorly along the posterior surface of the bladder (4) to cap the seminal vesicles which cannot be seen at this time (5). Posteriorly, the peritoneum lines the **rectovesi-**

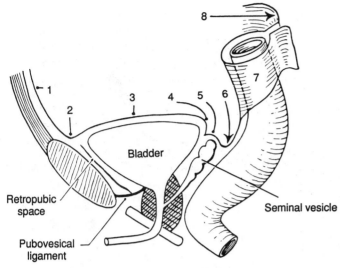

Figure 3.16. Peritoneum in male pelvis (paramedian plane).

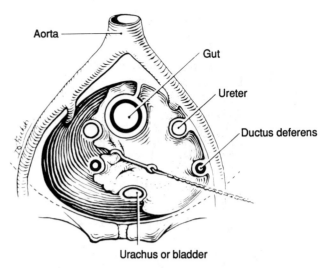

Figure 3.17. Pelvic structures adhering to peritoneum.

cal fossa (6) to the middle part of the rectum. At this level, it covers only the anterior portion of the rectum. However, at higher levels it gradually envelops the sides of the rectum as well (7). Finally, at the third sacral vertebra, the peritoneum becomes the sigmoid mesocolon (8). The **paravesical fossa,** a peritoneal fossa, is apparent on each side of the bladder (*Atlas*, 3.17). The peritoneal recess on each side of the rectum is called the **pararectal fossa** (*Atlas*, 3.17).

> As the bladder fills, the peritoneal reflection is elevated above the level of the pubic bones, and raised from the anterior abdominal wall. Thus, a filled bladder can be surgically approached through an incision just above the pubic bones without entering the peritoneal cavity.

Structures Adhering to Peritoneum. With your fingers, detach the peritoneum from the pelvic wall and note the following structures which adhere to the peritoneum (Fig. 3.17):

1. Rectum;
2. Ureter;
3. Ductus deferens;
4. Bladder.

Retropubic Space, Retrorectal Space, and Internal Iliac Vessels

Retropubic Space (prevesical space; space of Retzius; Fig. 3.4; *Atlas*, 3.8). This U-shaped space lies between the symphysis pubis and the bladder and extends dorsally on each side of the bladder. Posteriorly, the retropubic space is limited by the rectovesical fascia (*Atlas*, 3.8) that contains arteries and veins of the bladder and of the internal genital organs. The retropubic space is filled with fat

and loose areolar tissue that accommodates the expansion of the bladder. Place your fingers between the symphysis pubis and anterior border of the bladder. Move the fingers to each side of the bladder (Fig. 3.4). Inferiorly, the exploring finger is stopped by two cord-like thickenings of the pelvic fascia anchoring the neck of the bladder to the pubis: this is the **puboprostatic ligament** (*Atlas*, 3.8).

Retrorectal Space or Presacral Space (Fig. 3.10). The fused sacral vertebrae S3 to S5 and the coccyx are covered anteriorly with the rectum. Pass two fingers caudally behind the rectum and ease it off the sacrum and coccyx. Now, your fingers are in the deep retrorectal space. This space is limited inferiorly by a strong fascia investing the levator ani. Push your fingers inferiorly and verify by palpation the inferior limit of the retrorectal (presacral) space.

> Just as your fingers are limited inferiorly, so is the spread of an infection in this space. As a result of this fascial arrangement, an infection, e.g., a retrorectal abscess, cannot expand inferiorly. Instead, it is prone to rupture through the posterior wall of the rectum (which constitutes a lesser barrier) into the rectum.

Move your fingers laterally in the retrorectal space. Feel strands of **pelvic splanchnic nerves** (sacral parasympathetic outflow; *Atlas*, 3.11) on each side of the retrorectal space. These autonomic nerves branch off the ventral rami S2-S4 after traversing the corresponding anterior sacral foramina (Fig. 3.18; *Atlas*, 3.36)

> Since the pelvic splanchnic nerves (nervi erigentes; parasympathetic outflow of S2, S3, S4; Fig. 3.18) are closely related to the lateral aspects of the rectum, they can also be easily injured during rectal surgery, for example, when the rectum must be entirely removed because of cancer. Injury to or loss of the pelvic splanchnic nerves results in impairment of bladder control and sexual function (loss of penile erection).

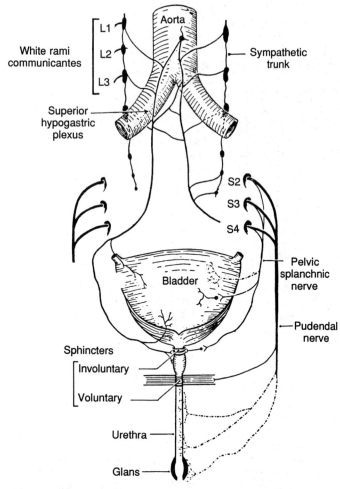

White rami communicantes

L1
L2
L3

Aorta

Sympathetic trunk

Superior hypogastric plexus

S2
S3
S4

Bladder

Pelvic splanchnic nerve

Pudendal nerve

Sphincters
Involuntary
Voluntary

Urethra

Glans

Figure 3.18. Diagram of nerve supply to bladder and urethra.

Realize that the common iliac artery divides into the external iliac artery and the internal iliac artery (*Atlas*, 5.6A). Study an iliac arteriogram (*Atlas*, 3.32). In the cadaver, follow the **internal iliac artery** and its branches to some extent (Fig. 3.19; *Atlas*, 3.31). A complete dissection of these vessels will be done when the pelvic cavity is more accessible. With your finger, palpate the **obturator canal** that traverses the superior aspect of the obturator membrane. Once you have identified the obturator canal, you will also be able to find the **obturator artery.** Follow this vessel proximally toward the internal iliac artery.

Usually (in about 70% of cases), the obturator artery arises directly from the internal iliac artery (*Atlas*, 3.30A). There is a slender anastomosis between obturator artery and inferior epigastric artery (a branch of the external iliac artery). However, in about 25% of cases, the obturator artery may receive the bulk of its blood supply directly from the inferior epigastric artery (*Atlas*, 3.30B; anomalous). Which vascular arrangement can you verify in the cadaver? Surgeons must be fully aware of this vascular arrangement. The "anomalous" obturator artery is very vulnerable and can be easily injured during surgical repair of a femoral hernia. Uncontrolled bleeding from this vessel can be dangerous.

Identify the **internal iliac vein** and some of its tributaries (*Atlas*, 3.29). Follow the vein to its junction with the **external iliac vein.** Here, the **common iliac vein** is formed. Note that the left common iliac vein lies directly posterior to the bifurcation of the aorta (*Atlas*, 2.85). This is of surgical importance, particularly in cases of abdominal aortic aneurysms.

On each side, identify the **ureter** as it crosses the external iliac vessels and the obturator vessels medially (Fig. 3.20; *Atlas*, 2.85, 3.29). Follow it toward the urinary bladder as far as possible. Subsequently, identify the **ductus deferens** (Fig. 3.20; *Atlas*, 3.29), and follow it for some distance on its way to the prostate. Remove fat and areolar tissue surrounding vessels and ducts. Clean the accessible parts of the bladder wall, but do *not* destroy its blood supply. Cleaning of the bladder wall will be facilitated by attaching a hemostat at its apex and pulling it taut. If in doubt whether or not the (collapsed) organ is really the bladder, make a small incision in the median plane and observe the lumen of this hollow organ. If the rectum interferes with the field of dissection, have your partner pull it to the left side. Frequently sponge the area to keep it clean. Moisten the dissecting field with mold-deterrent preservative fluid.

Pelvic Diaphragm

Lateral Wall of Pelvic Cavity. Once again, identify the obturator foramen and the obturator nerve and vessels passing through the obturator canal. The obturator foramen is closed internally by the **obturator internus muscle.** Realize that only the most superior portion of the muscle can be seen (*Atlas*, 3.60B): Superiorly, the fascia of the obturator internus is thickened and forms a **tendinous arch** stretching from ischial spine to pubic bone. The **levator ani** arises, in part, from this tendinous arch (Figs. 3.4, 3.21; *Atlas*, 3.19).

Pelvic Diaphragm and Levator Ani. These structures may only be observed, in part, because of the intervening pelvic organs. They will be completely dissected later after hemisection of the pelvis. However, it is important to have a conceptual understanding of these structures at this time. The **pelvic diaphragm** is funnel-shaped. The rectum is anchored to it in the middle (Fig. 3.10; *Atlas*, 3.60B). Realize that the muscular component of this funnel is the **levator ani** which consists of **three portions** (*Atlas*, 3.19, 3.60C):

1. **Pubococcygeus,** arising from the pubic bone;
2. **Iliococcygeus,** arising from the tendinous arch;
3. **Coccygeus** (ischiococcygeus), arising from the ischial spine.

The **pubococcygeus** is the thickened and most important part of the pelvic diaphragm. Fibers of the right and

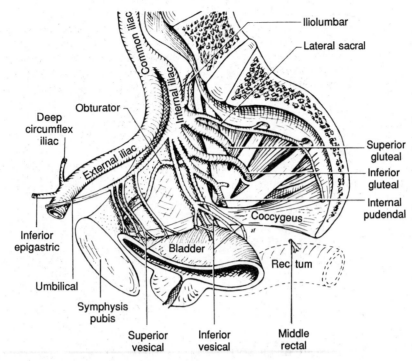

Figure 3.19. Internal iliac artery and its branches.

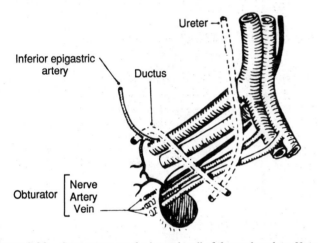

Figure 3.20. Structures on the lateral wall of the male pelvis. Note the medial position of the ureter and the ductus deferens.

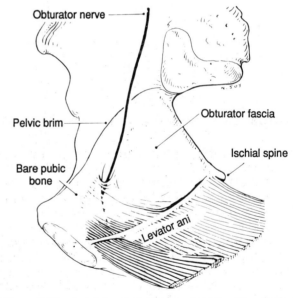

Figure 3.21. Lateral wall of pelvis and origin of levator ani.

the left pubococcygeus unite *posterior* to the rectum. This union of fibers creates a U-shaped "puborectal sling" (Fig. 3.22; *Atlas*, 3.12, 3.13, 3.15). This sling is responsible for the curvature at the anorectal junction. During defecation, the puborectal sling relaxes, the anorectal junction is straightened, and the expulsion of fecal matter is facilitated.

Review all structures of the male pelvis and perineum as dissected and seen so far. Make sure your laboratory partners have also participated in the review process. Subsequently, the pelvis will be sectioned in the midsagittal plane to facilitate more detailed studies of pelvic structures.

Hemisection

Before you begin . . .

Check with your instructor if you are allowed to proceed. The **goal** is to make a very careful midsagittal split of all (soft and bony) structures from the perineum up to the level of vertebra L3. Subsequently, the body will be transected at the vertebral level of L3 to L4. One lower extremity (preferably the left one) remains attached to the rest of

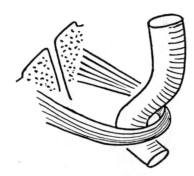

Figure 3.22. The "puborectal sling," the thickened portions of the right and left pubococcygeus uniting posterior to the rectum.

the body while the other side (preferably the right one) is mobilized. If this procedure is done with care, it will facilitate complete dissection and examination of the pelvis.

Section

Make sure you are using a new and sharp scalpel. Use this instrument to make a very precise split of all soft structures in the midsagittal plane (*Atlas*, 3.8):

1. Start precisely posterior to the symphysis pubis in the midsagittal plane. Carry this midsagittal section through the entire bladder wall. Sponge the interior of the urinary bladder. Continue to cut inferior to the bladder and split the prostate gland.
2. Subsequently, cut through the anterior and posterior walls of the rectum. Sponge it clean! Be careful *not* to cut into the sigmoid colon or any other loop of the GI tract! Now, the blade should have reached the anterior surface of the sacrum.
3. Finally, push the knife inferior to the symphysis pubis with the cutting edge directed posteriorly. In the midsagittal plane, cut through the pelvic diaphragm (*Atlas*, 3.59A, 3.60C) from symphysis pubis to coccyx.

Obtain a suitable handsaw and make two cuts in the midsagittal plane:

1. Cut through the symphysis pubis.
2. Start at the coccyx and extend the midline cut through the sacrum up to the third lumbar vertebra. Be careful *not* to injure the nerves of the cauda equina. During sawing, pull these nerves laterally for protection.

If you have decided to mobilize the right lower extremity (which is preferred), proceed as follows:

1. Cut horizontally through the right half of the intervertebral disc between L3 and L4 until this cut meets the superior extent of the midsagittal section of the vertebral column.

2. Cautiously mobilize the right lower extremity to some extent. Cut nerves and blood vessels connecting the right lower limb with the rest of the body. Section the ureter. Now, the right lower limb can be removed.

Continue with your studies of the *male* pelvic structures using either half of the hemisected pelvis. The pelvic structures are now readily accessible. Examine and dissect these structures and note their topographical relations:

Urethra (Fig. 3.15; *Atlas*, 3.8). The urethra is divided into **three portions: spongy, membranous, and prostatic.** The **spongy portion** (penile urethra) has been studied already together with the anatomical components of the penis. The **membranous urethra** (*Atlas*, 3.59B, C, and D) was seen earlier when the contents of the deep perineal space or pouch were explored. Now, in the bisected specimen, study the membranous urethra again. If the hemisection was done perfectly in the midsagittal plane, then the longitudinally opened halves of the membranous urethra should be present in each hemisectioned specimen. Otherwise, refer to the specimen that contains the membranous urethra. Note that it is only 1 to 2 cm long and traverses the urogenital diaphragm. Within the urogenital diaphragm, it is surrounded by a sphincter muscle, the **sphincter urethrae** (*Atlas*, 3.8). Be aware of the nerve supply to this important muscle (Fig. 3.18).

Prostate and Prostatic Urethra (*Atlas*, 3.8). In the bisected specimen, note that the prostate rests on the superior fascia of the urogenital diaphragm. Using a probe, identify the longitudinally sectioned **prostatic urethra.** Follow this structure proximally into the bladder. **Examine the interior of the prostatic urethra** (*Atlas*, 3.27):

a. Note its approximate length: 3 cm.
b. On the posterior wall, observe a median ridge, the **urethral crest.** The ovoid enlargement of the crest is the **colliculus seminalis.**
c. In the midline of the colliculus, find a small blind opening, the **utricle.**
d. On each side of the utricle, find the minute **orifice of the ejaculatory duct.** You may have to use a magnifying glass.
e. On each side of the urethral crest, observe a groove, the **prostatic sinus.** Here, the numerous ducts of the prostate open into the urethra.

Ductus (Vas) Deferens (Fig. 3.23; *Atlas*, 3.29). Pick up the ductus deferens as it crosses the external iliac vessels medially. Note that the ductus is closely related to the inferior epigastric vessels (*Atlas*, 3.38). Follow the ductus deferens inferiorly and observe that it crosses the obturator nerve and vessels medially (*Atlas*, 3.29). Next, follow the ductus toward the bladder. Near the posterolateral angle of the bladder, it crosses anterior to the ureter (Fig. 3.23). Subsequently, follow the duct along the posterior aspect of the bladder. Here it expands to form the **ampulla.** Lateral to each ampulla lies a **seminal vesicle.** Each seminal vesicle is a convoluted tube. Using a probe, carefully

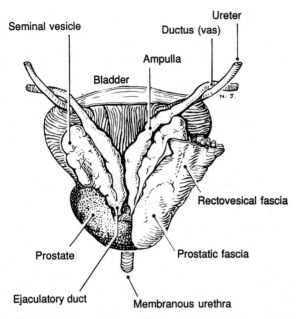

Figure 3.23. Ureter, ductus deferens, and seminal vesicles (dorsal view). The visceral pelvic fascia covers the bladder, prostate, and associated structures.

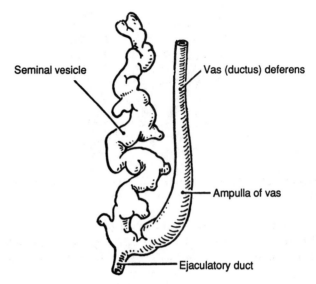

Figure 3.24. Ejaculatory duct: the union of ampulla of ductus deferens and seminal vesicle (unraveled).

expose the union of the ampulla and the **duct of the seminal vesicle** (Fig. 3.24; *Atlas*, 3.24). This is the beginning of the **ejaculatory duct**, which traverses the posterior half of the prostate gland (*Atlas*, 3.26) and terminates at the colliculus in the prostatic urethra (*Atlas*, 3.27, 3.28).

Ureter (Fig. 3.23; *Atlas*, 3.18). Pick up the ureter as it crosses the external iliac artery (*Atlas*, 3.29) and follow it to the posterolateral portion of the urinary bladder. Here, the ureter travels obliquely through the bladder wall (*Atlas*, 3.24).

Urinary Bladder. During section of the pelvis, the urinary bladder was completely opened and divided into right and left halves. Examine the **muscular coat** of the organ. It consists of bundles of smooth muscle. (This muscular coat is collectively called the detrusor urinae (L. *detrudere*, to thrust out). Examine the **interior of the bladder** (*Atlas*, 3.27):

a. The **trigone** is an equilateral triangle on the posterior wall (now divided). Its angles are formed by the **two orifices of the ureters** and the **internal urethral orifice**. The internal urethral orifice is situated at the lowest (most inferior) point of the bladder.
b. Note that the mucous membrane over the trigone is smooth. Over the other parts of the bladder, it lies in folds when the bladder is empty.
c. Pass a fine probe into the orifice of the ureter. Verify that the ureter traverses the muscular wall of the bladder in an oblique fashion.

Internal Iliac Artery and Branches (Fig. 3.19; *Atlas* 3.29, 3.31). You may not have time to dissect all 10 branches of the internal iliac artery. Demonstrate at least the following: Identify the **umbilical artery.** Note that it gives off 3 to 4 **superior vesical arteries** that supply the superior aspect of the bladder. The umbilical artery continues toward the anterior abdominal wall where it becomes the **medial umbilical ligament** (obliterated umbilical artery; *Atlas*, 3.20, 3.22). Verify these facts. Trace the **obturator artery** from its point of origin toward the superior aspect of the obturator foramen. Follow a branch of the internal iliac artery to the posteroinferior part of the bladder and to the region of the prostate and seminal vesicles. This is the **inferior vesical artery** (not present in the female). The **middle rectal artery** is a small vessel to the lateral aspect of the rectum. Follow the important **internal pudendal artery** (which is larger in the male than in the female) to the inferior part of the greater sciatic foramen. This artery is closely related to the sacrospinous ligament. The internal pudendal artery has been encountered earlier in the pudendal canal where it gives off branches to the ischioanal fossa and where it divides into its terminal branches, the deep artery of the penis and the dorsal artery of the penis. The **inferior gluteal artery** also passes through the inferior part of the greater sciatic foramen. This vessel passes between sacral nerves of the sacral plexus (*Atlas*, 3.34, 3.35). The **superior gluteal artery** is relatively large and runs in close relationship to the lumbosacral trunk. This vessel leaves the pelvis through the superior part of the greater sciatic foramen. Identify some of the branches of the internal iliac artery in an iliac arteriogram (*Atlas*, 3.32).

Observe the **rectal venous plexus**. Note the numerous veins on the surface of the rectum. Observe the **vesical venous plexus** at the base of the bladder. It receives blood from the **prostatic venous plexus,** which lies ventral and lateral to the prostate. Pick up the **deep dorsal vein of the penis** just inferior to the symphysis pubis and verify that it empties into the prostatic venous plexus. Do not dissect these complex pelvic venous plexuses. Remove all tributa-

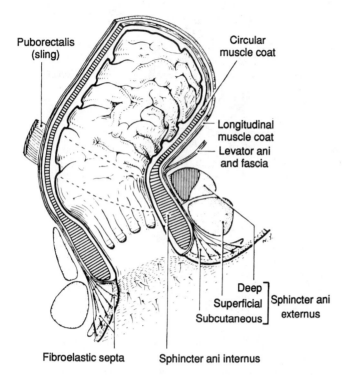

Figure 3.25. Rectum and anal canal (in sagittal section).

ries to the internal iliac vein so that the arterial distribution can be clearly demonstrated.

> The venous plexuses in the pelvis intercommunicate. This is of considerable clinical importance (e.g., transportation of tumor cells along vascular channels).
>
> The importance of the rectal venous plexus in cases of portal venous hypertension has been stressed earlier. Remember that the superior rectal vein originates from the rectal venous plexus (*Atlas*, 2.53, 2.54, 3.14). The rectal venous plexus is also drained by the middle and inferior rectal veins that, in turn, empty into the caval system of veins. In portal venous hypertension, blood flow in the superior rectal vein may be reversed: portal blood may be carried to the rectal plexus and, from there, shunted into the caval system. The resulting increased blood flow and pressure in the rectal venous plexus leads to the development of hemorrhoids. Thus, in case of hemorrhoids, the physician must always evaluate the condition of the portal venous system. The portal venous system has no valves. This fact explains why the blood flow in the portal system can be easily reversed.

Anal Canal (Fig. 3.25; *Atlas*, 3.8). During bisection of the pelvis, the anal canal has been opened. Clean it thoroughly. Examine the interior features (this may be difficult to demonstrate in some cadavers):

a. **Anal columns** (*Atlas*, 3.15). These are 5 to 10 longitudinal ridges of mucosa in the superior part of the anal canal. The terminal "branches" of the superior rectal vessels are contained in the anal columns. Here, the superior rectal veins of the portal system anastomose with middle and inferior rectal veins of the caval system (*Atlas*, 2.54). Abnormal increase in pressure in the valveless portal system leads to an enlargement of the veins contained in the anal columns, resulting in "internal hemorrhoids."

b. **Anal valves,** semilunar folds uniting the lower ends of the anal columns (*Atlas*, 3.15). If these anal valves are torn by hard fecal material, an infection can occur and spread from the injured anal valves into the wall of the anal canal.

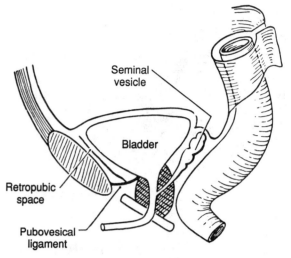

Figure 3.26. Topographic relations of rectum, prostate, and seminal vesicles.

Examine the **sphincter muscles of the anus** and the puborectal sling on section (Fig. 3.25; *Atlas*, 3.8, 3.15).

Place a gloved finger into the split anal canal and palpate topographically related structures (as if performing a digital rectal examination). Palpate the muscular wall formed by the sphincter ani externus. More superiorly, at the anorectal junction, feel the puborectalis (puborectal sling; part of levator ani). Verify that anterior to the finger (i.e., anterior to the rectum), the prostate and the seminal vesicles can be palpated (Fig. 3.26).

> **Rectal examination** is an important part of every physical examination. The size and consistency of the prostate gland can be assessed. Normally, the wall of the rectum can be moved against the prostate because of the intervening areolar tissue (Fig. 3.26; *Atlas*, 3.8). If this is not possible, one should suspect malignant tumor infiltration from prostate into rectum.
>
> Posteriorly, the anterior surface of sacrum and coccyx can be palpated. Laterally, the ischioanal fossa can be examined. Thus, a pathological process (e.g., abscess) in these regions may be detected by digital examination. Appreciate this unique opportunity to combine digital palpation with visual observation.

Levator Ani. The levator ani is funnel-shaped. In the middle of this funnel, the prostate is supported anteriorly (*Atlas*, 3.20, 3.25), and the rectum is positioned posteriorly (Fig. 3.26; *Atlas*, 3.60B and **C**). Study the **origin of the levator ani:** Identify the thickened fascia of the obturator internus stretching from pubic bone to ischial spine and

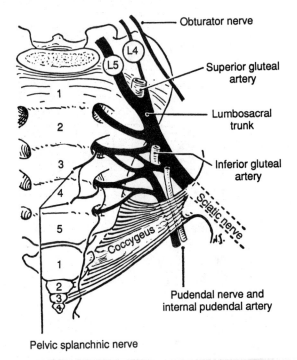

Figure 3.27. Sacral plexus and related vessels.

forming a tendinous arch. From this **tendinous arch** the levator ani takes origin (Fig. 3.21; *Atlas*, 3.19). Verify this. Identify the **three portions of the levator ani:** (1) The **pubococcygeus** arises from the pubic bone. It is the thickest and most important portion of the levator ani. Verify that it runs lateral and then posterior to the rectum and forms the "puborectal sling" as it unites with the same muscle from the other side posterior to the rectum (Fig. 3.22; *Atlas*, 3.12, 3.13). (2) The **iliococcygeus** is the relatively thin middle portion arising mainly from the tendinous arch. (3) Posteriorly, the **ischiococcygeus** contributes to the sacrospinous ligament.

Piriformis Muscle (*Atlas*, 3.34). Observe its origin from the pelvic or ventral surface of the sacrum at segments S2, S3, and S4. Note that the muscle fibers converge and pass through the greater sciatic foramen. The ventral nerve rami S2 and S3 emerge between the digitations of the piriformis.

Sacral Plexus. The sacral nervous plexus is closely related to the anterior surface of the piriformis. In the cadaver, verify the following (Fig. 3.27; *Atlas*, 3.33, 3.34, 3.35):

a. The **lumbosacral trunk** (L4, L5) contributes to the sacral plexus.
b. The ventral rami of S2 and S3 emerge between the digitations of the piriformis.
c. Ventral rami from L4 through S3 converge and form the large **sciatic nerve.** It passes through the greater sciatic foramen together with the piriformis.
d. Usually, the **gluteal arteries** (branches of the internal iliac artery) pierce the sacral plexus: Often, the lumbosacral trunk and S1 are separated by the superior gluteal artery. Occasionally, the superior gluteal artery in-

tervenes between L4 and L5. The inferior gluteal artery usually separates ramus S1 from S2.
e. Ventral rami S2, S3, and S4 contribute to the pudendal nerve (Fig. 3.27; *Atlas*, 3.39). Remember, ventral rami S2, S3, and S4 contain preganglionic parasympathetic fibers (sacral parasympathetic outflow; pelvic splanchnic nerves; *Atlas*, 3.16, 3.36). These autonomic nerves supply pelvic organs and the distal portion of the GI tract from left colic flexure to rectum.
f. Note the **sympathetic chain and its ganglia** medial to the sacral foramina (*Atlas*, 3.33, 3.34, 3.36). These ganglia give off gray rami communicantes to the ventral sacral rami. Review the entire innervation of the *male* pelvis (*Atlas*, 3.36).

Lymphatic Drainage of the Male Pelvis (*Atlas*, 3.37). Lymphatic channels are difficult to see unless injected with a dye. However, you may encounter lymph nodes in certain pelvic regions, particularly if there was a pelvic inflammatory or malignant process prior to death. Understand that penis, scrotum, and spongy urethra have a different lymphatic drainage than the testes and prostate. This is of considerable clinical significance. Be familiar with the lymphatic drainage of the rectum (*Atlas*, 3.37D).

Sections. Study **transverse sections through the male pelvis** (*Atlas*, 3.10). Identify important muscles such as the obturator internus and the levator ani. Realize that the prostate can be visualized using an ultrasound probe in the rectum. Be able to identify urinary bladder, rectum, prostate and seminal vesicles on section. Study a transverse section and a transverse MRI of the **male perineum** (*Atlas*, 3.63, 3.65). Identify important structures traversing the urogenital and anal triangles.

FEMALE PELVIS AND PERINEUM

Female Urogenital Region (Triangle)

General Remarks and Orientation

Understand the general arrangement of the *soft parts* of the female pelvis (Fig. 3.28; *Atlas*, 3.42, 3.43):

1. The **urethra** is short (3.5 to 4 cm). It pierces the anterior portion of the urogenital diaphragm.
2. The **vagina** is about 7 to 8 cm long. The vagina also traverses the urogenital diaphragm. The anterior wall of its middle part is in contact with the bladder. Its posterior wall is in contact with the rectum.
3. The **uterus** is about 7 cm long. It intervenes between bladder and rectum. The longitudinal axes of uterus and vagina are at almost a right angle.
4. **Fornix of vagina** (L. *fornix*, arch). This circular gutter surrounds the intravaginal part of the cervix uteri. It is divisible into *anterior*, *posterior*, and *lateral parts*. Posteriorly, the fornix is larger than anteriorly.
5. **Rectum** and **anal canal** are constructed as in the male.

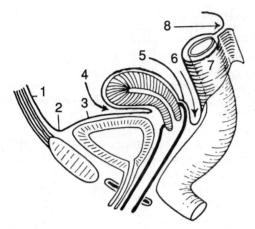

Figure 3.28. General arrangement of female pelvic organs. Peritoneal reflections (median section).

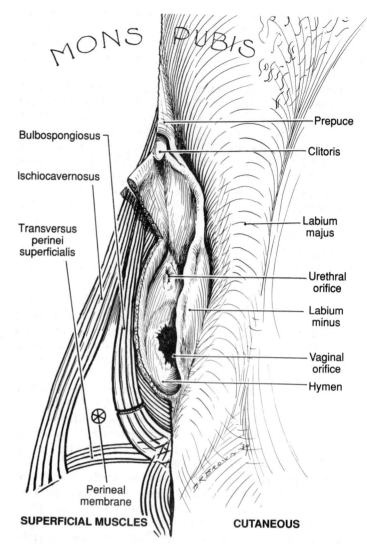

Figure 3.29. Female perineum. Right half of illustration: skin and external genitalia. Left half of illustration: superficial perineal muscles.

The **perineum** is the area between the thighs. It lies between vulva and anus. The perineal region is diamond-shaped and divided into two triangular areas, the **anal region** and the **urogenital region** (Fig. 3.3). The anal region has already been studied (see earlier part of this chapter). Now, the urogenital region (triangle) must be dissected. This will be done by using the so-called *"Traditional Approach,"* which is preferred by many anatomists: The cadaver is in the supine position (face up). The thighs are widely stretched apart. The dissector sits or stands in front of the exposed perineal region (just as a gynecologist would). Usually, only one student can work on the region at a given time. The lighting must be excellent.

Place the cadaver in the supine position. Stretch the thighs widely apart. This can be accomplished by using either wooden boards placed between the feet or by abducting the lower limbs with the aid of ropes.

Dissection

External Genitalia. First, identify the female external genitalia, collectively known as *vulva* (Fig. 3.29; *Atlas*, 3.59G): mons pubis, labia majora and minora, vestibule of the vagina (i.e., the space between the labia minora), clitoris, and prepuce of clitoris. In addition, identify the vaginal orifice and the external urethral orifice.

Skin Incisions. Make a transverse skin incision that passes between both ischial tuberosities and crosses the midline between anal and vaginal orifices. Make a midline incision from the just established transverse incision toward the pubic symphysis, encircling the labia majora.

Dissection. Reflect the skin flaps laterally and remove them. Raise the skin off the two labia majora, but leave the underlying mass of fat undisturbed. Place a finger into the ischioanal fossa and palpate the base of the urogenital triangle stretching between the ischial tuberosities via the perineal body. Realize that the **perineal body** is a fibromuscular node in the median plane where several perineal muscles converge and interlace (*Atlas*, 3.59F).

> Integrity of this fibromuscular node (perineal body) in the female is of clinical importance. When the perineal body is injured during parturition (childbirth), it must be carefully repaired to avoid weakness of the pelvic floor with all its consequences (prolapse of bladder, uterus, or rectum). Thus, the anatomy of this region should be studied carefully.

Study the mass of fat underlying each labium majus. Usually, it consists of a long finger-like process extending from the anterior abdominal wall and descending far into each labium majus (*Atlas*, 3.75). Closely related to this fat are the fascial bands of the distal part of the **round ligament of the uterus**. Lateral to the fat of the labium majus make a longitudinal cut. Using a probe, find the **posterior labial nerves and vessels** (*Atlas*, 3.75), branches of the pudendal nerve and the internal pudendal artery, respectively. Next, on both sides of the symphysis pubis, cut horizontally down to the bone and scrape away the fatty tissue (*Atlas*, 3.76). This will leave exposed the prominent and tough **suspensory ligament of the clitoris**. This suspensory ligament extends from the symphysis to the fixed part of the clitoris.

Superficial Perineal Space. Remove the fatty tissue of the labia majora (*Atlas*, 3.76). Cut and discard the branches of the posterior labial nerves and vessels. Flush with the vaginal orifice, cut away the two labia minora. Note that they do not contain fat. Clean the dissection field as thoroughly as possible. Incise the **superficial perineal fascia** and insert your finger deep to it. Your finger is now in the **superficial perineal space or pouch**. This space contains the greater vestibular glands and the superficial perineal muscles. These three paired muscles correspond to those in the male, but they are smaller.

Identify and clean the **three paired muscles** within the superficial perineal pouch (Fig. 3.29; *Atlas*, 3.59F, 3.76):

1. **Transverse perinei superficialis** (superficial transverse perineal muscle), a slender muscular slip passing from ischial tuberosity to the perineal body. Note that this **perineal body** (or central tendon) is a fibromuscular node in the median plane. At this point, several perineal muscles converge and interlace.

2. **Ischiocavernosus**, arising from inner surface of ischial tuberosity and covering the unattached surface of the crus of the clitoris. *Function*: Alters erection of the clitoris, once achieved, by forcing blood from the cavernous tissue of the crus of the clitoris into the distal corpus cavernosum of the clitoris.

3. **Bulbospongiosus.** It is a broad muscular band surrounding the vaginal orifice like a sphincter. Posteriorly, it blends with the perineal body and muscle fibers of the sphincter ani externus. Identify this muscle and its relations to the other perineal muscles. When separating the three superficial perineal muscles from each other, note a small triangular area of exposed perineal membrane (asterisk in Fig. 3.29; *Atlas*, 3.76). This perineal membrane is the inferior fascia of the urogenital diaphragm.

> The muscles of the female perineal region are of great obstetrical importance. Perineal lacerations during childbirth are common. Frequently, the external orifice of the birth canal is prophylactically widened by an episiotomy (surgical incision of perineum when laceration seems imminent during delivery). Intelligent repair of either lacerations or episiotomy wounds requires a good working knowledge of the female perineal region.

The **bulbospongiosus** muscle forces blood from the spongy tissue of the bulb of the vestibule into the glans clitoris after erection is achieved. The bulbospongiosus covers the vestibular bulb and the greater vestibular gland. To expose these deeper structures, the muscle must be divided or reflected. Therefore, cut the bulbospongiosus muscle and reflect it off the vaginal wall (Fig. 3.30; *Atlas*, 3.77). Now, the bulb of the vestibule and the greater

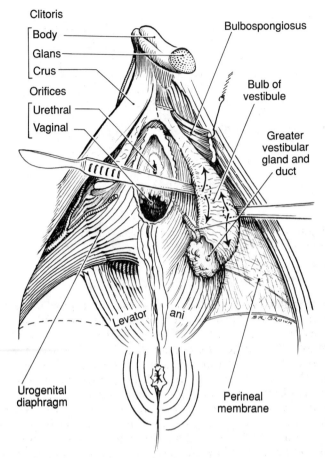

Figure 3.30. Female perineum. Right half of illustration: contents of superficial perineal space or pouch. Left half of illustration: contents of deep perineal pouch.

vestibular gland, adhering to the bulb, can be examined. The **bulbs of the vestibule** are two elongated (3 cm long) masses of erectile tissue on each side of the vaginal orifice. Anterior to the vaginal orifice, the two bulbs are united by a narrow band or commissure. Attached to each posterior end of the bulb is the **greater vestibular gland** (Bartholin's glands). Attempt to find the duct of one of these small glands (*Atlas*, 3.77). It opens into the vestibule in a groove between hymen and labium minus. The glands secrete lubricating mucus.

> Acute inflammation of the greater vestibular gland (Bartholinitis) is of gynecological importance. As can be expected from the anatomical position of the gland, such inflammation (or abscess) will manifest itself by a substantial swelling of the *lower* (posterior) half of the labium, up to 5 cm in diameter. Enlarged and infected glands may also be palpated during rectal examination.

With the handle of a scalpel, mobilize and free the **bulb of the vestibule** (Fig. 3.30), thereby tearing the blood vessels that enter and leave the erectile tissue of the bulb. Reflect the bulb. Now, the crura, body, and glans of the clitoris can be examined.

Clitoris (Fig. 3.30; *Atlas*, 3.78).   Identify the **glans,** which lies between two folds formed by labia minora. The anterior folds form the right and left sides of a hood over the glans, the **prepuce** of the clitoris (Fig. 3.29). The clitoris is homologous to the penis. It consists mainly of erectile tissue. Distinguish between its subdivisions: **glans, body, and crura.** Note that each crus is attached to the ischiopubic ramus. Realize that the clitoris has a rich blood and nerve supply (bilateral dorsal artery and nerve of clitoris; *Atlas*, 3.77).

The vulva is richly supplied with sensory nerve fibers. Thus, there is considerable pain when, during parturition, the head of the child is passing through the vulva and stretches its parts to the limit. The pain can be greatly diminished by locally anesthetizing the pudendal nerve bilaterally. This **pudendal block** is performed by injecting a local anesthetic in the vicinity of the pudendal nerve as it crosses the sacrospinous ligament near the ischial spine (Fig. 3.27 or *Atlas*, 3.35). Therefore, the ischial spine is palpated through the vagina, and the needle is aimed toward this important bony landmark. The pudendal block is also performed to anesthetize the perineum locally for surgical repairs of lacerations or an episiotomy incision.

Deep Perineal Space.   Make sure that all structures of the superficial perineal space (three superficial perineal muscles, bulb of vestibule, and greater vestibular glands) have been removed. Look for the thin triangular perineal membrane or **inferior fascia of the urogenital (U-G) diaphragm** (Fig. 3.29). This membrane is difficult to preserve. Probably it has been torn, thus opening the **deep perineal space or pouch.** Realize that this deep space must be traversed by the **urethra** and the **vagina** (*Atlas*, 3.59C). Also appreciate the fact that, during parturition, the child must pass through the vastly dilated deep perineal space. Identify the two striated muscles of the deep space (*Atlas*, 3.59C):

1. **Transversus perinei profundus** (deep transverse perineal muscle). This paired muscle originates at the pubic arch (*Atlas*, 3.79) and meets the opposite muscle in a tendinous raphe located just posterior to the vaginal wall. The muscle and its raphe are also attached to the perineal body. Examine the vagina in the deep perineal space together with the surrounding muscle.
2. **Sphincter urethrae.** This important muscle surrounds the female urethra in the deep perineal space (*Atlas*, 3.59C). When the muscle contracts, it compresses the urethra and stops the flow of urine. Injury of this muscle during parturition may lead to urinary incontinence.

Spread apart the muscle fibers of the deep perineal space and expose a small portion of the **superior fascia of the U-G diaphragm** (*Atlas*, 3.59B). Superiorly, the superior fascia is related to the levator ani (*Atlas*, 3.59A), particularly to its anterior portion, the **pubococcygeus** or "puborectal sling." Once more, note **branches of the inter-**

nal pudendal vessels. Identify **branches of the pudendal nerve,** which supply all muscles of the urogenital region (*Atlas*, 3.59D).

Review the various layers of the perineum in the female (*Atlas*, 3.59). Build up from deep to superficial (*A* through *F*).

Have all students of your group seen and studied the structures of the female urogenital triangle? If so, you may remove wooden boards and/or ropes used to spread the limbs apart. Now, return to the pelvic region.

Peritoneum in the Female Pelvis

Note: It is possible that the female cadaver under dissection does not have a uterus. The removal of the uterus (hysterectomy) with or without the ovaries is a common surgical procedure. Determine whether or not these organs are present in your specimen. If they have been surgically removed, examine these important organs in other cadavers.

Examine the peritoneum in the female pelvis (Fig. 3.28; *Atlas*, 3.42, 3.43, 3.45). The peritoneum descends from the anterior abdominal wall (1) to the level of the pubic bone (2) on to the superior surface of the urinary bladder (3). Next, it passes from bladder to uterus (4). Here it forms the **vesicouterine pouch** (*Atlas*, 3.45). The peritoneum covers the fundus and body of the uterus. It extends over the posterior fornix and the wall of the vagina (5). Between the uterus and the rectum, the peritoneum forms the deep **rectouterine pouch** (6). From the bottom of the rectouterine pouch, the peritoneum passes on to the anterior surface and sides of the rectum (7). Finally, at the 3rd sacral vertebra, the peritoneum becomes the sigmoid mesocolon (8). The **paravesical fossa,** a peritoneal fossa, is apparent on each side of the bladder (*Atlas*, 3.45). The peritoneal recess on each side of the rectum is called the **pararectal fossa.**

Adnexa (L., *adnexum, adnexa,* connected parts). This term is often used in clinical context. It refers to the **uterine appendages:** The ovaries, uterine tubes, and ligaments of the uterus.

Broad Ligament of the Uterus (Fig. 3.31; *Atlas*, 3.45, 3.46).   At the sides of the uterus, two layers of peritoneum (from the posterior and anterior aspects of the uterus) come together to form a broad fold, the **broad ligament of the uterus.** This peritoneal fold extends to the lateral wall of the pelvis. The **uterine tube** is contained within its free margin. The peritoneal fold that surrounds the uterine tube is called the **mesosalpinx** (Gr., *salpinx,* tube). The **ovary** is attached to the posterior aspect of the broad ligament (*Atlas*, 3.45, 3.52). The peritoneal fold that contains the ovary is the **mesovarium.** Mesovarium and mesosalpinx are, of course, just portions of the broad ligament. The loose fatty and areolar tissues enclosed between the two layers of the broad ligament are collectively called **parametrium** (Gr. *para,* beside; *metra,* womb, uterus).

Round Ligament of Uterus.   It is visible through the anterior layer of the broad ligament (*Atlas*, 3.45, 3.49). Observe its subperitoneal course over the pelvic brim toward

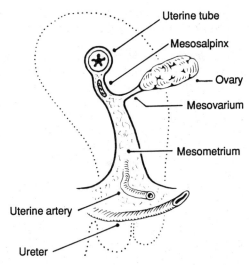

Figure 3.31. Broad ligament of uterus, its subdivisions and chief relations (paramedian section). Note the proximity of ureter and uterine artery.

1. Rectum;
2. Bladder;
3. Ureter;
4. Ovarian vessels;
5. Round ligament of uterus;
6. Uterus.

the deep inguinal ring. It terminates in the labium majus. The round ligament of the uterus corresponds to the ductus deferens in the male. It takes a similar subperitoneal course.

Other Ligaments (*Atlas*, 3.45, 3.52). The **ligament of the ovary** is a cord within the broad ligament connecting the ovary with the uterus at a point just below the uterine tube. The peritoneal fold covering the uterine tube extends laterally and posteriorly where it is continuous with the **suspensory ligament of the ovary**; this ligament contains the ovarian vessels. Once more, identify the **broad ligament of the uterus** as part of it stretches widely between the round ligament of the uterus anteriorly and the uterine tube posteriorly (*Atlas*, 3.45). Verify that the broad ligament separates the **vesicouterine pouch** from the **rectouterine pouch**.

Rectouterine Folds (*Atlas*, 3.45). They are sharp peritoneal folds containing true musculofascial ligaments, the **sacrouterine ligaments,** which anchor the uterus to the sacrum. Observe that the rectouterine folds curve dorsally from the superior part of the cervix of the uterus past the sides of the rectum to the sacrum. Together, the right and left folds form the brim of the rectouterine pouch. The rectouterine folds with their underlying sacrouterine ligaments can be palpated by digital rectal examination.

In the female, the pelvic fascia is substantially thickened at the sides of the cervix and vagina. This is the important **transverse cervical ligament** (lateral cardinal ligament; cardinal ligament; ligament of Mackenrodt). The ligament is triangular and holds the uterus in position by anchoring it to the lateral wall of the pelvis. Lateral to the uterus, push your finger inferiorly. Feel the stiff resistance and the firm support offered by the transverse cervical ligament.

Structures Adhering to the Peritoneum. With your fingers, detach the peritoneum from the pelvic wall (*Atlas*, 3.45, 3.49). Note the structures that adhere to the peritoneum:

Retropubic Space, Retrorectal Space, and Internal Iliac Vessels

Retropubic Space (prevesical space; space of Retzius; *Atlas*, 3.42). This U-shaped extraperitoneal space lies between the symphysis pubis and the bladder and extends dorsally on each side of the bladder. Posteriorly, the retropubic space contains arteries and veins of the bladder and of the internal genital organs. The retropubic space is filled with fat and loose areolar tissue, which accommodates the expansion of the bladder. Within this extraperitoneal space, place your fingers between the symphysis pubis and anterior border of the bladder. Inferiorly, the exploring finger is stopped by cord-like thickenings of the pelvic fascia anchoring the neck of the bladder to the pubis. This is the **pubovesical ligament** (*Atlas*, 3.42).

Retrorectal Space or Presacral Space. The fused sacral vertebrae S3 to S5 and the coccyx are covered anteriorly with the rectum. Pass two fingers caudally behind the rectum and ease it off the sacrum and coccyx. Now, your fingers are in the deep retrorectal space. This space is limited inferiorly by a strong fascia investing the levator ani. Push your fingers inferiorly and verify by palpation the inferior limit of the retrorectal (presacral) space.

Just as your fingers are limited inferiorly, so is the spread of an infection in this space. As a result of this fascial arrangement, an infection, e.g., a retrorectal abscess, cannot expand inferiorly. Instead, it is prone to rupture through the posterior wall of the rectum (which constitutes a lesser barrier) into the rectum.

Move your fingers laterally in the retrorectal space. Feel the strands of the **pelvic splanchnic nerves** (sacral parasympathetic outflow; *Atlas*, 3.11) on each side of the retrorectal space. These autonomic nerves branch off the ventral rami S2-S4 after traversing the corresponding anterior sacral foramina (Fig. 3.27; *Atlas*, 3.57)

Since the pelvic splanchnic nerves (parasympathetic outflow of S2, S3, S4) are closely related to the lateral aspects of the rectum, they can also be easily injured during rectal surgery; for example, when the rectum must be entirely removed because of cancer. Injury to or loss of the pelvic splanchnic nerves results in impairment of bladder control and sexual function (impairment of erectile tissue function).

Realize that the common iliac artery divides into the external iliac artery and the internal iliac artery (Fig. 3.32, *Atlas*, 5.6A). Study an iliac arteriogram (*Atlas*, 3.32). In the cadaver, follow the **internal iliac artery** and its branches to some extent (Fig. 3.32; *Atlas*, 3.55). A complete dissection of these vessels will be done when the pelvic cavity is more accessible. With your finger, palpate the **obturator canal** that traverses the superior aspect of the obturator membrane. Once you have identified the obturator canal, you will also be able to find the **obturator artery**. Follow this vessel proximally toward the internal iliac artery.

Usually (in about 70% of cases), the obturator artery arises directly from the internal iliac artery (*Atlas*, 3.30A). There is a slender anastomosis between obturator artery and inferior epigastric artery (a branch of the external iliac artery). However, in about 25% of cases, the obturator artery may receive the bulk of its blood supply directly from the inferior epigastric artery (*Atlas*, 3.30B; anomalous). Which vascular arrangement can you verify in the cadaver? Surgeons must be fully aware of this vascular arrangement. The "anomalous" obturator artery is very vulnerable and can be easily injured during surgical repair of a femoral hernia. Uncontrolled bleeding from this vessel can be dangerous.

Identify the **internal iliac vein** and some of its tributaries. Follow the vein to its junction with the **external iliac vein**. Here, the **common iliac vein** is formed. Note that the left common iliac vein lies directly posterior to the bifurcation of the aorta (*Atlas*, 2.85). This is of surgical importance, particularly in cases of abdominal aortic aneurysms.

On each side, identify the **ureter** as it crosses the external iliac vessels medially (*Atlas*, 3.45). Follow it inferiorly where it crosses the obturator vessels. Then trace it toward the urinary bladder as far as possible. Remove fat and areolar tissue surrounding vessels and ducts. Clean the accessible parts of the bladder wall, but do *not* destroy its blood supply. Cleaning of the bladder wall will be facilitated by attaching a hemostat at its apex and pulling it taut. If in doubt whether or not the (collapsed) organ is really the bladder, make a small incision in the median plane and observe the lumen of this hollow organ. If the rectum interferes with the field of dissection, have your partner pull it to the left side. Frequently sponge the area to keep it clean. Moisten the dissecting field with mold-deterrent preservative fluid.

Pelvic Diaphragm

Lateral Wall of Pelvic Cavity. Once again, identify the obturator foramen and the obturator nerve and vessels passing through the obturator canal. The obturator foramen is closed internally by the **obturator internus muscle**. Realize that only the most superior portion of the muscle can be seen (*Atlas*, 3.60B): Superiorly, the fascia of the obturator internus is thickened and forms a **tendinous**

arch stretching from ischial spine to pubic bone. The **levator ani** arises in part from this tendinous arch (Figs. 3.21; *Atlas*, 3.47, 3.60A and B).

Pelvic Diaphragm and Levator Ani. These structures may only be observed, in part, because of the intervening pelvic organs. They will be completely dissected later after hemisection of the pelvis. However, it is important to have a conceptual understanding of these structures at this time. The **pelvic diaphragm** is funnel-shaped. The rectum is anchored to it in the middle (*Atlas*, 3.60B). Realize that the muscular component of this funnel is the **levator ani** which consists of **three portions** (*Atlas*, 3.47, 3.60C):

1. **Pubococcygeus,** arising from the pubic bone;
2. **Iliococcygeus,** arising from the tendinous arch;
3. **Coccygeus** (ischiococcygeus), arising from the ischial spine.

The **pubococcygeus** is the thickened and most important part of the pelvic diaphragm. Fibers of the right and the left pubococcygeus unite *posterior* to the rectum. This union of fibers creates a U-shaped "puborectal sling" (Fig. 3.22; *Atlas*, 3.15). This sling is responsible for the curvature at the anorectal junction. During defecation, the puborectal sling relaxes, the anorectal junction is straightened, and the expulsion of fecal matter is facilitated. In the female, portions of the pubococcygeus muscle are inserted into the terminal portion of the vagina (*Atlas*, 3.47).

The pubococcygeus, particularly the portions supporting the vagina and rectum, are frequently injured during childbirth. The supporting ligaments of the pelvic fascia (e.g., the cardinal ligament) may also be torn during parturition. As a consequence, the pelvic viscera are no longer adequately supported by the pelvic diaphragm. Pelvic organs may push downward and prolapse through the weakened vaginal wall (prolapse of bladder, cystocele; prolapse of rectum, rectocele), or the uterus may descend down the vaginal canal (prolapse of uterus).

Review all structures of the female pelvis and perineum as dissected and seen so far. Make sure your laboratory partners have also participated in the review process. Subsequently, the pelvis will be sectioned in the midsagittal plane to facilitate more detailed studies of pelvic structures.

Hemisection

Before you begin . . .

Check with your instructor to determine if you are allowed to proceed. The **goal** is to make a very careful midsagittal split of all (soft and bony) structures from the perineum up to the level of vertebra L3. Subsequently, the body will be transected at the vertebral level of L3 to L4. One lower extremity (preferably the left one) remains attached to the rest of the body while the other side (preferably the right one) is mobilized. If this procedure is done with care, it will facilitate complete dissection and examination of the pelvis.

Section

Make sure you are using a new and sharp scalpel. Use this instrument to make a very precise split of all soft structures in the midsagittal plane (*Atlas*, 3.42):

1. Start precisely posterior to the symphysis pubis in the midsagittal plane. Carry this midsagittal section through the entire bladder wall. Sponge the interior of the urinary bladder. Continue to cut inferior to the bladder until you have reached the urogenital diaphragm.
2. Next, carry the midsagittal cut through the uterus. Include in this section the cervix of the uterus and the superior portion of the vagina.
3. Subsequently, cut through the anterior and posterior walls of the rectum. Sponge it clean! Be careful *not* to cut into the sigmoid colon or any other loop of the GI tract! Now, the blade should have reached the anterior surface of the sacrum.
4. Finally, push the knife inferior to the symphysis pubis with the cutting edge directed posteriorly. In the midsagittal plane, cut through the pelvic diaphragm (*Atlas*, 3.59A; 3.60C) from symphysis pubis to coccyx.

Obtain a suitable handsaw and make two cuts in the midsagittal plane:

1. Cut through the symphysis pubis.
2. Start at the coccyx and extend the midline cut through the sacrum up to the 3rd lumbar vertebra. Be careful *not* to injure the nerves of the cauda equina. During sawing, pull these nerves laterally for protection.

If you have decided to mobilize the right lower extremity (which is preferred), proceed as follows:

1. Cut horizontally through the right half of the intervertebral disc between L3 and L4 until this cut meets the superior extent of the midsagittal section of the vertebral column.
2. Cautiously mobilize the right lower extremity to some extent. Cut nerves and blood vessels connecting the right lower limb with the rest of the body. Section the ureter. Now, the right lower limb can be removed.

Continue with your studies of the *female* pelvic structures using either half of the hemisectioned pelvis. The pelvic structures are now readily accessible. Examine and dissect these structures and note their topographical relations:

Urethra (*Atlas*, 3.42).   If the hemisection was done perfectly in the midsagittal plane, then the longitudinally opened halves of the urethra should be present in each hemisectioned specimen. Otherwise, refer to the specimen that contains the urethra. Verify that the female urethra is a short muscular tube, about 5 to 6 mm in diameter and 3.5 to 4 cm in length. Trace the sectioned urethra anteroinferiorly from the urinary bladder to the **external urethral orifice.** Note that the urethra lies *anterior* to the vagina; therefore, the urethral orifice must also be located *anterior* to the vaginal orifice. Examine the portion of the urethra that passes through the **urogenital diaphragm.** Note the solid **sphincter urethrae muscle** that is located in the deep perineal space. Close-up examination of the urethral mucosa with a magnifying glass will reveal numerous tiny orifices of the periurethral glands. The two largest of these glands open at the paraurethral orifice (orifice of Skene's duct), which lies just posterior to the urethral opening on either side of the midline.

Ureter.   Pick up the ureter as it crosses the external iliac artery (*Atlas*, 3.48). Verify that the ureter descends on the lateral wall of the true pelvis (pelvis minor) to a point close to the ischial spine. Here, the **uterine artery** crosses superior to the ureter. Next, the ureter passes close to the lateral fornix of the vagina. At this point, the vaginal artery crosses inferior to the ureter. Trace the ureter to the posterosuperior angle of the bladder. Here, the ureter travels obliquely through the bladder wall (*Atlas*, 3.49).

Urinary Bladder.   During section of the pelvis, the urinary bladder was completely opened and divided into right and left halves. Examine the **muscular coat** of the organ. It consists of bundles of smooth muscle. (This muscular coat is collectively called the detrusor urinae (L. *detrudere*, to thrust out). Examine the **interior of the bladder** which is not different from the male urinary bladder (*Atlas*, 3.27):

a. The **trigone** is an equilateral triangle on the posterior wall (now divided). Its angles are formed by the **two orifices of the ureters** and the **internal urethral orifice.** The internal urethral orifice is situated at the lowest (most inferior) point of the bladder.
b. Note that the mucous membrane over the trigone is smooth. Over the other parts of the bladder, it lies in folds when the bladder is empty.
c. Pass a fine probe into the orifice of the ureter. Verify that the ureter traverses the muscular wall of the bladder in an oblique fashion (*Atlas*, 3.48).

Vagina (L. *vagina*, sheath).   In the sectioned specimen, observe that the anterior vaginal wall is about 7.5 to 8 cm long. The posterior wall is slightly longer to accommodate the posterior vaginal fornix. Once again, examine the relationship of posterior fornix to rectouterine pouch (*Atlas*, 3.42). Observe the close topographical relations of lateral vaginal fornix and uterine artery (*Atlas*, 3.48, 3.56). In the living, particularly in the pregnant woman, the pulsations of the uterine artery may be felt through the lateral fornices. Realize that the vagina is so distensible that it

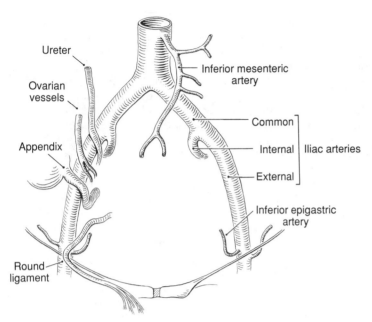

Ureter

Ovarian vessels

Appendix

Round ligament

Inferior mesenteric artery

Common

Internal | Iliac arteries

External

Inferior epigastric artery

Figure 3.32. Structures crossing the iliac arteries to enter or leave the pelvis.

can accommodate head and shoulders of a baby passing through the birth canal.

Uterus (*Atlas*, 3.42). Note its normal anteverted position. Observe that the longitudinal axes of uterus and vagina are at an angle of approximately 90°. Realize that the position of the uterus must change when the bladder is full, or in pregnancy. Identify the following features of the uterus (*Atlas*, 3.54):

a. **Cervix,** protruding into the vaginal canal. The **cervical canal** opens through the ostium uteri (external os) into the vagina. Review the strong ligamentous attachments that hold the cervix in place (sacrouterine ligament; transverse cervical or cardinal ligament).

b. **Body of uterus.** Identify the **vesical surface** facing the vesicouterine pouch, and the **superior surface** facing the rectouterine pouch. Note that the **lateral surfaces** are attached to the **broad ligament** (*Atlas*, 3.52). Structures to and from the uterus are contained in the loose areolar tissue between the two layers of the broad ligament. This tissue is the **parametrium.** Identify the **uterine cavity.** In sagittal section, it is a mere slit (*Atlas*, 3.42). In coronal section, it is triangular in shape (*Atlas*, 3.54). Make a coronal section through the sectioned half of the uterus. Explore the uterine cavity and its continuation with the cervical canal and the uterine tube. The uterine mucosa is called **endometrium.** Observe the thick uterine wall composed of smooth musculature, the **myometrium.** Understand clinically important terms: *Endometrium* (Gr. *endon*, within; *metra*, uterus); *myometrium* (Gr. *mys*, muscle); *parametrium* (Gr., *para*, beside). The **fundus** is the rounded part of the uterus which lies above the entrances to the tubes (*Atlas*, 3.54).

Uterine Tube (fallopian tube; oviduct). With a pair of scissors, open one uterine tube longitudinally. Note the funnel-shaped **infundibulum** with its **fimbriae** (*Atlas*, 3.52). Observe the narrow medial one-third of the uterine tube, the **isthmus.** Realize that the uterine tubes provide an open channel from the outside into the peritoneal cavity. With a probe, follow this channel from vagina via cervical canal, uterine cavity, and uterine tubes into the abdominal cavity. At this point, correlate your gross anatomical observations with the interpretation of a hysterosalpingogram (*Atlas*, 3.53).

Ovary (*Atlas*, 3.42, 3.52). In nulliparous women, each ovary lies in a shallow depression bounded by ureter, external iliac vein, and uterine tube. If not already done, dissect the ovarian vessels throughout their course. Incise one ovary. The structure of the ovary varies with age. If the age of subject is under 40 to 50 years, look for follicles.

> In assessing certain pathological conditions, the topographic anatomical relations between lower urinary tract and vagina should always be remembered (*Atlas*, 3.42). The vagina lies posterior to the base of the bladder. Thus, a finger placed into the vagina can exert pressure on the posterior bladder wall. The close relationship between vagina and posterior bladder wall has clinical implications: As a consequence of injuries sustained during labor and delivery, the bladder may be insufficiently supported by the muscular pelvic floor. Under this condition and especially in the upright position, the full bladder may push downward and against the anterior vaginal wall. Eventually, a bulge appears in the anterior vaginal wall caused by the prolapsed bladder. This rather common condition is known as cystocele. Similarly, the female urethra can prolapse, a condition known as urethrocele. The urethrocele, which is usually accompanied by a cystocele, occurs with weakening of the normal supporting structures of the pelvic floor; e.g., following birth trauma. As a result of postsurgical trauma, a urethrovaginal fistula can develop. This pathological communication between urethra and vagina allows urine to discharge constantly through the vagina, a most miserable although not life-threatening condition.

Internal Iliac Artery and Branches (Fig. 3.32). The internal iliac artery supplies most of the blood to the pelvic viscera. In many cases, the arterial distribution of certain branches is identical with that in the male; in these instances, *Atlas figure references for male* specimens may be cited. Arterial branches that supply the *female* reproductive organs are summarized in *Atlas*, 3.55. You may not have time to dissect all branches of the internal iliac artery. Demonstrate at least the following: Identify the **umbilical artery.** Note that it gives off 3 to 4 **superior vesical arteries** that supply the superior aspect of the bladder. The umbilical artery continues toward the anterior abdominal wall where it becomes the **medial umbilical ligament** (obliterated umbilical artery; *Atlas*, 3.20, 3.22). Verify these facts. Trace the **obturator artery** from its point of origin to the superior aspect of the obturator foramen.

Next, identify the origin of the **uterine artery** (*Atlas*, 3.55). Usually, it arises directly from the internal iliac artery. Follow it to the inferior margin of the broad ligament and into the parametrium, i.e., into the areolar tissue be-

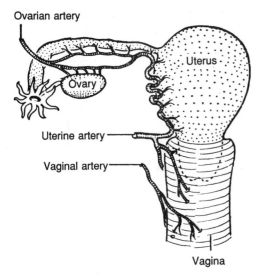

Figure 3.33. Arterial supply of uterus, ovary, and vagina.

tween the two layers of the broad ligament. Subsequently, trace it to the lateral aspect of the uterus, specifically to the isthmus, i.e., the region between body and cervix of the uterus (*Atlas*, 3.54, 3.56). Note that the uterine artery divides into a large superior branch to the body and fundus of the uterus, and into a smaller branch to the cervix and vagina (Fig. 3.33; *Atlas*, 3.56). Be aware of the **anastomosis between uterine and ovarian arteries.** Identify and trace the **vaginal artery** (Fig. 3.33; *Atlas*, 3.56). Follow some of its branches to the vagina and the posteroinferior parts of the urinary bladder. Note that the **ureter** is interposed between vaginal and uterine arteries (*Atlas*, 3.49). Pay particular attention to the relation between ureter and uterine artery (Fig. 3.31; Atlas, 3.46). Verify that the uterine artery crosses the ureter near the lateral fornix of the vagina (*Atlas*, 3.48).

> The close proximity of ureter and uterine artery near the lateral fornix of the vagina is of considerable clinical importance. During hysterectomy, the uterine artery is tied off and cut. Inadvertently, the ureter may also be clamped, tied off, and severed. This will have serious consequences for the corresponding kidney.

Other Branches of the Internal Iliac Artery (*Atlas*, 3.55). The **middle rectal artery** is a small vessel to the lateral aspect of the rectum. Follow the important **internal pudendal artery** (which is smaller in the female than in the male) to the inferior part of the greater sciatic foramen. This artery is closely related to the sacrospinous ligament. The internal pudendal artery has been encountered earlier in the pudendal canal where it gives off branches to the ischioanal fossa and where it divides into its terminal branches, supplying the muscles of the U-G diaphragm and the erectile tissue of the clitoris. The **inferior gluteal artery** also passes through the inferior part of the greater sciatic foramen. This vessel passes between sacral nerves of the sacral plexus (*Atlas*, 3.55). The **superior gluteal artery** is relatively large and runs in close relationship to the

lumbosacral trunk (*Atlas*, 3.34, 3.35). This vessel leaves the pelvis through the superior part of the greater sciatic foramen.

Pelvic Venous Plexuses. These plexuses are networks of veins that are located around the bladder, the uterus, and the rectum. The plexuses intercommunicate and eventually drain into the internal iliac vein. Do not dissect these complex pelvic venous plexuses. Remove all tributaries to the internal iliac vein so that the arterial distribution in the female pelvis can be clearly demonstrated.

> The venous plexuses in the pelvis intercommunicate. This is of considerable clinical importance (e.g., transportation of tumor cells along vascular channels). The importance of the rectal venous plexus in cases of portal venous hypertension has been stressed earlier. Remember that the superior rectal vein originates from the rectal venous plexus (*Atlas*, 2.53, 2.54, 3.14). The rectal venous plexus is also drained by the middle and inferior rectal veins that, in turn, empty into the caval system of veins. In portal venous hypertension, blood flow in the superior rectal vein may be reversed: portal blood may be carried to the rectal plexus and, from there, shunted into the caval system. The resulting increased blood flow and pressure in the rectal venous plexus leads to the development of hemorrhoids. Thus, in case of hemorrhoids, the physician must always evaluate the condition of the portal venous system. The portal venous system has no valves. This fact explains why the blood flow in the portal system can be easily reversed.

Anal Canal (Fig. 3.25; *Atlas*, 3.42). During bisection of the pelvis, the anal canal has been opened. Clean it thoroughly. Examine the interior features (this may be difficult to demonstrate in some cadavers):

a. **Anal columns** (*Atlas*, 3.15). These are 5 to 10 longitudinal ridges of mucosa in the superior part of the anal canal. The terminal "branches" of the superior rectal vessels are contained in the anal columns. Here, the superior rectal veins of the portal system anastomose with middle and inferior rectal veins of the caval system (*Atlas*, 2.54). Abnormal increase in pressure in the valveless portal system leads to an enlargement of the veins contained in the anal columns, resulting in "internal hemorrhoids."

b. **Anal valves,** semilunar folds uniting the lower ends of the anal columns (*Atlas*, 3.15). If these anal valves are torn by hard fecal material, an infection can occur and spread from the injured anal valves into the wall of the anal canal.

Examine the **sphincter muscles of the anus** and the puborectal sling on section (Fig. 3.25; *Atlas*, 3.15, 3.42).

Digital Examination of Rectum and Vagina. Perform digital examination of the female pelvic organs *per rectum*. Place a gloved finger into the split anal canal and palpate topographically related structures (as if performing a digital rectal examination). Palpate the muscular wall formed by the sphincter ani externus. More superiorly, at the anorectal junction, feel the puborectalis (puborectal sling; part of levator ani). Verify that anterior to the finger the posterior wall of the vagina and cervix of the uterus can be palpated. Place one finger of the other hand in the rectouterine fossa and note that the anterior wall of the rectum intervenes between the two fingers. Laterally, feel the sharp rectouterine fold.

Next, perform digital examination of the pelvic organs *per vaginam*. Place one or two gloved fingers into the split vagina and palpate topographically related structures (as if performing a vaginal examination). Place the fingers of the other hand in the pelvis. Between the two hands, palpate and observe: urinary bladder, cervix of uterus, rectouterine pouch, and uterus.

> Digital rectal and vaginal examinations are very important procedures in assessing the disposition and condition of pelvic organs. Under pathological conditions, one can palpate the enlarged or displaced broad ligament, enlarged ovaries, and uterine tubes (inflammatory processes, tumors, cysts, ectopic pregnancies, etc.).
>
> Note that only the posterior fornix of the vagina intervenes between the peritoneal cavity (rectouterine pouch of Douglas) and the outside (Fig. 3.28; *Atlas*, 3.42). Therefore, a needle can be pushed through the posterior vaginal fornix to aspirate pathological contents from the rectouterine pouch. Also, a culdoscope can be introduced through the posterior vaginal fornix into the abdominal cavity. The culdoscope allows visual observations of uterine tubes, ovaries, posterior surface of uterus, and anterior surface of rectum.

Levator Ani. The levator ani is funnel-shaped. In the middle of this funnel, the vagina and uterus are supported anteriorly, and the rectum is positioned posteriorly (Fig. 3.28; *Atlas*, 3.47, 3.60, 3.80). Study the **origin of the levator ani**: Identify the thickened fascia of the obturator internus stretching from pubic bone to ischial spine and forming a tendinous arch. From this **tendinous arch**, the levator ani takes origin (Fig. 3.21; *Atlas*, 3.47). Verify this. Identify the **three portions of the levator ani**: (1) The **pubococcygeus** arises from the pubic bone. It is the thickest and most important portion of the levator ani. Verify that it runs lateral and then posterior to the rectum and forms the "puborectal sling" as it unites with the same muscle from the other side posterior to the rectum (Fig. 3.22; *Atlas*, 3.12, 3.13). (2) The **iliococcygeus** is the relatively thin middle portion arising mainly from the tendinous arch. (3) Posteriorly, the **ischiococcygeus** contributes to the sacrospinous ligament.

Piriformis Muscle (*Atlas*, 3.34). Observe its origin from the pelvic or ventral surface of the sacrum at segments S2, S3, and S4. Note that the muscle fibers converge and pass through the greater sciatic foramen. The ventral nerve rami S2 and S3 emerge between the digitations of the piriformis.

Sacral Plexus. The sacral nervous plexus is closely related to the anterior surface of the piriformis. In the cadaver, verify the following (Fig. 3.27; *Atlas*, 3.33, 3.34, 3.35):

a. The **lumbosacral trunk** (L4, L5) contributes to the sacral plexus.
b. The ventral rami of S2 and S3 emerge between the digitations of the piriformis.
c. Ventral rami from L4 through S3 converge and form the large **sciatic nerve**. It passes through the greater sciatic foramen together with the piriformis.
d. Usually, the **gluteal arteries** (branches of the internal iliac artery) pierce the sacral plexus: Often, the lumbosacral trunk and S1 are separated by the superior gluteal artery. Occasionally, the superior gluteal artery intervenes between L4 and L5. The inferior gluteal artery usually separates ramus S1 from S2.
e. Ventral rami S2, S3, and S4 contribute to the pudendal nerve (Fig. 3.27). Remember, ventral rami S2, S3, and S4 contain preganglionic parasympathetic fibers (sacral parasympathetic outflow; pelvic splanchnic nerves; *Atlas*, 3.16, 3.57). These autonomic nerves supply the female pelvic organs and the distal portion of the GI tract from left colic flexure to rectum.
f. Note the **sympathetic chain and its ganglia** medial to the sacral foramina (*Atlas*, 3.33, 3.34, 3.36). These ganglia give off gray rami communicantes to the ventral sacral rami. Review the entire innervation of the *female* pelvis (*Atlas*, 3.57).

Lymphatic Drainage of the Female Pelvis (*Atlas*, 3.58). Lymphatic channels are difficult to see unless injected with a dye. However, you may encounter lymph nodes in certain pelvic regions, particularly if there was a pelvic inflammatory or malignant process prior to death. Understand that the external genitalia have a different lymphatic drainage than the uterus and the ovaries. This is of considerable clinical significance. Be familiar with the lymphatic drainage of the rectum (*Atlas*, 3.58D).

Sections. Study a **transverse section of the female pelvis** (*Atlas*, 3.82) and correlate it with a corresponding MRI (*Atlas*, 3.82B). Identify important muscles such as the obturator internus and the puborectalis. Be able to identify urinary bladder or urethra, uterus or vagina, and rectum on section. Study a transverse section of the **female perineum** (*Atlas*, 3.81), and identify important structures traversing the urogenital and anal triangles. Review the female pelvis in coronal section (*Atlas*, 3.49), and correlate pertinent anatomical structures with coronal magnetic resonance images (*Atlas*, 3.50, 3.51).

CHAPTER 4

THE BACK

Muscles of the Back

General Remarks

The muscles of the back are divided into three groups: superficial, intermediate, and deep. The **superficial group** acts on the upper limb. These muscles anchor the upper limb to the axial skeleton. This anchorage extends from the skull to the pelvic girdle. The **intermediate group** functions in respiration. The **deep group** consists of intrinsic or "native" muscles of the back (dorsum). These are supplied by dorsal nerve rami (see Fig. 4.7; *Atlas*, 1.20). Embryologically, the superficial and intermediate groups migrated from the ventrum and hence are supplied by ventral nerve rami.

Bony Landmarks

Refer to the skull, the skeleton, and to the cadaver, which must be in the prone position (face down). Identify the following bony landmarks:

1. **Occipital bone** (Fig. 4.1 or *Atlas*, 7.32A). Note the **external occipital protuberance or inion** and the **nuchal lines.**
2. **Mastoid process** (Fig. 4.1 or *Atlas*, 7.2).
3. **Scapula** (*Atlas*, 6.1B). Identify its **spine.** Trace it from the medial border to the **acromion.** Palpate the **superior** and the **inferior angle.** Palpate the **medial or vertebral border** of the scapula.
4. **Iliac crest** (*Atlas*, 5.1B). It terminates posteriorly in the **posterior superior iliac spine** (*Atlas*, 5.39). Here, the overlying skin often shows a dimple, since there are no fleshy muscle fibers (*Atlas*, 4.47).
5. Examine the **vertebral column** (*Atlas*, 4.1, 4.2). Realize that it consists of seven cervical vertebrae, 12 thoracic vertebrae, five lumbar vertebrae, the sacrum (five fused pieces), and the coccyx.
6. Study a **lumbar** and a **thoracic vertebra** (*Atlas*, 4.7). It consists of a weight-bearing body and a protective vertebral arch that is made up of two rounded **pedicles** (roots) and two flat plates or **laminae.** At the junction of pedicle and lamina, a **transverse process** projects laterally, and **articular processes** project superiorly and inferiorly. At the junction of the two laminae, a **spinous process** projects posteriorly in the median plane. The bodies and transverse processes of the thoracic vertebrae have facets for the ribs (Fig. 4.2; *Atlas*, 4.8).
7. Two adjacent vertebral bodies are united by a fibrocartilaginous **intervertebral disc.** This is a joint of the symphysis variety (Fig. 4.3; *Atlas*, 4.35A and B).
8. Two adjacent vertebral arches are united by their articular processes (Fig. 4.3).
9. An **intervertebral foramen** is completed between the pedicles of two adjacent vertebrae. It transmits the spinal nerve of the corresponding segment (Fig. 4.3).
10. The head of a rib articulates typically with two vertebral bodies and the intervening disc. The tubercle of a

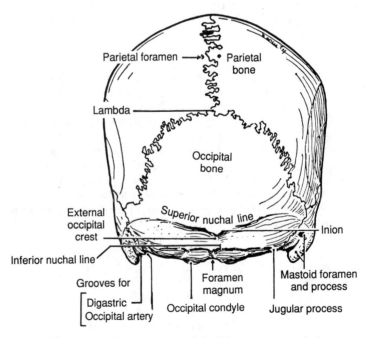

Figure 4.1. Posterior view of skull (norma occipitalis).

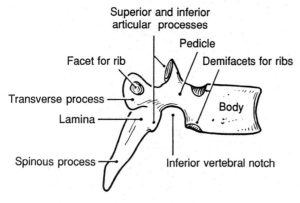

Figure 4.2. Typical thoracic vertebra (lateral view).

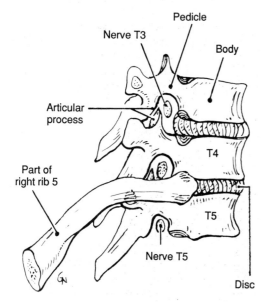

Figure 4.3. Part of vertebral column in thoracic region: intervertebral disc, intervertebral foramen with spinal nerve, and rib attachment.

rib articulates with the transverse process of the vertebra with the same segmental number (Fig. 4.3). The head of rib 5 articulates with vertebral bodies T4 and T5. The tubercle of rib 5 articulates with the transverse process of T5.

11. Examine the **cervical vertebrae** (*Atlas*, 4.10, 4.12, 4.14). Identify the right and left **transverse process**, each containing a characteristic opening, the **foramen transversarium.** Identify the **spinous processes** of all cervical vertebrae. Usually, the 7th cervical spine is the most prominent of the cervical spines. In the cadaver, run the finger down in the dorsal midline from external occipital protuberance, until it is arrested by the 7th cervical spine. Study radiographs of the cervical spine, particularly of the important lateral cervical spine (*Atlas*, 4.11, 4.13).

12. The **atlas** (C1) does not have a spinous process. The **first thoracic spine** belongs to the *axis* (C2). It may be more prominent than the spine of C7 (*Atlas*, 4.1A).

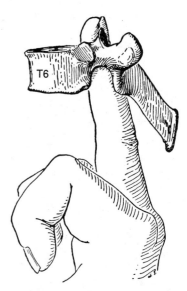

Figure 4.4. A vertebral foramen is not larger than a finger ring. In the articulated vertebral column, the vertebral foramina collectively form the vertebral canal.

13. Place your index finger into the **vertebral foramen** of a vertebra (Fig. 4.4). Observe that the size of the vertebral foramen is not larger than a finger ring and that the diameter of the vertebral foramina differs from vertebra to vertebra (*Atlas*, 4.14, 4.17B, 4.18). In the articulated vertebral column, the vertebral foramina collectively form a bony tube, the **vertebral canal**. This canal encloses and protects the important spinal cord. Understand that access to the contents of the spinal canal is possible by surgical removal of the laminae (laminectomy).

14. Be aware that there are **primary and secondary curvatures** of the spinal column (*Atlas*, 4.3). Identify these curvatures in a skeleton.

> With an imaginary line, connect the highest points of the left and right iliac crests. This line crosses the vertebral column at the 4th lumbar spine. The 3rd lumbar interspace is between the 3rd and 4th lumbar spines. A needle is usually introduced into the 3rd lumbar interspace to obtain cerebrospinal fluid (CSF) from the subarachnoid space (spinal tap or lumbar puncture) for diagnostic purposes.

Before you begin . . .

To save time, skin and superficial fascia of the back will be removed together. The muscles of the superficial and intermediate groups will be reflected. Subsequently, the deep group will be studied. The dorsal aspect of the vertebral column will be exposed. The vertebral canal will be opened, and the spinal cord and its coverings will be studied. Finally, the muscles and nerves of the suboccipital region will be examined.

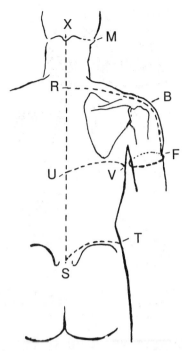

Figure 4.5. Skin incisions.

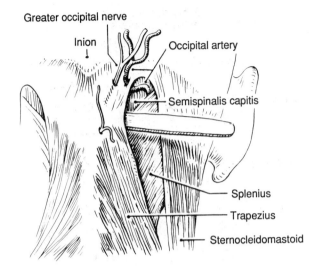

Figure 4.6. Greater occipital nerve and occipital artery.

Skin Incisions

Refer to Figure 4.5. In the midline, make a vertical skin incision from the external occipital protuberance (*X*) to the level of the posterior superior iliac spines (*S*). Carry out the following transverse incisions:

1. From *S* to *T* (if not already done for the dissection of the gluteal region);
2. From *U* to *V*, at the level of the inferior scapular angle;
3. From *R* to *B*, superior to the scapula and to the tip of the acromion, and on to point *F*. Here, make a complete circular skin incision at the root of the arm.
4. From the external occipital protuberance (*X*) laterally to the base of the mastoid process (*M*).

Dissection

Begin dissection with reflection of the skin in the area bounded by points *X*, *M*, and *R* (Fig. 4.5). In the underlying subcutaneous tissue, attempt to locate the **greater occipital nerve** and the accompanying **occipital artery** (Fig. 4.6; *Atlas*, 4.47). The nerve pierces the trapezius muscle about 3 cm inferolateral to the inion. The artery lies lateral to the nerve. The deep fascia in this area is very dense and tough. Therefore, it may be difficult to find the nerve, even though it is large. With scissors, split the deep fascia parallel to the expected course of the nerve. If you find the occipital artery first, look for the nerve medial to it. Limit your time searching for the nerve. Check with your instructor. It is possible that you

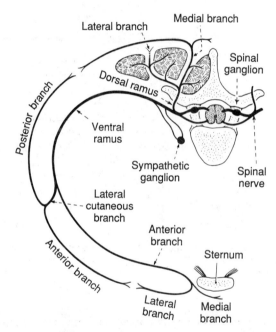

Figure 4.7. Schema of spinal nerve. Note distribution of dorsal ramus to deep back muscles and to skin of back.

may have removed the distal portion of this cutaneous nerve with the skin. In that case, you will later encounter the proximal portion of the nerve at it passes through the semispinalis capitis or as it emerges inferior to the obliquus capitis inferior (see Fig. 4.12; *Atlas*, 4.56, 4.57).

Realize that the greater occipital nerve is the dorsal ramus of C2. Read an account of the **dorsal primary divisions or dorsal rami** of the spinal nerves (Fig. 4.7 or *Atlas*, 1.20). To save time, make no deliberate effort to display other cutaneous branches of the dorsal rami. However, several of these nerves may be seen piercing the trapezius or latissimus dorsi to enter the superficial fascia (*Atlas*, 4.47).

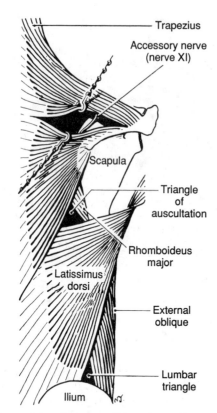

Figure 4.8. Exposure of dorsal scapular region.

Reflect skin and superficial fascia of the back together. In doing this, you will also remove the medial and lateral cutaneous branches of the dorsal rami (Fig. 4.7). These cutaneous branches course in the superficial fascia (or subcutaneous fat). Be careful **not** to incise the superficial fascia along the anterior border of the trapezius. Here, the spinal accessory nerve and other structures are in danger of being cut. The spinal accessory nerve and branches of ventral rami C2 to C4 supply the large trapezius muscle.

Clean two extensive muscles of the superficial group: **trapezius** and **latissimus dorsi** (Fig. 4.8; *Atlas*, 4.47). Notice that they cover almost the entire back. Observe two triangles associated with the latissimus dorsi: triangle of auscultation, and lumbar triangle.

> The **triangle of auscultation** (Fig. 4.8) is bounded by latissimus dorsi, trapezius, and rhomboid major together with the vertebral border of the scapula. Here, ribs 6 and 7 and intercostal space 6 are free of overlying muscles. Thus, this area is particularly suited for auscultation (listening to sounds produced by thoracic viscera).
>
> The **lumbar triangle** (of Petit) is bounded by the latissimus dorsi, external oblique of the abdomen, and iliac crest (Fig. 4.8; *Atlas*, 4.47, 4.48). Its floor is formed by the internal oblique of the abdomen. On rare occasions, this weak triangular space is the site of a "lumbar hernia."

Trapezius (Fig. 4.8; *Atlas*, 4.47).   Observe the origin of this triangular muscle from the external occipital protuberance (inion), the ligamentum nuchae, and the spinous processes of C7 and T1 to T12. Note that different parts of the muscle take different fiber courses:

1. Fibers of the **superior portion** run inferolaterally and are inserted into the lateral third of the clavicle (*Atlas*, 8.2, 8.3).
2. Fibers of the **middle portion** run transversely. These are inserted into the acromion and spine of the scapula (*Atlas*, 4.47).
3. Fibers of the **inferior portion** run superolaterally. These fibers converge into an aponeurosis near the medial end of the spine of the scapula.

The trapezius must be reflected in such a manner as (a) to allow complete access to underlying structures; and (b) to preserve its blood and nerve supply.

Ask your partner to push the shoulder backward (posteriorly). This relaxes the trapezius. Pass your hand under the free lateral and inferior border of the muscle. Feel the loose fat and areolar tissue separating the trapezius from other muscles. Now, detach the muscle from its origin very close to the spinous processes. Start inferiorly. Carefully carry the detachment toward the inion. Frequently define and loosen the muscle with a finger before you proceed with the cutting. Then, detach the trapezius from its insertion into the spine and acromion of the scapula. Do this with a scalpel, cutting very close to the bone. Now, the muscle is attached only to the clavicle. Reflect the muscle laterally.

Study the deep surface of the trapezius (*Atlas*, 4.47). In the loose fatty tissue, find blood vessels and nerves. Using blunt dissection and a probe, identify the **spinal accessory nerve** as it is attached to the anterior border of the muscle (*Atlas*, 8.2). Realize that the nerve passes though the posterior triangle of the neck. However, do not follow the nerve into the triangle at this time. Keep the triangle undisturbed. This area will be dissected later with other head and neck structures (*Note:* If your dissection sequence was such that the posterior triangle of the neck has already been dissected, then establish the continuity of the accessory nerve in the triangle). Follow the accessory nerve inferiorly and note that it sends numerous twigs into the musculature of the trapezius muscle (*Atlas*, 4.47).

Latissimus Dorsi (Fig. 4.8; *Atlas*, 4.47).   Verify the following:

1. Its thin superior border extends laterally from the spinous processes of T6 and T7.
2. Its most lateral fibers interdigitate with those of the external oblique below the origin of the serratus anterior (*Atlas*, 2.7).
3. The muscle arises from the vast thoracolumbar fascia (lumbodorsal fascia) that covers the deep (intrinsic) musculature of the back.
4. Superiorly, the muscle fibers of the latissimus dorsi converge (*Atlas*, 4.47). They form a broad tendon which is inserted into the humerus. Close to the tendon, the muscle receives its nerve supply (*Atlas*, 6.26). Do not

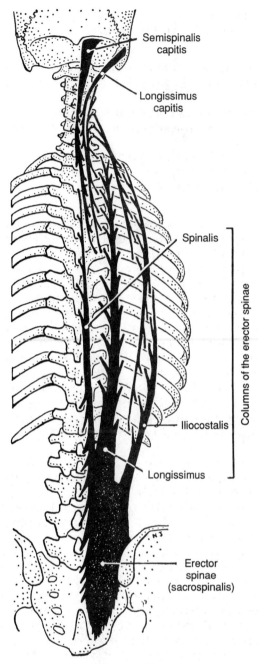

Figure 4.9. Deep muscles of the back: erector spinae and semi-spinalis capitis.

explore either tendinous insertion or nerve supply at this time.

Place your hand deep to the latissimus dorsi and lift it up slightly. With a scalpel, cut through its tendinous origin from the thoracolumbar fascia (*Atlas*, 4.47). Avoid cutting too close to the lumbar spinous processes. Reflect the muscle laterally.

Next, study the three remaining muscles of the superficial group: **rhomboideus major, rhomboideus minor,** and **levator scapulae.** They are inserted into the medial border of the scapula (*Atlas*, 4.47). Place your finger deep to the

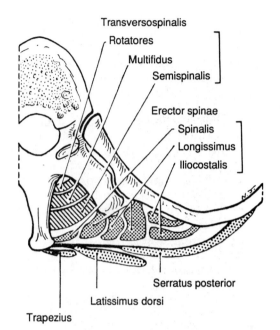

Figure 4.10. Schematic transverse section of muscles of the back.

two rhomboids. Then, detach these muscles from the spinous processes. Reflect them laterally. On the deep surface of the muscles, look for nerves and blood vessels. Leave the levator scapulae undisturbed. However, observe three or four slips arising from the transverse processes of the upper four cervical vertebrae (*Atlas*, 4.48). Realize that all muscular attachments (with the exception of the levator scapulae) of the shoulder girdle to the vertebral column have been severed. As a result, the shoulder will easily fall forward (anteriorly).

Now, the **intermediate muscle group** is readily accessible. Observe the thin sheets of the **serratus posterior superior** and **serratus posterior inferior.** These muscles are respiratory in action. Note their insertions into the ribs. Cut through the thin aponeuroses of both muscles at their origins from the spinous processes (*Atlas*, 4.48). Reflect the muscle laterally. Now, only the muscles of the deep group remain (*Atlas*, 4.49).

The **muscles of the deep group** to be studied at this time include (Figs. 4.9, 4.10; *Atlas*, 4.49): **splenius capitis and cervicis, semispinalis capitis,** and the enormous musculature collectively called the **erector spinae** and **transversospinalis.** Deep to the semispinalis capitis lie the small muscles of the suboccipital region. The suboccipital region will be studied at the end of this chapter.

Splenius Capitis and Cervicis (Gr. *splenion*, bandage; L., *caput*, head; *cervix*, neck; *Atlas*, 4.49). Identify the splenius capitis which is inserted into the occipital bone and the mastoid process. The splenius cervicis is inserted into the transverse processes of the upper cervical vertebrae. On one side only, detach the splenius where it arises from the ligamentum nuchae and spinous processes. Reflect the muscle laterally. Now, the semispinalis capitis is fully exposed.

The **semispinalis capitis** (*Atlas*, 4.49, 4.57) arises from the transverse processes of the upper thoracic vertebrae. It is inserted into the occipital bone between the nuchal lines. Note that it is traversed by the greater occipital nerve.

Erector Spinae or Sacrospinalis (Figs. 4.9, 4.10; *Atlas,* 4.49, 4.50). This bilateral structure is formed by long, vertically running muscle bundles on each side of the vertebral column. In the well developed specimen, it is a prominent and massive muscular bulge stretching from the pelvis to the skull. Distinguish **three columns** of the erector spinae: **iliocostalis, longissimus,** and **spinalis.**

The **iliocostalis** is the **lateral column of the erector spinae** (Fig. 4.9). As its name appropriately suggests, it arises from the ilium (iliac crest) and inserts into ribs (L. *costa,* rib). Identify the three parts of the iliocostalis: (1) Its *lumbar part, iliocostalis lumborum,* arising from the iliac crest and inserting into the angles of the lower six ribs. (2) Its *thoracic part, iliocostalis thoracis,* arising from the six lower ribs and inserting into the six upper ribs. Its *cervical part, iliocostalis cervicis,* arising from the upper six ribs and inserting into the transverse processes of the lower cervical vertebrae. Identify these structures.

The **longissimus** (L., meaning the longest) is the **middle column of the erector spinae.** It is characterized by the fact that it gives muscles slips to the transverse processes of the thoracic and cervical vertebrae (Fig. 4.9). Identify these *thoracic and cervical portions* of the longissimus. Note that its most *superior portion, the longissimus capitis,* inserts into the mastoid process of the skull.

Now identify the **spinalis** which forms the **medial column of the erector spinae.** It is relatively thin (about 2 cm). As the name implies, it is connected to the *spinous processes* of lumbar, thoracic and cervical vertebrae (Fig. 4.9).

Function. Appreciate the fact that all three columns of the erector spinae extend the vertebral column if both sides work together. If only one side is active, the three columns bend the vertebral column laterally. Are you familiar with the nerve supply to the erector spinae?

On one side of the cadaver, remove the spinalis and the longissimus. This removal will expose the space between spinous processes and transverse processes of the vertebrae. A number of short muscles (*semispinalis, multifidus, rotatores*) can be seen filling the groove between transverse and spinous processes (Fig. 4.10; *Atlas,* 4.51, 4.53, 4.55). These muscles are collectively called the **transversospinalis.** If required to define and dissect these short, obliquely running muscles, please refer to *Atlas,* 4.53.

Spinal Cord

Exposure of the Spinal Canal. Place a block under the pelvis to reduce the concavity of the lumbar region. Remove all the dorsal musculature from T6 to L5. Scoop out the muscles that fill the groove between transverse and spinous processes (Fig. 4.10; *Atlas,* 4.55A and **B**). In the lower thoracic (T6) region or in the lumbar (L1) region, remove several spinous processes with bone pliers. Note that

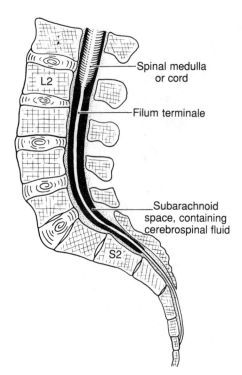

Figure 4.11. Diagram of vertebral canal and lower portion of spinal cord.

the spines are attached to each other by **supraspinous and interspinous ligaments** (*Atlas,* 4.39). After removing the spinous processes, observe the strong and elastic **ligamenta flava** (*Atlas,* 4.39). These ligaments connect the laminae of adjacent vertebrae. They extend laterally to the intervertebral foramina and bound them posteriorly.

Remove the **laminae** (laminectomy) of several vertebrae. Do this about 1 cm from the midline, using a saw inclined to enter the vertebral canal. Remove individual pieces of bone with bone pliers. Protect your eyes from flying chips of bone.

Identify the **epidural or extradural space.** Remove the fatty tissue and venous plexus from it (*Atlas,* 4.40). Expose the **dura mater** of the spinal cord. Next, carefully incise the dura mater in the dorsal midline. Try to do this without incising the **arachnoid mater**: i.e., without opening the subarachnoid space (*Atlas,* 4.66A). In the living subject (but usually not in the embalmed cadaver), the subarachnoid space contains cerebrospinal fluid (Fig. 4.11). After identifying the arachnoid, open the subarachnoid space. Note the following (*Atlas,* 4.66B):

1. **Spinal cord.** It is completely surrounded with delicate pia mater.
2. On each side of the cord, the pia mater forms strong pointed prolongations. These are the **denticulate ligaments.** They secure the spinal cord to the dura mater (*Atlas,* 4.64, 4.65). Usually, there are 21 points of attachment on each side.
3. **Ventral and dorsal roots** (*Atlas,* 4.65, 4.66B, 4.70). Using a probe, follow a ventral and a dorsal root to the

point where they pierce the dura and enter the intervertebral foramen.

4. In the thoracic region, place a probe into an **intervertebral foramen** to protect the nerve within it. Using bone pliers, remove the articular processes lying posterior to this foramen (Fig. 4.3). Expose the **spinal ganglion** or dorsal root ganglion (*Atlas*, 4.66A). If you are careful enough, you can see the spinal nerve dividing into ventral and dorsal rami (*Atlas*, 4.66A).

It will be unnecessary to expose the entire spinal cord if demonstration or museum specimens are available. Consult with your instructor. In either the dissected or in a specially prepared museum specimen study the following:

1. **Cervical enlargement of spinal cord** from C3 to T2, corresponding to the large nerve supply of the upper limb.
2. **Lumbar enlargement of spinal cord** from T9 to T12, corresponding to the large nerve supply of the lower limb. (Realize that these levels T9 to T12 are vertebral levels. They do not correspond to spinal cord segmental levels.)
3. **Conus medullaris**, the end of the spinal cord, between L1 and L2 (*Atlas*, 4.66B). Of pediatric importance: at birth, the conus medullaris lies at the level of L3.
4. **Filum terminale** (Fig. 4.11; *Atlas* 4.66B, 4.67). It is a delicate filament continuous with the pia mater. Its intradural portion ends at S2 where it is attached to the end of the dural sac. Its extradural prolongation ends at the coccyx.
5. **Cauda equina** (L., tail of horse). It is a collection of ventral and dorsal roots caudal to the termination of the spinal cord (*Atlas*, 4.66B; transverse section 4.38).
6. Realize that there are 31 pairs of spinal nerves (eight cervical; 12 thoracic; five lumbar; five sacral; one coccygeal).

In relationship to the spinal cord, **review the following:**

1. **Nerve plexuses** (*Atlas*, 4.75).
2. Distribution of a **spinal nerve** (Fig. 4.7; *Atlas*, 1.20).
3. **Dermatomes and myotomes** (*Atlas*, 4.71, 4.72).
4. **Sympathetic chain** and its connections with spinal nerves (Fig. 4.7; *Atlas*, 1.82, 3.33).

Review the **articulated vertebral column.** Once more, examine all seven cervical vertebrae (*Atlas*, 4.10, 4.12). Correlate your observations with corresponding radiographs (*Atlas*, 4.11, 4.13). In a lateral radiograph of the cervical spine (also called lateral C-spine), identify the following (*Atlas*, 4.13):

1. **Posterior arch of atlas** (C1); note that there is only a **posterior tubercle** but no spinous process (compare *Atlas*, 4.14). Realize that the **posterior arch,** in part, surrounds the cervical spinal cord.
2. **Anterior arch and anterior tubercle of atlas** (C1).
3. **Dens (odontoid process) of axis** (C2). Note that the dens is closely related to the anterior arch of C1 (compare *Atlas*, 4.14, 4.15).
4. **Spinous process of axis** (C2).
5. Study the clinically important **atlantoaxial joint** and correlate your observations with a radiograph (*Atlas*, 4.15, 4.16A).

Review the **lumbar vertebral column** (*Atlas*, 4.1, 4.2). Correlate your findings with an anteroposterior (AP) and lateral radiograph of the lumbosacral spine (*Atlas*, 4.20, 4.21). Pay special attention to **lumbar vertebrae L4 and L5** and the space between them. This is the location of the **intervertebral disc.** Intervertebral discs at L4/L5 are particularly prone to injuries (prolapsed nucleus pulposus with resulting compression of the cauda equina and corresponding neurological impairment; compare *Atlas*, 4.39).

Suboccipital Region

Students may or may not be required to dissect the suboccipital region. Check with your instructor. At any rate, the following description will aid you in either dissecting this region or in understanding a prosected specimen.

Bony Landmarks

Refer to a skull and a vertebral column. Identify the following pertinent landmarks:

1. On the occipital bone: the two **nuchal lines** and the area between them (Fig. 4.1; *Atlas*, 4.56); **foramen magnum** (*Atlas*, 7.35).
2. On the **1st cervical vertebra or atlas** (*Atlas*, 4.10, 4.12, 4.14): **posterior arch** with **posterior tubercle; transverse process; foramen transversarium** for the trans-

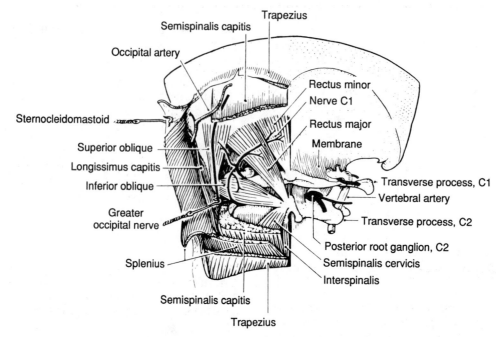

Occipital artery

Sternocleidomastoid

Superior oblique

Longissimus capitis

Inferior oblique

Greater occipital nerve

Splenius

Semispinalis capitis

Trapezius

Semispinalis capitis

Trapezius

Rectus minor

Nerve C1

Rectus major

Membrane

Transverse process, C1

Vertebral artery

Transverse process, C2

Posterior root ganglion, C2

Semispinalis cervicis

Interspinalis

Figure 4.12. Diagram of suboccipital region.

mission of the vertebral artery; **groove for the vertebral artery.**
3. On the **2nd cervical vertebra or axis** (*Atlas*, 4.10, 4.12, 4.14): spinous process; transverse process; foramen transversarium.

Dissection

Once again, identify the **semispinalis capitis** (*Atlas*, 4.56, 4.57). If not already done, detach the semispinalis capitis bilaterally close to its attachment to the occipital bone. Carefully reflect the muscle inferiorly. Be cautious not to tear the **greater occipital nerve.** Follow this nerve through the muscle. Deep to the muscle, follow the nerve, as a guiding structure, to the lower border of the inferior oblique (Fig. 4.12; *Atlas*, 4.56).

The **obliquus capitis inferior** (inferior oblique) forms the lower limit of the suboccipital region. Verify that this muscle extends from the spinous process of the axis (C2) to the transverse process of the atlas (C1).

Suboccipital Triangle (Fig. 4.12; *Atlas*, 4.56 through 4.59).   Identify and clean three muscles bounding the triangle:

1. **Obliquus capitis** (inferior oblique). It bounds the triangle inferiorly.
2. **Rectus capitis posterior major** (rectus major). It bounds the suboccipital triangle medially. Follow it from the spinous process of the axis superolaterally to the inferior nuchal line. (The rectus minor lies medial to the rectus major. It originates from the posterior tubercle of the atlas.)

3. **Obliquus capitis superior** (superior oblique). It bounds the triangle laterally. It lies deep. Follow it from the transverse process of the atlas to the occipital bone.

With the suboccipital triangle well defined, identify the nerves of the region (Fig. 4.12). The **greater occipital nerve** (dorsal ramus of C2; cutaneous) has already been identified. Note that it emerges between vertebrae C1 and C2. Find the **suboccipital nerve** (dorsal ramus of C1) within the suboccipital triangle. Note that the nerve emerges between the occipital bone and vertebra C1. The suboccipital nerve is motor to the muscles of the suboccipital region.

Next, find the **vertebral artery** (Fig. 4.12; *Atlas*, 4.60). On one side of the body, cut all dorsal musculature away from the transverse processes of C1 and C2. Identify the vertebral artery as it passes through the **foramina transversaria** of axis and atlas. On the same side, scrape clean the **posterior arch of the atlas.** Note the thin **posterior atlanto-occipital membrane** that stretches from this arch to the posterior margin of the foramen magnum. Observe that the vertebral artery curves around the superior articular process of the atlas. Follow it in its groove on the arch of the atlas. Finally, the artery passes through a hiatus in the posterior atlanto-occipital membrane. (Later, after removal of the membrane and a wedge of occipital bone, the artery will be followed in its course through the foramen magnum into the cranial cavity; see Chapter 7, "Head and Neck"). The tortuous course of the vertebral artery can be demonstrated in a vertebral arteriogram. Such a radiograph looks complicated and may be difficult to understand unless the topographic anatomy of the vertebral artery is fully understood.

CHAPTER 5

THE LOWER LIMB

Introductory Remarks

The essential functional requirements of the lower limb are: (a) weight bearing; (b) locomotion; and (c) maintenance of equilibrium. Anatomically, the lower limb is divided into three segments:

1. **Thigh,** the segment between hip and knee;
2. **Leg,** specifically the segment between knee and ankle;
3. **Foot.**

It is advantageous to dissect the lower limb in the following sequence: first, the superficial veins and nerves and the deep investing fascia of the entire lower limb will be examined. Next, the anterior and the medial regions of the thigh will be dissected. Subsequently, the gluteal region, back of thigh, and popliteal fossa will be explored. Finally, the three crural compartments of the leg will be dissected, and their contents will be followed onto the dorsum and into the sole of the foot.

Note: Remember that this manual is intended to guide you with the **dissection** of the human body. It is **not** the purpose of *Grant's Dissector* to provide you with a list of all muscles, their origins, insertions, and functions. However, you may find it advantageous to prepare or to copy such a list and to bring it to the laboratory for systematic review of all muscles of the lower limb you are held responsible for in your laboratory course.

Before you begin . . .

Do *not* dissect at this time. Realize that **superficial veins** and cutaneous nerves are contained in the **superficial fascia.** The first objective is to study these structures (superficial fascia; superficial veins; cutaneous nerves) of the entire lower limb as a whole. To accomplish this, the entire lower extremity will be skinned in an initial dissecting effort. The subcutaneous connective tissue and fat will be removed, leaving the more important superficial veins and nerves intact. Subsequently, the **deep fascia** will be demonstrated. The deep or investing fascia surrounds the various muscle compartments as well as the **deep system of veins.** Special attention will be paid to the clinically important **perforating veins,** which *perforate* the deep fascia and provide anastomoses between the deep and the superficial system of veins.

Skin Incisions

With the cadaver in the supine position (face up), make skin incisions according to Figure 5.1. Be sure to cut only through the thickness of the skin. Do not cut into or remove the superficial fascia.

Make skin incisions as indicated by the *dotted lines* in Figure 5.1A: anteriorly, vertically, and in the midline of the lower limb, starting inferior to the inguinal ligament, passing over the patella (knee cap), along the anterior portion of the leg and onto the dorsum of the foot. Make as many transverse skin incisions as needed to speed up the skinning process or to allow other students to participate. Cut transversely across the foot at the webs of the toes. Cut along the midline of each toe. Put traction on the skin as it is being removed, and keep the sharp knife directed against it to make the skinning process as efficient as possible. Leave the superficial fascia intact. Turn the skin flaps as far laterally as possible.

Eventually, you must turn the cadaver into the prone position (face down) in order to remove the skin from the posterior aspect of the lower limb. As shown in Figure 5.1B, make a vertical cut, beginning inferior to the gluteal region, along the middle of the thigh and leg down to the heel. Extend the previously made transverse skin incisions posteriorly. If not already done (during the dissection of the pelvis), remove the skin from the gluteal region.

While the previously described skinning is under way, another student can remove the skin from the sole of the foot as indicated in Figure 5.1C.

The next objective is to remove the superficial fascia while leaving intact the superficial veins and nerves. With the cadaver still in the prone position, examine the structures contained in the **superficial fascia of the posterior aspect of the lower limb.** Familiarize yourself with the expected course of **superficial veins** (*Atlas,* 5.4) and **superficial nerves** (*Atlas,* 5.7B).

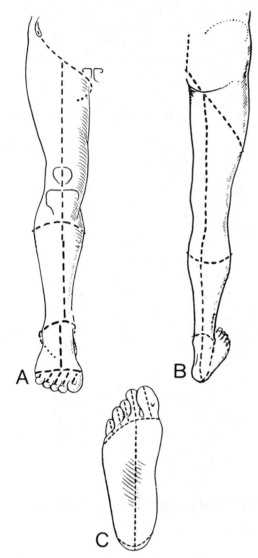

Figure 5.1. Skin incisions.

branches to the posterior aspect of the thigh pierce the fascia. Isolate at least one of the terminal twigs. Examine the cutaneous nerves in the gluteal region (these nerves may have been removed earlier during the dissection of the perineum and pelvis). Be aware that the **posterior cutaneous nerve of the thigh** sends cutaneous branches to the gluteal region around the inferior border of the gluteus maximus (*Atlas*, 5.7**B**). Superiorly, the skin of the gluteal region is supplied by **cutaneous branches of dorsal rami L1, L2, and L3.**

Now, **remove** all connective tissue and fat of the **superficial fascia** from the posterior aspect of the leg, thigh, and gluteal region, leaving intact the deep fascia and the principal superficial nerves and veins. Be very careful with tissue removal around the superficial veins. Demonstrate that the **superficial veins** are connected to **perforating veins,** which pierce the deep fascia and anastomose with the deep venous system (*arrows* in *Atlas*, 5.4, 5.5).

Next, turn the cadaver over into the supine position (face up). First, the **superficial veins** of the anterior and medial aspects of the lower limb will be examined. Start with the **great saphenous vein,** the longest vein in the body (Gr., *saphenous*, manifest; visible). Pick it up at the medial aspect of the knee, and follow it inferiorly along the medial side of the leg and anterior to the medial malleolus (medial ankle; same side as the great toe). Identify veins on the dorsum of the foot and note that the **dorsal venous arch of the foot** is the main tributary to the **great saphenous vein** (*Atlas*, 5.4, 5.100). Follow this vein from the medial aspect of the knee superolaterally to a point just inferior to the inguinal ligament (*Atlas*, 5.10). Here, the vein passes through an oval aperture in the deep fascia, the **saphenous opening or fossa ovalis,** to end in the femoral vein (*Atlas*, 5.4**B**). This region will be dissected later following removal of the superficial fascia. Slit open the proximal portion of the great saphenous vein and observe one or two of its valves (*Atlas*, 5.13**A** and **B**). There are 10 to 20 valves along the entire course of the vein. Gently remove the superficial fascia around the great saphenous vein, pull on the vein at various locations, and demonstrate again the existence of **perforating veins.**

Pick up the **small saphenous vein** as it passes posterior to the lateral malleolus (ankle) and ascends toward the popliteal fossa (posterior to the knee). Note the numerous tributaries and communications with other superficial veins. Pay particular attention to the venous communications with the **great saphenous vein,** which runs at the medial aspect of the leg and knee.

Observe that the **small saphenous vein** pierces the deep fascia in the popliteal fossa (at a deeper level, this vessel joins the popliteal vein). Identify two cutaneous nerves related to the course of the small saphenous vein (*Atlas*, 5.4, 5.7**B**): (1) Isolate the **sural nerve** that pierces the deep fascia near the middle of the posterior aspect of the leg. Follow this nerve inferiorly as it courses together with the small saphenous vein posterior to the lateral malleolus toward the lateral aspect of the foot (*Atlas*, 5.5). (2) Note the terminal branch of the **posterior cutaneous nerve of the thigh** emerging in the popliteal fossa. Realize that the more proximal portion of the posterior cutaneous nerve of the thigh runs deep to the investing fascia (*Atlas*, 5.7**B**); however, terminal cutaneous

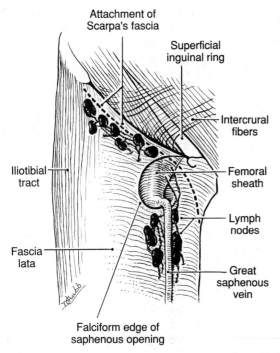

Figure 5.2. Fascia lata with saphenous opening, femoral sheath, and superficial inguinal lymph nodes.

Next, the **superficial nerves** of the anterior aspect of the lower limb will be examined (*Atlas*, 5.7A). Identify the **saphenous nerve** as it pierces the deep fascia on the medial aspect of the knee. Verify that the nerve supplies the anterior and medial aspects of the leg and that it accompanies the great saphenous vein to the dorsum of the foot to supply the medial aspect of the foot (note the clinical comment—screened material). As seen previously, the lateral side of the foot, including the small (5th) toe, is supplied by terminal branches of the sural nerve. Locate the **superficial peroneal** nerve as it pierces the deep fascia in the lateral distal third of the leg (*Atlas*, 5.7A). Follow it distally and verify that it supplies the dorsum of the foot and sends **dorsal digital nerves** to most of the skin of the toes. (It should be noted here that the skin between the 1st toe or big toe and the 2nd toe is innervated by a terminal branch of the deep peroneal nerve, a matter of importance in the neurological assessment of nerve injuries in the leg.) Next, explore the nerve supply of the anterior and medial aspects of the thigh. These cutaneous nerves pierce the deep fascia along the line of the sartorius, a slender, strap-like muscle crossing the front of the thigh obliquely from the anterior superior iliac spine to the medial side of the knee (*Atlas*, 5.7A). Identify the **cutaneous nerves of the thigh: lateral, intermediate, and medial.** Inferior to the saphenous ring and medial to the great saphenous vein, attempt to find the **cutaneous branch of the obturator nerve.**

Inguinal Lymph Nodes. Lymph vessels from the lower limb, lower anterior abdominal wall, gluteal region, perineum, and external genitalia drain into the **superficial inguinal lymph nodes** (Fig. 5.2; *Atlas*, 5.9B). Identify **two groups of superficial nodes:** (1) A horizontal group lies about 2 cm below the inguinal ligament. (2) A vertical group is applied to both sides of the great saphenous vein. Realize that the superficial nodes are connected with one to three **deep inguinal nodes** that lie at a deeper level on the medial side of the femoral vein (they cannot be seen at this time). Correlate your anatomical observations and knowledge with the radiographic image of a lymphangiogram (*Atlas*, 5.9A).

Remove all superficial fascia, leaving intact the superficial inguinal lymph nodes, the deep fascia, and the principal superficial nerves and veins.

Deep Fascia. Now, the full extent of the **deep fascia** of the lower limb can be appreciated. The deep fascia is a strong, dense layer of connective tissue that keeps the muscles in their various compartments much like a firm stocking. In the thigh, the deep fascia is referred to as **fascia lata** (L., *latus*, broad). The lateral portion of the fascia lata is particularly strong and known as the **iliotibial tract.** Inferiorly, the deep fascia of the thigh is continuous with the deep fascia of the leg (area between knee and ankle). The thick and strong deep fascia of the leg is also known as the **crural fascia.** Underlying muscles may originate from the deep fascia (e.g., the tibialis anterior). The deep fascia may also form strong bands that hold muscles or tendons in place (e.g., extensor retinacula). There are areas where the deep fascia is absent because it is not needed (e.g., over the subcutaneous part of the medial surface of the tibia). Obviously, the deep fascia will have to be incised and removed in order to explore the deep structures of the lower limb.

Anterior and Medial Regions of Thigh

Landmarks

Refer to a skeleton and study the following landmarks (*Atlas*, 5.1A and B):

1. **Anterior superior iliac spine;**
2. **Anterior inferior iliac spine;**
3. **Pubic tubercle** (remember: the *inguinal ligament* stretches from the anterior superior iliac spine to the pubic tubercle);
4. **Greater trochanter of femur;**
5. **Lesser trochanter of femur;**
6. **Lateral condyle** and **epicondyle** of femur;
7. **Medial condyle** and **epicondyle** of femur;
8. **Adductor tubercle** located on the medial epicondyle; the adductor tubercle is close to the *epiphyseal plate*, where most of the growth in length of the femur takes place;
9. **Linea aspera;**
10. **Patella;**
11. **Tuberosity** (tubercle) **of tibia.**

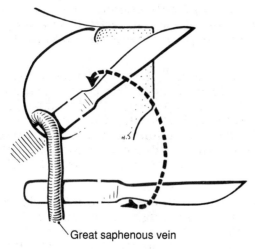

Figure 5.3. Find the inferior margin of the saphenous opening with the handle of the scalpel.

Before you begin . . .

The saphenous opening and its relation to the saphenous vein and femoral vein will be studied. Subsequently, the femoral sheath, canal, and ring will be explored. The femoral triangle will be defined, and some of its contents will be followed into the adductor canal. The muscles of the anterior and medial regions of the thigh will be displayed.

Dissection

Saphenous Opening. Clean the fascia lata (deep fascia) in the vicinity of the **saphenous opening** or fossa ovalis (*Atlas*, 5.11). Insert the handle of the knife into the opening (Fig. 5.3) and ease back the underlying femoral sheath without injuring it. With the handle, clean the pectineal fascia (deep fascia covering the pectineus muscle) medial to the saphenous opening and posterior to it (*Atlas*, 5.12). Note the femoral sheath that envelops the femoral vein, femoral artery, and deep lymph nodes. Trace the great saphenous vein proximally to the femoral vein. Clean the vessels at their junction. Observe that the great saphenous vein hooks over the free inferior margin of the saphenous opening (*Atlas*, 5.11, 5.12). Occasionally, the two vessels join slightly higher. Enlarge the saphenous opening by freely removing the deep fascia in its vicinity. This will widely expose the **femoral sheath.**

Femoral Sheath and Contents (*Atlas*, 5.11, 5.12, 5.14). This delicate sheath envelops the femoral artery, femoral vein, and some deep lymph vessels or nodes. Notice that the femoral sheath is shaped like a short cone (Fig. 5.4). The sheath is subdivided by two delicate vertical partitions into **three compartments** (Fig. 5.5; *Atlas*, 5.15). In the midline of each compartment, make a vertical cut (*Atlas*, 5.12). In the **lateral compartment**, observe the femoral artery. In the **middle compartment**, identify the femoral vein. Slit the vein open and demonstrate a valve (*Atlas*, 5.13A and B). The **medial compartment** of the femoral

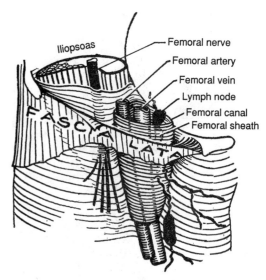

Figure 5.4. The femoral sheath and its three compartments.

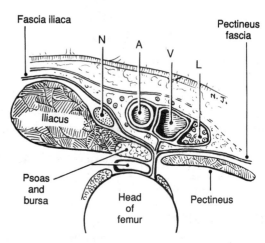

Figure 5.5. The femoral sheath and its three compartments on transverse section. *N*, femoral nerve; *A*, femoral artery in lateral compartment; *V*, femoral vein in middle compartment; *L*, lymphatics in medial compartment.

sheath is the **femoral canal**, which contains lymphatics and loose areolar tissue. Pass a probe up into the femoral canal and study the topographical relations of its mouth, the **femoral ring**. These relations are (*Atlas*, 5.12):

1. Anteriorly, the inguinal ligament;
2. Posteriorly, the pectineus and its fascia;
3. Laterally, the femoral vein;
4. Medially, the sharp lateral edge of the lacunar ligament.

The femoral ring is a potentially weak area in the lower portion of the anterior abdominal wall. Knowledge of the femoral ring and canal is important in understanding the mechanism of **femoral hernia.** A femoral hernia is a protrusion of parts of abdominal viscera through the femoral ring into the femoral canal. Study Figure 5.5 and understand the following facts: by necessity, a femoral hernia must be relatively small since it is contained in the limited femoral canal; it can usually be palpated below the inguinal ligament; it is frequently strangulated due to the rigid boundaries of the fem-

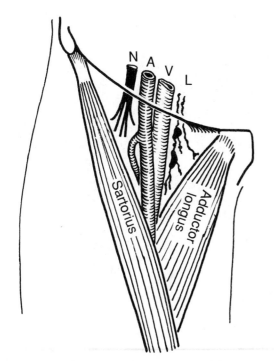

Figure 5.6. Femoral triangle and contents: *N*, femoral nerve; *A*, femoral artery; *V*, femoral vein; *L*, lymphatics.

oral ring and the tightness of the closely related inguinal and lacunar ligaments. Strangulation implies that the blood supply of the herniated bowel is impaired, and that tissue death (gangrene) is imminent. Femoral hernias are more common in women since the femoral ring in females is wider.

Femoral Triangle

The **femoral triangle** is bounded superiorly by the **inguinal ligament,** laterally by the medial border of the **sartorius,** and medially by the medial border of the **adductor longus** (Fig. 5.6; *Atlas,* 5.16A and B).

The femoral triangle contains the clinically important femoral vessels. The pulse of the femoral artery can be easily palpated about 3 cm inferior to the midpoint of the inguinal ligament.

Within the triangle, the femoral vessels are also frequently approached for diagnostic radiographic purposes. A special catheter can be inserted into either the femoral artery or the femoral vein. Catheters in the femoral artery can be advanced proximally into the aorta or selectively into aortic branches, such as the renal arteries or the mesenteric arteries. The catheter can be pushed via the aortic arch into the coronary arteries to obtain a coronary angiogram. In a similar fashion, a catheter in the femoral vein can be pushed through the inferior vena cava into the right atrium of the heart.

Clean the **femoral artery and vein** within the limits of the femoral triangle. Just inferior to the inguinal ligament, the artery gives rise to superficial branches of the abdominal wall and scrotum or labium majus (*Atlas,* 5.10,

5.12). Pay particular attention to the following three substantial arteries; these may arise from a large common stem, or they may arise independently (*Atlas,* 5.6):

1. **Profunda femoris artery.** It pursues the same general direction as the femoral artery, but on a more posterior plane. It is accompanied by the profunda femoris vein.
2. **Lateral femoral circumflex artery.**
3. **Medial femoral circumflex artery.** This artery is clinically important since it supplies the bulk of blood to the head and neck of the femur (*Atlas,* 5.6, 5.46).

Note that these three arteries are accompanied by corresponding veins. The largest of the veins is the **profunda femoris vein,** which drains into the femoral vein within the limits of the femoral triangle. Preserve the principal veins (femoral; profunda femoris; great saphenous). In order to clarify the dissection field, remove all other smaller veins. Display the **floor of the femoral triangle** by removing fat and fascia, particularly from the **pectineus** and **adductor longus** (*Atlas,* 5.16A). Open the interval between the contiguous borders of **iliopsoas** and **pectineus.** The **medial femoral circumflex vessels** pass dorsally between these two muscles (*Atlas,* 5.22).

Just lateral to the femoral artery, cut vertically through the fascia iliaca and expose the **femoral nerve** (*Atlas,* 5.14). Follow the nerve inferiorly and notice numerous branches of the nerve (*Atlas,* 5.16A). Identify the **intermediate** and the **medial cutaneous nerve of the thigh.** These nerves follow the medial border of the sartorius. Also, identify **motor branches to the sartorius** and to the **rectus femoris.** Usually, the **pectineus** is supplied by the femoral nerve. Find the small motor branch (*Atlas,* 5.24). Occasionally, the pectineus may have dual nerve supply by receiving an additional branch from the obturator nerve.

Adductor Canal

In the middle third of the thigh, the femoral vessels and the saphenous nerve are contained in the **adductor canal** (Hunter's canal). The adductor canal is a narrow fascial tunnel that begins at the **apex of the femoral triangle** (*Atlas,* 5.20). It ends at the **adductor hiatus,** which is a slit-like opening or hiatus in the tendon of the **adductor magnus** (*Atlas,* 5.6, 5.24). The femoral vessels pass through the adductor canal to reach the popliteal fossa (posterior to the knee). Note that the adductor canal lies deep to the **sartorius muscle.** Lift this muscle out of its bed and cut it transversely near the apex of the femoral triangle. Reflect the inferior part of the sartorius inferiorly. Now the adductor canal is exposed and can be studied.

Beginning at the apex of the femoral triangle, pass a probe into the canal and gently push it inferiorly. Slit open the fascial roof of the adductor canal. Study the **walls of the canal** (*Atlas,* 5.24): it is bounded laterally by the **vastus medialis,** posteromedially by the **adductor longus and magnus,** and anteriorly by the **sartorius.** Verify these relations on transverse section (Fig. 5.7; *Atlas,* 5.52A).

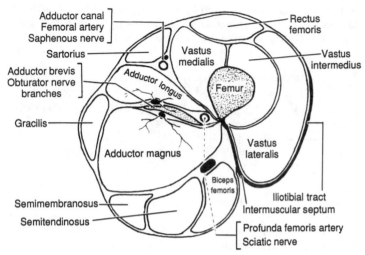

Figure 5.7. Transverse section of thigh. Boundaries and contents of adductor canal.

Study the whole length of the femoral vessels within the adductor canal. The **femoral vein** lies posterior to the **femoral artery.** Trace the femoral artery to the point where it passes through the **adductor hiatus** (*Atlas*, 5.6, 5.34A and B). Here, the artery changes its name to **popliteal artery.** Note that the **saphenous nerve** accompanies the femoral vessels; however, it does not pass through the adductor hiatus. Instead, it runs anterior to the adductor magnus tendon (*Atlas*, 5.24) toward the medial aspect of the knee (*Atlas*, 5.7A). Follow the saphenous nerve inferiorly to the point where it pierces the deep fascia. This area is usually located between the tendons of the **sartorius** and the **gracilis** muscles.

Fascia Lata

Once more, study the deep fascia of the thigh, referred to as **fascia lata.** In the lateral region of the thigh, the **fascia lata** is strong and dense (*Atlas*, 5.14, 5.16A). Immediately posterior and inferior to the anterior superior iliac spine, the fascia lata encases a muscle, the **tensor fasciae latae** (*Atlas*, 5.20, 5.27A). Identify it. Verify that the muscle pulls on a strap-like, longitudinal thickening of the fascia lata, the **iliotibial tract** (*Atlas*, 5.20, 5.27A). Split the fascia lata longitudinally between rectus femoris and vastus lateralis. Retract the iliotibial tract from the underlying vastus lateralis (*Atlas*, 5.20). With your fingers and the handle of the knife, follow the fascia lata posteriorly. Here, it is continuous with a very strong **intermuscular septum,** which is attached to the **linea aspera** on the posterior aspect of the femur (*Atlas*, 5.1B, 5.52A).

Muscles of Front of Thigh

Define the **rectus femoris** in the middle of the anterior thigh (Fig. 5.8; *Atlas*, 5.20). Observe that the flattened inferior tendon of the muscle is inserted into the patella. Identify and examine the **three vasti muscles**. The **vastus lateralis** lies on the lateral side of the thigh. The **vastus**

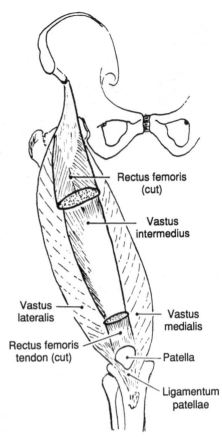

Figure 5.8. Quadriceps femoris. The vastus intermedius is covered by the rectus femoris.

medialis covers the medial aspect of the thigh. Positioned between the vastus medialis and lateralis is the **vastus intermedius.** Expose the vastus intermedius by pulling the overlying rectus femoris either laterally or medially. Identify motor branches of the femoral nerve supplying the sartorius, rectus femoris, and the vasti muscles (*Atlas*, 5.8A, 5.24). Study the vasti muscles on transverse section (Fig. 5.7; *Atlas*, 5.52A and B). Realize that their attachments include large parts of the shaft of the femur (*Atlas*, 5.28).

The **four muscles** of the anterior thigh (vastus lateralis, medialis, intermedius, and rectus femoris) are collectively known as the **quadriceps femoris.** Observe that the tendons of all four heads of the quadriceps unite to form a strong tendon. This tendon is inserted into the patella, and it continues inferiorly to the tibial tuberosity as the **ligamentum patellae or patellar tendon** (Fig. 5.8; *Atlas*, 5.20, 5.21).

Tapping the **patellar tendon** (inferior to the patella) normally leads to the elicitation of the **quadriceps reflex** (patellar reflex; knee jerk). The tapping activates muscle spindles in the quadriceps. Afferent impulses from these muscle spindles travel in the femoral nerve to spinal segments L2, L3, and L4 (*Atlas*, 5.8A). From here, efferent impulses are mediated in motor fibers of the femoral nerve to the quadriceps, resulting in a jerk-like contraction of this muscle group. Obviously, intelligent clinical evaluation of the quadriceps reflex depends on thorough knowledge of the underlying anatomical substrate.

Verify that both the sartorius and rectus femoris muscles span two joints, the hip joint and the knee joint. Thus, motion in these two joints is likely to occur during contraction of the sartorius and rectus femoris muscles. Examine each muscle individually and determine its action. The three remaining muscles of the quadriceps group (vastus medialis, vastus intermedius, vastus lateralis) act only on one joint, the knee joint. Verify this fact. Once again, examine the insertion of the ligamentum patellae into the tuberosity of the tibia. Palpate the patella (kneecap). It can be considered a sesamoid bone, developed and contained within the ligamentum patellae (*Atlas*, 5.60A).

Medial Side of Thigh

Remove any remaining deep fascia from the medial side of the thigh in order to display the **adductors**. Observe that **pectineus, adductor longus,** and **gracilis** originate from a curved line on the pubic bone (*Atlas*, 5.22, 5.21, 5.23, 5.25). On the medial aspect of the thigh, follow the slender, strap-like **gracilis** inferiorly to its insertion into the tibia. Trace the **pectineus** and **adductor longus** muscles as they fan out to their insertions along the linea aspera on the posterior aspect of the femur (*Atlas*, 5.23B). Note that the **profunda femoris vessels** pass between the two muscles (*Atlas*, 5.22). Now, separate the adjacent borders of pectineus and adductor longus. Cut the adductor longus 5 cm inferior from its origin and reflect it (*Atlas*, 5.24). The **adductor brevis** can now be seen at a deeper plane. On transverse section, verify that the adductor brevis lies posterior to the adductor longus (Fig. 5.7; *Atlas*, 5.52A and B).

Examine the **adductor brevis**. Realize that part of it is covered by the pectineus (*Atlas*, 5.21, 5.23B and C). In order to expose the adductor brevis more fully, carefully reflect the pectineus close to its origin. Clean the adductor brevis. Do *not* damage nerves and vessels anterior to the muscle. Identify the nerves as branches of the **obturator nerve** (*Atlas*, 5.24). If in doubt, gently pull on the obturator nerve within the pelvis, or pass your probe along the nerve through the obturator foramen (*Atlas*, 3.40, 3.41). Realize that the obturator nerve supplies motor fibers to the adductor muscles (*Atlas*, 5.8A).

Examine a transverse section of the thigh (Fig. 5.7; *Atlas*, 5.52A and B) and verify that some branches of the obturator nerve run anterior to the adductor brevis; others run posterior to the adductor brevis. Once more, examine the *anterior* nerve branches in your cadaver specimen (*Atlas*, 5.24). Next, verify that the *posterior* nerve branches pass between the **adductor brevis** and **adductor magnus.** Separate the two muscles with your fingers.

Now, study the **profunda femoris artery** and its distribution (*Atlas*, 5.6). To clarify the dissecting field, sacrifice the accompanying veins. Note that the profunda femoris artery arises from the femoral artery 2 to 5 cm below the inguinal ligament. Clean the artery and some of its branches. Identify one or two of the **perforating arteries,** which encircle the femur and supply the adjacent musculature.

Cut the adductor brevis close to its origin in order to display the whole length of the **adductor magnus** (*Atlas*, 5.23D). At this point, identify the **obturator externus** as it covers the external surface of the obturator membrane (*Atlas*, 5.42A). Also note the anterior and posterior divisions of the obturator nerve. The accompanying arteries are branches of the obturator artery. Now, examine the **adductor magnus.** Once again, define the **hiatus** in the adductor magnus tendon through which the femoral vessels pass to become the popliteal vessels (*Atlas*, 5.6, 5.22, 5.34A). Medial to the hiatus, trace the adductor tendon to its insertion into the **adductor tubercle** on the medial epicondyle (*Atlas*, 5.23D). Realize that the bulk of the adductor magnus is inserted by means of a broad aponeurosis into the **linea aspera**. Note that the adductors of the thigh (with exception of the slender gracilis muscle) span only one joint, the hip joint. The gracilis spans two joints by inserting into the medial surface of the tibia. Therefore, this muscle acts on the hip joint (adduction) and on the knee joint (flexion and medial rotation). Verify this fact.

Review the **obturator nerve.** Study its motor branches (*Atlas*, 5.8A) and its cutaneous branch (*Atlas*, 5.7A). Observe that the proximal portion of the obturator nerve is accompanied by branches of the obturator artery (*Atlas*, 5.6).

Gluteal Region

General Remarks

The gluteal (buttock) region was considered, in part, during the dissection of the perineum and pelvis (Chapter 3). The gluteus maximus was partially reflected so that: (a) the greater and lesser sciatic foramina could be defined; and (b) the nerve and blood supply to the perineal region could be traced.

If the prescribed dissections of your gross anatomy course conform with the particular sequence of chapters in this manual, the previously mentioned procedures have been already performed. If you have not as yet dissected the perineum and pelvis, the gluteal region will be intact. At any rate, the area has already been skinned, the deep fascia has been demonstrated, and the cutaneous nerves of the region have been studied.

Important Landmarks

Refer to the skeleton and an articulated pelvis with intact ligaments. Identify the following landmarks:

1. **Greater sciatic notch** (*Atlas*, 5.1B);
2. **Lesser sciatic notch;**
3. **Ischial spine** separating the greater and lesser sciatic notches;
4. **Ischial tuberosity;**
5. **Sacrotuberous ligament** (Fig. 5.9);
6. **Sacrospinous ligament;**

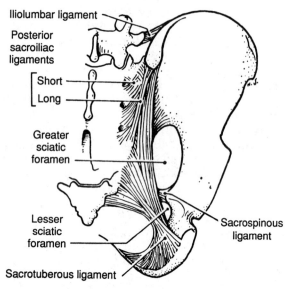

Iliolumbar ligament

Posterior sacroiliac ligaments

Short

Long

Greater sciatic foramen

Lesser sciatic foramen

Sacrotuberous ligament

Sacrospinous ligament

Figure 5.9. Ligaments of the pelvis.

7. Understand how these two ligaments (5 and 6) contribute to the formation of the **greater sciatic foramen** and the **lesser sciatic foramen;**
8. **Greater trochanter of femur;**
9. **Intertrochanteric crest** (*Atlas*, 5.1B);
10. **Trochanteric fossa,** a deep depression at the medial side of the greater trochanter.

Before you begin . . .

The large gluteus maximus will be studied. The muscle will be reflected to allow access to the deeper plane of the gluteal region. The greater and lesser sciatic foramina are key areas. It will be demonstrated that these foramina are traversed by important nerves, vessels, and muscles.

Dissection

Define the superior and inferior borders of the vast, rhomboidal **gluteus maximus,** the largest muscle in the body (*Atlas*, 5.31). Carefully clean and define the inferior border of the muscle. Do not cut too deep, or you may sever the posterior cutaneous nerve of the thigh (*Atlas*, 5.7B). Midway between ischial tuberosity and greater trochanter, make a 5-cm longitudinal incision through the deep fascia of the posterior aspect of the thigh, just inferior to the inferior border of the gluteus maximus. Find the **posterior cutaneous nerve of the thigh.** Make sure that it will not be severed during subsequent dissection. Now, remove the deep fascia from the entire gluteal region. Demonstrate the coarse muscle fibers of the gluteus maximus and their oblique direction.

A portion of the **gluteus medius** can be seen superior to the gluteus maximus (*Atlas*, 5.31). Identify it. Push your fingers into the space between gluteus medius and maximus (if the pelvis and perineum have been dissected previously, you will find the gluteus maximus reflected from

its origin). In the heretofore undissected gluteal region, proceed as follows:

1. Refer to a bony pelvis and familiarize yourself with the sites of origin of the gluteus maximus from the iliac crest and the external surface of the ilium, the dorsal surfaces of the sacrum and coccyx, and from the sacrotuberous ligament (*Atlas*, 5.28B, 5.35A, 5.39).
2. Detach the superior and medial portions of the muscle by cutting through its fibers very close to the posterior surfaces of the ilium, sacrum, and coccyx.
3. Place your fingers under the inferior portion of the muscle. Realize that it is attached to the sacrotuberous ligament. Using a pair of scissors or a scalpel, carefully detach the muscle from this ligament.
4. Gently reflect the muscle laterally. Observe the inferior gluteal nerve and vessels entering the muscle near its center. Cut the nerve and vessels close to the muscle, but leave a small button of the muscle attached to the nerve (to serve as an identifying indicator). Now, completely reflect the muscle laterally (*Atlas*, 5.33).

Observe the insertions of the gluteus maximus: the lower deeper quarter of the muscle is attached to the **gluteal tuberosity of the femur** (*Atlas*, 5.35A, 5.48B); the remaining three-quarters of the muscle are inserted into the **iliotibial tract** (*Atlas*, 5.34A).

The gluteus maximus slides over the **greater trochanter of the femur.** To protect the muscle from pressure and wear, it is separated from the greater trochanter by a bursa. Open this **trochanteric bursa,** which is the largest in the body (*Atlas*, 5.36). Observe another smaller bursa between the gluteus maximus and the ischial tuberosity.

Now, the deeper structures of the gluteal region are suitably exposed for examination. Identify the **sciatic nerve,** the largest nerve in the body. Verify that the nerve is located midway between the ischial tuberosity and the greater trochanter (*Atlas*, 5.33, 5.39). Follow the nerve proximally to the point where it appears in the gluteal region inferior to the **piriformis muscle** (*Atlas*, 5.36). Be aware of the fact that a different relationship between piriformis and sciatic nerve may exist (*Atlas*, 5.32). In the majority of cases, both the tibial and fibular (peroneal) divisions of the nerve pass together inferior to the piriformis. However, these nerve divisions may emerge separately at different levels of the piriformis muscle.

The **piriformis** occupies a key position in the gluteal region. Verify that this muscle passes through the greater sciatic foramen and divides it (Fig. 5.10; *Atlas*, 5.39). A number of vessels and nerves from the pelvis traverse the greater sciatic foramen to reach the gluteal region. Some of these structures enter the gluteal region above the piriformis; others enter below the piriformis (Fig. 5.11).

At the *superior border* of the piriformis (Fig. 5.11; *Atlas*, 5.37), identify the stems of the **superior gluteal nerve and vessels.** These structures are more or less covered by the **gluteus medius** (*Atlas*, 5.36).

At the *inferior* border of the piriformis (Fig. 5.11; *Atlas*, 5.36, 5.37), identify the following structures:

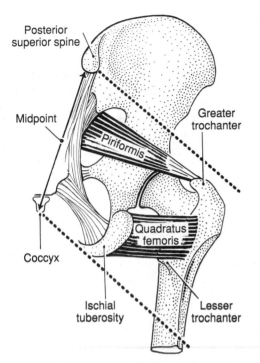

Figure 5.10. The reference line in the gluteal region is the readily defined inferior border of the piriformis muscle. The position of the gluteus maximus is indicated by *dotted lines*.

1. **Inferior gluteal nerve and vessels** (which were cut during the reflection of the gluteus maximus).
2. **Sciatic nerve**, the largest nerve in the body. Verify that the inferior gluteal artery supplies a small branch to the sciatic nerve. Be aware that this important nerve has a rich blood supply via a continuous anastomotic chain of arteries (*Atlas*, 5.38).
3. **Posterior cutaneous nerve of thigh**, running parallel to the sciatic nerve.
4. **Pudendal nerve** and **internal pudendal vessels.**

The **pudendal nerve and internal pudendal vessels** originate in the pelvis and appear only briefly in the gluteal region, entering through the **greater sciatic foramen.** They exit through the **lesser sciatic foramen** (Figs. 5.11, 5.12) to reach structures in the anal and urogenital regions. Push a probe along these structures through the lesser sciatic foramen into the **pudendal canal.**

Identify the **obturator internus**, which traverses the lesser sciatic foramen (*Atlas*, 5.37, 5.41). Clean the broad tendon of the obturator internus as inserts into the medial surface of the greater trochanter of the femur. Notice that the tendon lies between the fleshy **gemelli.** The *superior gemellus* arises from the ischial spine; the *inferior gemellus* from the ischial tuberosity. Inferior to the inferior gemellus, identify the **quadratus femoris** that stretches from ischial tuberosity to intertrochanteric crest of femur (Fig. 5.10; *Atlas*, 5.39). Search with a probe near the greater trochanter and in the interval between the quadratus femoris and the inferior gemellus; there, locate

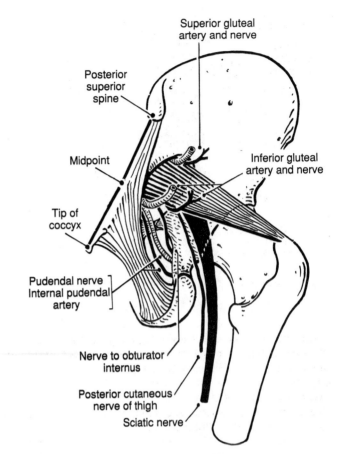

Figure 5.11. Structures passing through the greater sciatic foramen superior and inferior to the piriformis.

the **obturator externus tendon,** where it is inserted into the trochanteric fossa of the femur (*Atlas*, 5.41).

Identify the dense deep fascia covering the fan-shaped **gluteus medius.** Some of its fibers arise from this fascia (*Atlas*, 5.35C). Verify this fact by vertically incising the deep fascia overlying the gluteus medius. In addition, a portion of the muscle arises from the external surface of the ilium (*Atlas*, 5.28B, 5.35B). Observe the gluteus medius tendon at its area of insertion into the lateral surface of the greater trochanter of the femur (Fig. 5.13). Understand that contraction of this muscle will lead to abduction of the thigh (abduction of hip joint). In walking and standing, the gluteus medius is the primary stabilizer of the hip joint.

Once again, identify the **superior gluteal nerve and vessels** superior to the piriformis. Follow these vessels by sweeping your fingers deep to the gluteus medius. Your fingers are now in the plane between gluteus medius and minimus (*Atlas*, 5.35C). Sever the **gluteus medius** about 3 cm superior to its insertion into the **greater trochanter** of the femur (*Atlas*, 5.37). Gently reflect the proximal portion of the muscle superiorly and observe motor branches of the superior gluteal nerve entering the muscle. Reflect the gluteus medius completely and identify the underlying **gluteus minimus.** Occasionally, the medius and minimus are not well differentiated. The reason for this occasional fusion of the two muscles is the fact that they share a very

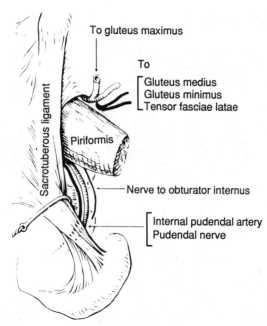

Figure 5.12. The pudendal nerve and internal pudendal artery entering the gluteal region via the greater sciatic foramen and leaving it via the lesser sciatic foramen.

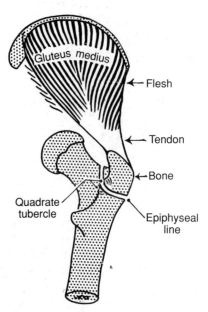

Figure 5.13. Fleshy and tendinous portions of the gluteus medius; insertion into the greater trochanter of femur.

similar fiber course and function. Observe the insertion of the gluteus minimus into the greater trochanter of the femur (*Atlas*, 5.35**D**). Note branches of the superior gluteal nerve entering the muscle. Now, clean the entire **superior gluteal nerve** and follow a branch laterally to the **tensor fasciae latae** (*Atlas*, 5.34A, 5.37).

Refer to a skeleton and the dissected specimen at the same time. **Study the functions of muscles in the gluteal region** (*Atlas*, 5.35). *Extend* the femur of the skeleton; this movement is accomplished by the gluteus maximus. *Abduct the femur;* this movement depends on the functional integrity of the three abductors of the hip joint: gluteus medius, gluteus minimus, and tensor fasciae latae.

> **Intragluteal Injections.** The gluteal region is commonly used for intramuscular injections of drugs. These injections should always be made superolaterally in the *superior lateral quadrant.* Why? Divide the gluteal region into four quadrants. Realize that injections into the two inferior quadrants will endanger and possibly paralyze the important sciatic nerve, or nerves and vessels entering the gluteal region inferior to the piriformis muscle (*Atlas*, 5.36). Injections into the superior medial quadrant may injure the stems of the superior gluteal nerve and vessels (*Atlas*, 5.37) or an abnormally high peroneal division of the sciatic nerve (*Atlas*, 5.32C). Intragluteal injections into the *superior lateral quadrant* are relatively safe since the superior gluteal nerve and vessels are well ramified in this region. Be sure the injection needle never deviates inferiorly or medially toward the greater sciatic foramen with its important structures.

Study the continuity of nerves, vessels, and muscles observed in the gluteal region. Within the pelvis (*Atlas*, 3.34), review the gluteal vessels, the piriformis muscle, and es-

sential components of the sacral plexus. Identify the fleshy part of the obturator internus covering the obturator foramen and membrane.

Back of Thigh and Popliteal Fossa

Before you begin . . .

The hamstring muscles and the sciatic nerve will be demonstrated. Subsequently, the dissection will be extended into the diamond-shaped popliteal fossa. The muscular boundaries of the fossa will be established, and the important contents of the popliteal fossa (nerves, vessels) will be identified. The proximal and distal continuity of these structures will be explored.

Back of Thigh

Review the field of sensory innervation of the **posterior cutaneous nerve of the thigh** (*Atlas*, 5.7B). Remove the deep fascia covering the posterior aspect of the thigh. Identify the posterior cutaneous nerve of the thigh; then reflect it superiorly. Clean the **sciatic nerve** and its branches to the hamstring muscles (*Atlas*, 5.36).

Define the hamstring muscles and separate them from one another (*Atlas*, 5.31, 5.33). These muscles are the **semitendinosus, semimembranosus,** and the **long head of the biceps femoris.** Verify that these muscles have a **common site of origin: the ischial tuberosity.** On the medial side of the thigh, identify the **semitendinosus** (meaning "half tendon") with its round and remarkably long tendon of insertion. Separate the semitendinosus from the **semimembranosus**

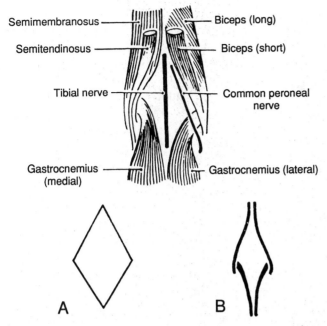

Semimembranosus — Biceps (long)

Semitendinosus — Biceps (short)

Tibial nerve — Common peroneal nerve

Gastrocnemius (medial) — Gastrocnemius (lateral)

A B

Figure 5.14. Boundaries of the diamond-shaped popliteal fossa.

(meaning "half membrane") with its substantial membranous tendon of origin.

At this point, verify that the most medial portion of the adductor magnus also arises from the ischial tuberosity. Identify its thick, fleshy mass descending almost vertically (*Atlas*, 5.34A). Note that its rounded tendon is inserted into the adductor tubercle of the medial condyle of the femur. This **hamstring part of the adductor magnus** is innervated by the sciatic nerve, which also supplies the other hamstring muscles (*Atlas*, 5.8D). In contrast, the larger remaining part of the adductor magnus is innervated by the obturator nerve.

On the lateral side of the thigh, identify the **long head of the biceps femoris.** Verify that the **short head** of this muscle arises from the shaft of the femur (*Atlas*, 5.28B, 5.34A). In contrast, the true hamstring muscles arise from the ischial tuberosity. For this reason and the fact that it also has a different nerve supply, the short head of the biceps femoris does not belong to the hamstring muscles.

Understand that the hamstring muscles span two joints, the hip joint and the knee joint. Verify that the biceps femoris tendon is inserted into the head of the fibula (*Atlas*, 5.63, 5.64). The semimembranosus has its insertion into the medial condyle of the tibia. The semitendinosus is inserted into the medial aspect of the tibia (*Atlas*, 5.65, 5.66). Understand that the principal actions of the hamstrings are flexion of the leg and extension of the thigh, especially during walking.

Look for arteries supplying the hamstring muscles (*Atlas*, 5.36). Most of the blood is derived from the **perforating branches** of the profunda femoris artery, the chief artery of the thigh (*Atlas*, 5.6).

Display the **sciatic nerve,** the largest nerve in the body. Observe branches of the sciatic nerve as they enter the hamstring muscles (*Atlas*, 5.8D, 5.36, 5.37).

Popliteal Fossa

Define the superior angle of the popliteal fossa (Fig. 5.14): on the lateral side is the **biceps femoris.** On the medial side, identify the round **semitendinosus** and the fleshy **semimembranosus.** Define the lower angle of the popliteal fossa: here, the two bellies of the **gastrocnemius** are closely applied to each other.

Place a block under the dorsum of the foot to relax the **gastrocnemius.** Incise the deep fascia at the medial and lateral borders of this muscle. At the lower angle of the popliteal fossa, insert your two index fingers between the contiguous bellies of the gastrocnemius, raise them, and pull them apart for a distance of about 5 to 10 cm. Now, underlying parts of the **soleus, popliteus,** and **plantaris** muscles can be seen (*Atlas*, 5.54).

Follow the **sciatic nerve** in the thigh distally toward the popliteal fossa. Note that it divides into two major branches, the **common peroneal nerve** and the **tibial nerve** (Fig. 5.14; *Atlas*, 5.54, 5.55). Identify these two nerves within the popliteal fossa. Trace the **tibial nerve** to the lower limit of the fossa. Notice that it passes through a gap in the origin of the soleus muscle (*Atlas*, 5.54). Display the nerve.

Observe the dense **vascular sheath** that envelops the **popliteal artery and popliteal vein** (*Atlas*, 5.55). Push a probe through the adductor hiatus, and establish the continuity of the femoral with the popliteal vessels (*Atlas*, 5.6, 5.40, 5.55). Within the popliteal fossa, open the vascular sheath by incising it vertically. Extend the incision superiorly and inferiorly. Separate the popliteal artery from the popliteal vein. Cut away tributaries of the vein. This will clarify the dissection field. Retract the plantaris muscle laterally in order to expose fully the **popliteal artery** and some of its branches.

Spend a few minutes studying and understanding the elaborate arterial anastomoses around the knee joint (*Atlas*, 5.40, 5.57). Understand that these collateral vessels ensure adequate blood supply of the knee in case of injury. At this time, only the **superior lateral genicular artery** and the **superior medial genicular artery** can be seen (*Atlas*, 5.55). The inferior genicular arteries are still covered by the bellies of the gastrocnemius.

Verify that three slender muscles converge to an apex on the medial side of the proximal end of the tibia (*Atlas*, 5.25, 5.26), essentially forming an inverted "tripod." These muscles are the **sartorius, gracilis, and semitendinosus.** Each muscle belongs to a different muscle group; thus each has a different nerve supply and a different site of origin on the hip bone. All three muscles span (i.e., act on) two joints, the hip joint and the knee joint.

Now, **review the principal muscle groups** of the thigh and their respective **nerve territories** (Fig. 5.15; *Atlas*, 5.52B). The posteriorly located **hamstring muscles** are supplied by the **sciatic nerve.** The medially positioned **adductors** belong to the **obturator nerve** territory. The **femoral nerve** supplies the **sartorius and the quadriceps group** anteriorly and laterally to the femur. Correlate your anatomical observations with a transverse MRI of the thigh (*Atlas*, 5.52C).

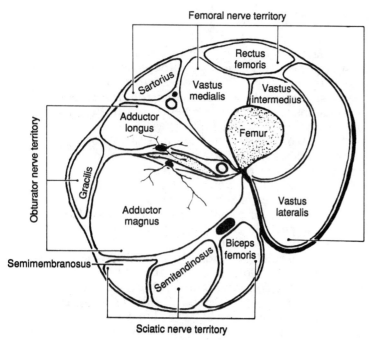

Figure 5.15. The three principal muscle groups of the thigh and their respective motor nerve territories.

Leg (or Crus)

General Remarks

The morphological organization and function of the leg will be best understood if a transverse section is studied and analyzed (Fig. 5.16; *Atlas*, 5.97A). Before attempting dissection, understand the following facts:

1. The two bones of the leg are unequal in size. The larger **tibia** lies medial; its medial surface is subcutaneous. The smaller **fibula** is deeply placed. Tibia and fibula are connected by an **interosseous membrane.**
2. The investing deep fascia reaches the fibula by means of septa, the **anterior and posterior crural septa.**
3. The two bones, their interosseous membrane, and the crural septa serve to divide the leg into **three compartments: anterior, lateral or peroneal, and posterior.** Each compartment contains a synergistic muscle group. A nerve supplying these muscles runs in each compartment.
4. The muscles in the **anterior crural compartment** are mainly concerned with **dorsiflexion of the foot** (turning of the foot upward) and with extension of the toes. The nerve within this compartment is the **deep peroneal nerve** (Fig. 5.16). It is a branch of the common peroneal nerve that passes around the lateral side of the neck of the fibula (*Atlas*, 5.79, 5.80). The deep peroneal nerve is accompanied by the **anterior tibial artery** that enters the anterior compartment through a gap above

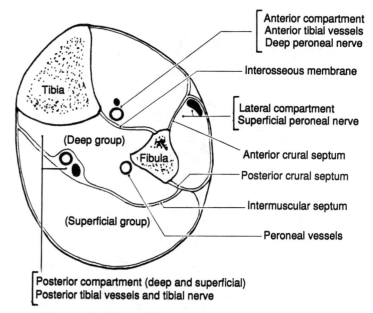

Figure 5.16. Schematic transverse section through the leg. Two bones, septa, and three crural compartments with contents.

the proximal border of the interosseous membrane (*Atlas*, 5.6, 5.80).

5. The **lateral crural compartment or peroneal compartment** contains two muscles for **plantar flexion and eversion of the foot.** The nerve within this compartment is the **superficial peroneal nerve** (Fig. 5.16). It is a branch of the common peroneal nerve (*Atlas*, 5.79) that, in turn, is the smaller of the two terminal branches of the sciatic nerve.
6. The **posterior crural compartment** contains several muscles whose principal function is **plantar flexion of the foot** and toes (turning foot downward). The muscles are divided into a **superficial group** and a **deep group** by an intermuscular septum. Note that the nerve of the posterior compartment runs between the superficial and deep groups (Fig. 5.16). This nerve is the **tibial nerve,** the larger of the two terminal branches of the sciatic nerve. Study its ramifications (*Atlas*, 5.8D). The nerve is accompanied by the **posterior tibial artery,** a branch of the popliteal artery (*Atlas*, 5.6, posterior view).

Important Landmarks

Refer to an articulated lower limb of a skeleton. Identify the following landmarks (Fig. 5.17; *Atlas*, 5.1):

1. **Medial condyle** and **lateral condyle of tibia;**
2. **Anterior border of tibia,** descending from the tibial tuberosity; note that its proximal portion is sharp and prominent;
3. **Head of fibula;**
4. **Medial malleolus,** the large medial prominence at the ankle;

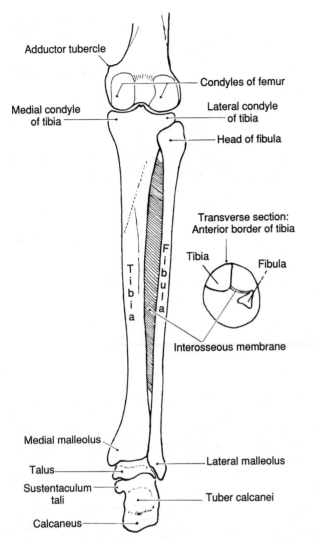

Figure 5.17. Posterior view of right lower limb: bones and important landmarks.

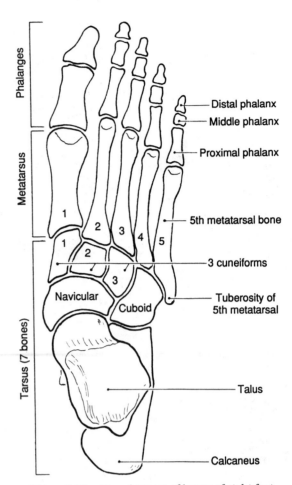

Figure 5.18. Dorsal aspect of bones of right foot.

5. **Lateral malleolus,** the lateral prominence at the ankle;
6. In the articulated foot (Fig. 5.18; *Atlas,* 5.83), identify the **tarsus,** which consists of seven tarsal bones: **talus** (L., ankle bone); **calcaneus** (L. *calx,* heel); **navicular** (L., little ship); **cuboid** (Gr., cube-shaped); and the **three cuneiforms** (L., wedge-shaped); 1st, 2nd, and 3rd. On the **calcaneus,** identify the **tuber calcanei** (tuberosity) for attachment of the tendo calcaneus or Achilles tendon (*Atlas,* 5.88), and a groove below the **sustentaculum tali** for the passage of the flexor hallucis longus tendon (*Atlas,* 5.101, 5.120**B**). Identify the **five metatarsals** and the tuberosity of the 5th metatarsal (Fig. 5.18). Note that the 1st toe has two **phalanges,** whereas the other toes have three.

Before you begin . . .

After reflecting the skin, the crural compartments (anterior; lateral; posterior) will be dissected. The derivation and course of blood vessels and nerves will be explored,

and their continuation onto the dorsum or into the sole of the foot will be demonstrated. The muscles of the crural compartments will be followed to their insertions in the foot.

Anterior Crural Compartment and Dorsum of Foot

The superficial nerves and veins have already been dissected. Review the **deep fascia.** Demonstrate that muscle fibers of the **tibialis anterior** arise from this deep fascia: make a vertical cut through the fascia just below the lateral tibial condyle, lift the edges of the deep fascia, and see the muscle fibers arising from the fascia (Fig. 5.19). Since the muscle takes origin from the fascia, this fascia must be strong and thick. Verify that the fascia is attached to the sharp anterior border of the tibia.

The superior and inferior **extensor retinacula** are transversely directed thickenings of the deep fascia that hold tendons in place (Fig. 5.20; *Atlas,* 5.82**B**, 5.86, 5.88). The **superior extensor retinaculum** extends across the tendons superior to the ankle joint. The **inferior extensor retinaculum** is Y shaped. The stem of the Y is fixed to the calcaneus in front of the lateral malleolus. Laterally, the stem of the inferior extensor retinaculum is in broken con-

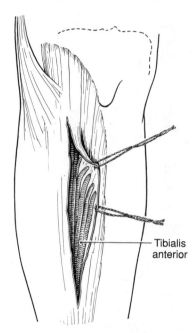

Figure 5.19. Deep fascia (incised) giving, in part, origin to the tibialis anterior muscle. Therefore, the fascia is aponeurotic, thick, and creates lines on the tibia.

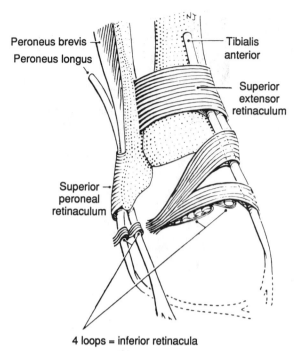

4 loops = inferior retinacula

Figure 5.20. Retinacula.

tinuity with the **inferior peroneal retinaculum.** Define these retinacula and understand their function. What would happen if tendons were not held in place by these retinacula? Subsequently, cut vertically through the deep fascia overlying the anterior crural compartment.

The structures of the anterior crural compartment cross the ankle anteriorly (*Atlas,* 5.82**B**). From the medial to the lateral side they are: **Tibialis anterior, extensor hallucis longus, deep peroneal nerve** together with **anterior tibial vessels, and extensor digitorum longus.** The lateral lower fleshy part of the extensor digitorum longus is the **peroneus tertius** (*Atlas,* 5.82**B**, 5.86). Separate the muscles from each other and trace them to their origins. Correlate your observations with a transverse section through the anterior crural compartment and a corresponding MRI (*Atlas,* 5.97**A** and **B**). Subsequently, trace the tendons of the three muscles of the anterior crural compartment inferiorly to their insertions in the foot (*Atlas,* 5.82**B**). Pull on the tibialis anterior tendon and confirm that the action of this muscle is dorsiflexion and inversion of the foot. Pull on the tendons of the extensor hallucis longus and the extensor digitorum longus. Observe that these muscles basically extend the digits and assist in dorsiflexion of the foot.

Study the **anterior tibial artery** and the **deep peroneal nerve** (*Atlas,* 5.78). Observe that artery and nerve occupy the median plane and have two tendons on each side of them. Trace the artery proximally to the point where it passes over the superior border of the interosseous membrane. Review the **anterior tibial artery** and its ramifications (*Atlas,* 5.6). Understand the course and connections of the **perforating branch** of the peroneal artery that passes distal to the interosseous membrane. Occasionally, this perforating branch is large and may replace the dorsalis pedis artery. Usually, the **dorsalis pedis artery** (L.

pes, pedis, foot) is the continuation of the anterior tibial artery onto the dorsum of the foot. Note the **arcuate artery** across the base of the metatarsal bones. The **dorsal digital arteries** originate from it (*Atlas,* 5.6, anterior view). A deep plantar branch connects to the plantar arch in the sole of the foot (*Atlas,* 5.6, posterior view). In the cadaver specimen, demonstrate the various branches of the anterior tibial artery (*Atlas,* 5.80). Note that the dorsalis pedis artery and its branches lie on the skeletal plane; there they remain intact even if all muscles are torn away (*Atlas,* 5.84). Identify the **medial malleolar artery** to the medial ankle and the **lateral malleolar artery** to the lateral ankle. Note **tarsal branches** to the tarsus. Usually, the lateral tarsal artery connects with the arcuate artery.

Examine the **deep peroneal nerve,** the nerve of the anterior crural compartment. Verify that this nerve is a branch of the common peroneal nerve: Identify and pull on the common peroneal nerve posterior to the head of the fibula (Fig. 5.21). Follow the nerve into the anterior crural compartment (*Atlas,* 5.80). Note the muscular branches (*Atlas,* 5.78). Follow the deep peroneal nerve onto the dorsum of the foot (*Atlas,* 5.80). Note the nerve branches to the two short extensors of the toes, **extensor digitorum brevis** and **extensor hallucis brevis.** Examine these muscles. They take origin from the calcaneus and are inserted into the extensor expansions of the toes (*Atlas,* 5.82**B**).

Lateral Crural Compartment and Lateral Side of Ankle

Open the **deep fascia** overlying the **lateral (peroneal) compartment.** This compartment contains two muscles, the **peroneus longus and peroneus brevis** (*Atlas,* 5.97**A**).

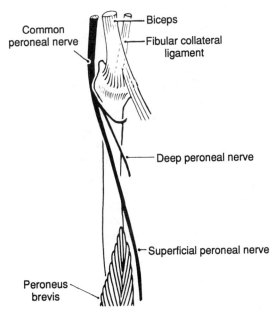

Figure 5.21. Common peroneal nerve and its branches in contact with fibula.

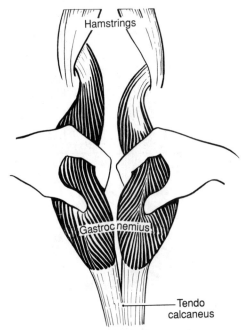

Figure 5.22. Pull the two bellies of the gastrocnemius forcibly apart to expose the underlying soleus.

Distinguish these two muscles from each other. The peroneus brevis is inserted into the tuberosity of the 5th metatarsal bone (*Atlas*, 5.76, 5.77). The peroneus longus hooks around the cuboid and travels medially in the sole of the foot. The sole of the foot will be dissected later.

Examine how the tendons of the two muscles are held in place (*Atlas*, 5.88): The **superior peroneal retinaculum** retains the tendons posterior to the **lateral malleolus;** the **inferior peroneal retinaculum** holds them to the calcaneus. Follow the **peroneus longus tendon** to the point where it disappears into the sole of the foot. Realize (without dissection at this time) that this tendon is indeed long: it reaches as far as the undersurface of the 1st metatarsal bone (*Atlas*, 5.128). Follow the tendon of the peroneus brevis muscle to the tuberosity of the 5th metatarsal (*Atlas*, 5.88). Pull on the peroneal muscles. Understand and verify that they evert the foot.

Identify the nerve of the lateral crural compartment, the **superficial peroneal nerve.** It lies along the anterior border of the peroneus brevis (*Atlas*, 5.77, 5.80). Follow the nerve distally. Its cutaneous branches to the dorsum of the foot have been examined earlier (*Atlas*, 5.7A). Trace the nerve proximally and verify that it is a branch of the **common peroneal nerve** (Fig. 5.21; *Atlas*, 5.80). Push a probe parallel to the nerve as it passes between the fibula and peroneus longus. You may carefully divide this muscle over the probe to establish continuity of the common, superficial, and deep peroneal nerves.

> Of all nerves in the body, the **common peroneal nerve** is the most frequently injured. Once again, observe the superficial position of the nerve in relation to the head and neck of the fibula (Fig. 5.21; *Atlas*, 5.80). The nerve may be readily damaged by superficial wounds, prolonged pressure by hard objects during sleep, anesthesia, and chronic illness, or by compression against the opposite patella while sitting with the knees crossed.

> What are the neurological findings of common peroneal nerve lesions? The nerves of the lateral and anterior crural compartments are affected. Consequently, eversion, extension (dorsiflexion) of the foot, and extension of the toes will be impaired. There is a "foot drop" resulting in a characteristic steppage gait. There may be some sensory loss on the dorsum of the foot and toes (compare *Atlas*, 5.7A).
>
> Sudden overuse of the anterior tibial muscles may lead to swelling and edema in the anterior crural compartment. This painful condition is known as "shin splints" in lay terminology.

Posterior Crural Compartment and Medial Side of Ankle

Review the contents of the **posterior crural compartment** on transverse section (Fig. 5.16; *Atlas*, 5.97A). Turn the cadaver into the prone position (face down). Review the **deep fascia.** Cut it vertically from popliteal fossa to calcaneus, and reflect it laterally.

Identify the **gastrocnemius** (*Atlas*, 5.93). Pull the **two bellies (heads) of the gastrocnemius** apart (Fig. 5.22). Follow them to the **tendo calcaneus** (Achilles tendon), the common tendon for the gastrocnemius and underlying **soleus.** Cut across the two bellies of the gastrocnemius well inferior to the entrance of their nerves (*Atlas*, 5.94). Reflect the proximal and distal portions of the bellies, and expose the underlying soleus. Verify that the two heads of the gastrocnemius originate from the medial and lateral condyles of the femur (*Atlas*, 5.91). Now you can easily identify the **popliteus.** It is a flat, triangular muscle positioned deep in the popliteal fossa and covered by the heads of the gastrocnemius (*Atlas*, 5.55, 5.57A).

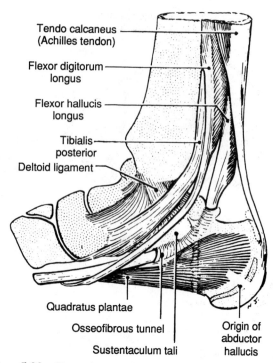

Tendo calcaneus
(Achilles tendon)

Flexor digitorum
longus

Flexor hallucis
longus

Tibialis
posterior

Deltoid ligament

Quadratus plantae

Osseofibrous tunnel

Sustentaculum tali

Origin of
abductor
hallucis

Figure 5.23. Deep structures on the medial side of the ankle.

Look for the long and thin tendon of the **plantaris**. This tendon is located on the medial border of the tendo calcaneus. The small plantaris muscle runs obliquely between gastrocnemius and soleus. Occasionally, it is absent.

An **intermuscular septum** separates the superficial from the deep muscles of the posterior compartment (Fig. 5.16; *Atlas*, 5.97A). The **tibial nerve** and **posterior tibial vessels** are closely related to the intermuscular septum. To obtain access to the plane of this septum, the soleus must be reflected. Proceed as follows:

Cut the **tendo calcaneus** (Achilles tendon) about 5 cm superior to its insertion into the tuber calcanei (*Atlas*, 5.95). Reflect the tendon superiorly together with the fleshy parts of gastrocnemius and soleus. Pass two fingers superiorly between soleus and the loose intermuscular septum. Palpate the horseshoe-shaped origin of the soleus from tibia and fibula (*Atlas*, 5.91, 5.95). Carefully detach the soleus from its tibial origin, but leave it attached to the fibula. Turn the muscle laterally. Now, the **intermuscular septum** is in full view. Slit the loose layer vertically to expose the **posterior tibial vessels** and the **tibial nerve** (*Atlas*, 5.95).

Three muscles comprise the **deep group** of the posterior crural compartment. To aid in identification, it is useful to correlate a transverse section (*Atlas*, 5.97A) with a figure showing the origin of the muscles (Atlas, 5.91). Note:

1. The **flexor digitorum longus** lies medial. It is closely attached to the tibia.
2. The **flexor hallucis longus** lies lateral. It is closely attached to the fibula.

3. The **tibialis posterior** lies in the middle. It takes origin from the tibia, fibula, and the interosseous membrane.

Identify these three muscles (*Atlas*, 5.95, 5.96). Their insertions will be demonstrated later during dissection of the sole of the foot (*Atlas*, 5.107). Without dissection at this time, understand the following facts: the **flexor digitorum longus** lies medial in the posterior compartment; it is inserted into the four lateral toes. The **flexor hallucis longus** lies lateral in the posterior compartment; it is inserted into the most medial (1st) toe. Therefore, by necessity, the two tendons must cross each other (*Atlas*, 5.107).

Identify the **flexor hallucis longus** in the posterior compartment of the leg. Follow its tendon distally until it disappears in an **osseofibrous tunnel** (Fig. 5.23; *Atlas*, 5.101, 5.102). Push a probe into the tunnel, then open it. Note that the tendon is surrounded by a synovial sheath. Temporarily lift out the tendon of the flexor hallucis longus. Verify that it runs in a **groove** below the **sustentaculum tali**, using the sustentaculum as a pulley. The **flexor digitorum longus tendon** passes along the medial border of the sustentaculum. Observe that the tendons of flexor digitorum longus and flexor hallucis longus cross each other (Fig. 5.23; *Atlas*, 5.101).

Pulling on tendons and observing the resulting action is often informative. However, this maneuver may be difficult in cadavers with very stiff tissues. Pull on the flexor digitorum longus tendon. Understand that this muscle flexes the terminal phalanges of the four small toes (toes 2, 3, 4, 5) and also assists in plantar flexion and inversion of the foot. Pull on the tendon of the flexor hallucis longus. Observe flexion of the great toe (toe 1). The flexor hallucis longus also assists in plantar flexion and inversion of the foot. Verify that the **tibialis posterior** tendon passes superior to the sustentaculum tali. Pull on the tendon. Understand that the muscle inverts the foot and assists in plantar flexion.

Explore the vascular distribution in the back of the leg (Fig. 5.24; *Atlas*, 5.6, posterior view). Clean the **posterior tibial artery** and the accompanying **tibial nerve** (*Atlas*, 5.95, 5.96). Note that the artery is accompanied by two or more veins. The largest branch of the posterior tibial artery is the **peroneal artery**. Identify the peroneal vessels in the interval between tibialis posterior and flexor hallucis longus (*Atlas*, 5.95, 5.97A). Note again that at least two veins accompany the artery. Positively identify the peroneal artery. Distally, search for its *communicating branch* and its *perforating branch* (Fig. 5.24). Note the motor branches of the tibial nerve to the muscles of the posterior compartment (*Atlas*, 5.96).

Now, review the **muscle groups** of the three crural compartments and their respective **nerve territories** (Fig. 5.25): the **muscles** in the **anterior compartment** (tibialis anterior, extensor hallucis longus, extensor digitorum longus, and peroneus tertius) are supplied by the **deep peroneal nerve**. The two muscles in the **lateral compartment** (peroneus brevis, peroneus longus) belong to the territory of the **superficial peroneal nerve**. All muscles of the **posterior compartment** (superficial: gastrocnemius, soleus, plantaris; deep: tibialis posterior, flexor digitorum

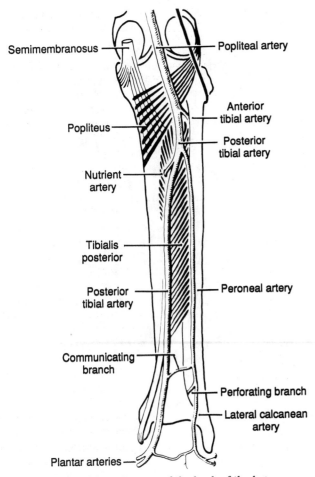

Figure 5.24. Arteries of the back of the leg.

Labels for Figure 5.24:
Semimembranosus — Popliteal artery
Popliteus — Anterior tibial artery
Nutrient artery — Posterior tibial artery
Tibialis posterior
Posterior tibial artery — Peroneal artery
Communicating branch
Perforating branch
Lateral calcanean artery
Plantar arteries

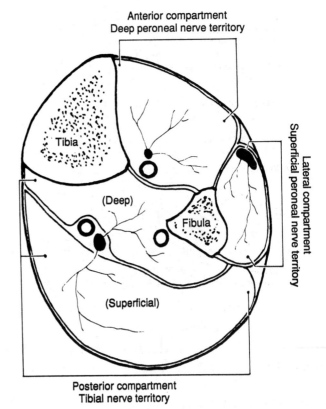

Figure 5.25. Three crural compartments and their respective motor nerve territories.

Labels for Figure 5.25:
Anterior compartment
Deep peroneal nerve territory
Tibia
(Deep)
Fibula
Lateral compartment
Superficial peroneal nerve territory
(Superficial)
Posterior compartment
Tibial nerve territory

longus, flexor hallucis longus, popliteus) are supplied by branches of the **tibial nerve.**

Review the compartmental organization of the leg by studying a transverse section (*Atlas*, 5.97A). Correlate your anatomical observations with an appropriate MRI of the leg (*Atlas*, 5.97B).

Sole of Foot (Planta)

General Remarks

Understand the following important facts:

1. The **foot is arched longitudinally** (Fig. 5.26). Viewed from the medial side, the arch appears high. Viewed from the lateral side, the longitudinal arch is low. Can these facts be recognized in a footprint?
2. The **bearing points** of the foot are the calcaneus posteriorly, and the heads of the five metatarsal bones anteriorly (Figs. 5.26, 5.27; *Atlas*, 5.115). These bearing points are the ends of the longitudinal arches.
3. The **plantar aponeurosis** (fascia) acts as a strong tie for the maintenance of the longitudinal arches.

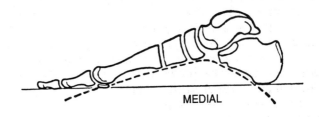

MEDIAL

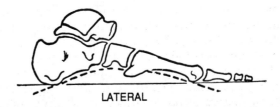

LATERAL

Figure 5.26. Medial and lateral longitudinal arches of the foot.

Therefore, it is logical that the plantar aponeurosis stretches from the calcaneus posteriorly to the five digits anteriorly (*Atlas*, 5.103). The plantar aponeurosis must be of considerable **strength** to perform its function. The aponeurosis is covered with thick skin. The toughness of the tissues in the sole of the foot often makes dissection difficult. Be aware of this fact in alloting your time.

4. Deep to the plantar aponeurosis are **four layers of muscles.** These will be described later.

5: T h e L o w e r L i m b

105

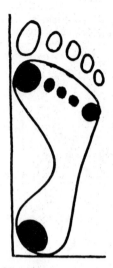

Figure 5.27. Bearing points of the foot.

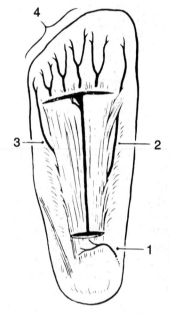

Figure 5.28. Incisions in plantar aponeurosis.

5. The posterior tibial vessels are continuous with the **plantar vessels** in the sole of the foot (*Atlas*, 5.6, 5.104).
6. The tibial nerve sends two branches into the sole: The **medial plantar nerve** and the **lateral plantar nerve** (*Atlas*, 5.100, 5.112A).

Dissection

When dissecting the **plantar aponeurosis,** certain cutaneous nerves and vessels are easily cut. Therefore, attempt to secure these structures in the beginning (Fig. 5.28, *Atlas*, 5.103). In a longitudinal direction, cut through the thick fatty fascia and a film of deep fascia (Fig. 5.28). Find the following nerves:

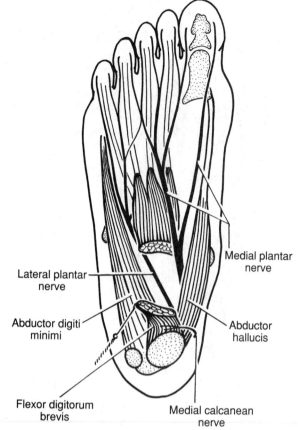

Figure 5.29. Sole of foot. First layer of muscles and plantar nerves.

1. **Medial calcanean nerve** (*1* in Fig. 5.28; *Atlas*, 5.7B, 5.103), which supplies the skin of the heel.
2. **Digital branches of the medial plantar nerve** (and artery); in part to the medial side of the great toe.
3. **Digital branches of the lateral plantar nerve** (and artery); in part to the lateral side of the little toe.
4. **Other digital nerves** (*4* in Fig. 5.28) may be traced now or later.

Plantar Aponeurosis (Fig. 5.28; *Atlas*, 5.103). Scrape the superficial fascia off the plantar aponeurosis. Note its proximal attachment to the calcaneus. Define the five diverging aponeurotic bands that pass to each toe. To expose the underlying muscles, split the plantar aponeurosis longitudinally throughout its length (Fig. 5.28). Then, carefully cut it transversely close to the calcaneus and in the anterior third of the foot. Reflect the flaps medially and laterally (*Atlas*, 5.105A). Separate the flaps from the **flexor digitorum brevis** that originates, in part, from the central portion of the plantar aponeurosis.

First Layer of Muscles (Fig. 5.29; *Atlas*, 5.105A). Medial to the plantar aponeurosis, expose the **abductor hallucis.** Note its origin from the calcaneus. Understand its function. Be careful not to destroy the plantar digital nerve and artery to the medial side of the big toe.

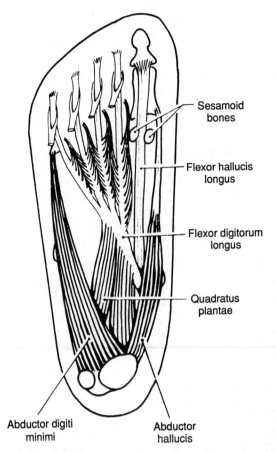

Figure 5.30. Sole of foot. Second layer of muscles displayed by removal of flexor digitorum brevis.

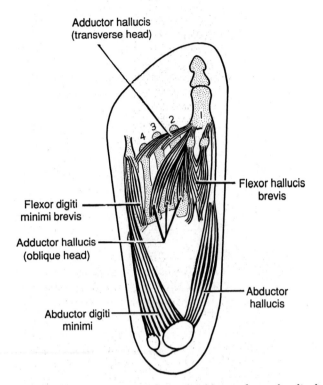

Figure 5.31. Sole of the foot. Third layer of muscles displayed by reflection of flexor digitorum longus, quadratus plantae, and lumbricals.

On the lateral side, expose and clean the **abductor digiti minimi.** Free the muscle and follow it to its origin and insertion. Understand its function.

In the middle between the two abductors, identify the **flexor digitorum brevis.** Trace its tendons forward to digits 2, 3, 4 (and sometimes 5). In doing so, remove piecemeal the remaining and interfering distal part of the plantar aponeurosis. Subsequently, cut the flexor digitorum brevis close to the calcaneus and reflect it anteriorly.

Establish the continuity of the posterior tibial artery and the tibial nerve with plantar structures. Follow nerve and artery into the sole by pushing a probe deep to the abductor hallucis (*Atlas*, 5.112A). Carefully cut the muscle overlying the probe, and demonstrate the distribution of the **plantar nerves and arteries** (Fig. 5.29; *Atlas*, 5.105A).

Second Layer of Muscles (Fig. 5.30; *Atlas*, 5.107, 5.108). Reflect the flexor digitorum brevis as described previously. To make reflection easier, you may sacrifice some of the digital nerves and vessels (check with your instructor!). Identify the **quadratus plantae** (flexor accessorius), a sheet of fleshy muscle in the posterior half of the foot. Note that the muscle arises from the calcaneus and is inserted into the tendon of the **flexor digitorum longus.** Now is the time to explore the distal portion of the flexor digitorum longus tendon in the sole of the foot. Note that it divides into four slips for toes 2, 3, 4, and 5. Four delicate **lumbricals** arise from the tendinous slips. Note that these slips perforate the tendons of the flexor digitorum brevis. A similar arrangement of perforating tendons can be observed in the hand.

Third Layer of Muscles (Fig. 5.31; *Atlas*, 5.112A). Cut through the flexor digitorum longus tendon where it is joined by the quadratus plantae. Reflect the distal part of the tendon anteriorly together with the lumbricals. Look for the small nerves supplying them. Now, the short muscles that occupy the anterior half of the foot are exposed. Identify the **flexor hallucis brevis.** This muscle covers the 1st metatarsal. It has two heads (medial and lateral) and two tendons. A **sesamoid bone** is attached to each of the tendons (*Atlas*, 5.113). Observe that the **tendon of the flexor hallucis longus** runs between the two sesamoid bones that form a guiding bony ridge for the tendon (*Atlas*, 5.108). Verify that the tendon of the flexor hallucis longus is inserted into the bases of the distal phalanx of the great toe (*Atlas*, 5.83, 5.113). Follow the tendons of the flexor hallucis longus and flexor digitorum longus proximally toward the medial ankle. Once more, verify that the tendons cross each other (*Atlas*, 5.107).

Identify the **adductor hallucis** for the big toe. It consists of a transverse head and an oblique head. This muscle helps to maintain the transverse arch of the foot. Observe the **flexor digiti minimi** to the 5th digit.

Fourth Layer of Muscles (*Atlas*, 5.113). This layer consists of a compact muscular mass, the **interossei.** The four dorsal interossei are abductors, the three plantar interossei are adductors of the toes. The reference axis for abduction and adduction passes through the 2nd toe. The arrangement and action of the interossei is similar to that in the hand. Adduction and abduction of digits is more important in the hand than in the foot. Therefore, the interossei are more thoroughly discussed in the section for the hand. At this point, trace the peroneus longus tendon distally toward its insertion into the base of the 1st metatarsal and the medial cuneiform bone (*Atlas*, 5.113, 5.114). Similarly, follow the tibialis posterior tendon distally and verify its multiple insertions into the navicular, cuneiforms, cuboid, and the bases of the 2nd, 3rd, and 4th metatarsals (*Atlas*, 5.113, 5.114, 5.128).

Identify the **plantar arterial arch**. Understand the essentials of the blood supply to the foot (*Atlas*, 5.6, 5.104, 5.106). Identify one or two of the **perforating branches** that connect the plantar arch with the dorsalis pedis artery. Find these branches in the intervals between the metatarsal bones.

Review the **medial side of the ankle** and its related tendons (*Atlas*, 5.107). Posterior to the medial malleolus, note the tibialis posterior, flexor digitorum longus, and flexor hallucis longus. Anterior to the medial malleolus observe the tibialis anterior. Next, review the **lateral side of the ankle** (*Atlas*, 5.86, 5.88). Posterior to the lateral malleolus, identify the peroneus brevis and peroneus longus.

Joints of the Lower Limb

General Remarks

It is advantageous to dissect the joints only in one lower limb. Keep the soft structures of the other limb intact for review purposes.

Refer to the articulated bones of the lower limb. Identify the following important joints that should be dissected:

1. **Hip joint;**
2. **Knee joint;**
3. **Ankle joint;**
4. **Joints of inversion and eversion.**

If time permits, you may dissect additional joints of the lower limb. Refer to Appendix II for a detailed text on the following joints:

5. Tibiofibular joints;
6. Various joints between the tarsal bones;
7. Joints of the digits.

Hip Joint

Review the essential bony features of the hip joint and its vicinity (*Atlas*, 5.1A, 5.1B, 5.43).

Anterior Relations of the Hip Joint. Realize that the **sartorius** projects across the neck of the femur (*Atlas*, 5.16B). The **femoral artery** and the inguinal ligament project in relation to the head of the femur or the acetabulum.

Cut and reflect the sartorius, rectus femoris, pectineus, and the femoral nerve and vessels. Identify the **iliopsoas muscle** (*Atlas*, 5.21). Trace its tendon to the lesser trochanter, and sever it close to this bony landmark. Reflect it superiorly.

Study the anterior portion of the hip joint (*Atlas*, 5.42A). Moisten the strong and dense fibrous capsule of the hip joint to make it more pliable. Identify the ligaments that contribute to the formation of the fibrous capsule. Note the exceedingly strong **iliofemoral ligament**. Verify that the base of this triangular ligament is attached to the intertrochanteric line of the neck of the femur; its apex is attached to the anterior inferior iliac spine. Produce various motions of the femur and determine what movements render the exposed ligament taut and what movements make it flaccid. Extend the hip joint and observe that the iliofemoral ligament becomes taut. Thus, this ligament prevents overextension of the hip joint.

Open the **joint capsule** anteriorly by making a vertical incision along a line indicated by the former position of the psoas tendon. Inside the capsule, observe the extensive **articular area of the head of the femur** (*Atlas*, 5.42A). Rotate the limb laterally: note that you can see more of the articular surface. Rotate the limb medially: observe that the articular surface disappears in the acetabulum.

At this stage, define the **obturator externus** (*Atlas*, 5.42A). Once again, examine the obturator nerve as it enters the thigh.

Posterior Relations of the Hip Joint. Turn the cadaver into the prone position (face down). Review the essential features of the gluteal region (*Atlas*, 5.30 to 5.41). Cut and remove all muscles that hold the femur close to the hip bone: piriformis, obturator internus with gemelli, quadratus femoris, gluteus medius and minimus, and obturator externus (*Atlas*, 5.41). Cut and reflect the obturator internus tendon to expose the posterior aspect of the hip joint fully (*Atlas*, 5.42B).

Clean the posterior aspect of the fibrous joint capsule. Identify the **ischiofemoral ligament** as it runs from acetabular rim to the neck of the femur (*Atlas*, 5.42B). Relax the capsule by rotating the lower limb in the appropriate direction. Extend the hip joint and medially rotate the femur. Observe that the ischiofemoral ligament becomes taut, thus resisting hyperextension of the hip joint.

Open the joint cavity by incising the capsule vertically. Insert a probe, and explore the limits of the synovial cavity. Appreciate the thickness of the joint capsule.

The next objective is to dislocate the hip joint, i.e., to remove the head of the femur from its socket. Proceed as follows:

1. Have the specimen in the prone position.
2. Position the pelvis at the end of the table. Let the lower limb hang over the end of the table.
3. Let your partner hold the pelvis steady.
4. Simultaneously, flex the hip joint and forcibly rotate the femur medially. Persist in this maneuver until the *ligament of the head of the femur* ruptures (*Atlas*, 5.49, 5.51A). Subsequently, the head of the femur will

pass out of the acetabulum onto the dorsum of the ilium.

Examine the head and neck of the femur. Observe the articular surface and the reflections of the synovial membrane (*Atlas*, 5.48, 5.49, 5.51). Note the pit for the ligament of the head or the stump of the torn ligament.

Socket for Head of Femur or Acetabulum (*Atlas*, 5.43, 5.47). Identify the smooth **lunate articular surface.** Note the torn **ligament of the head of the femur** (ligamentum teres). Observe that the **acetabular fossa** contains a fatpad that is lined with synovial membrane. With a probe, break through the synovial membrane and examine the underlying fatpad. Expose the blood vessels of the acetabular fossa (*Atlas*, 5.44); these are the acetabular branches of the obturator vessels. Note that a branch runs with the ligament of the head of the femur. This small branch contributes to the blood supply of the head of the femur.

Reflect the ischiofemoral ligament from the femur. Attempt to find a small branch of the medial femoral circumflex artery (*Atlas*, 5.46). Search for fine arterial twigs as they pass through tiny nutrient foramina to supply the neck and the head of the femur. In a similar fashion, a small branch of the lateral femoral circumflex artery supplies the more anterior portions of the head and neck of the femur. Study the clinically important blood supply to the head of the femur (*Atlas*, 5.46).

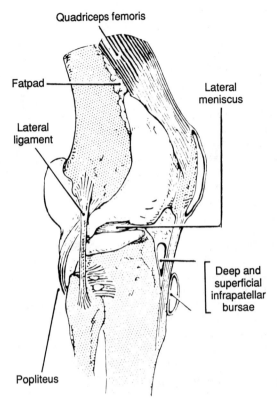

Figure 5.32. Distended synovial capsule of knee joint (lateral view).

> Understand that a fracture of the femoral neck, particularly if it is close to the head, can disrupt the vital blood supply to the head. If the blood supply via the ligament of the head is minimal or also interrupted (as in a ruptured ligament), the head will become necrotic. Such necrosis is a common complication in femoral neck fractures of the elderly. The condition can be assessed radiologically. An injured or diseased hip joint may be surgically replaced by a hip prosthesis.

Turn the specimen into the supine position. Notice that the strong **iliofemoral ligament** is still intact in spite of the dislocation procedure. Palpate its substantial thickness.

Study a radiograph of the hip (*Atlas*, 5.50) and correlate it with a coronal section through the hip joint (*Atlas*, 5.49). In addition, study a transverse section of the hip joint (*Atlas*, 5.51A).

Knee Joint

Review the bony landmarks related to the knee joint (*Atlas*, 5.1A, 5.1B).

Medial Aspect of Knee Joint. On the **medial aspect,** detach the tendons of the sartorius, gracilis, and semitendinosus from their insertions (*Atlas*, 5.25, 5.26, 5.65, 5.66). Reflect the muscles and tendons. Remove the deep fascia. Deep to the tendons of the three muscles, identify the **tibial collateral ligament** of the knee (*Atlas*, 5.65). With a probe, explore the relations between the ligament and the

medial meniscus. Realize that the deeper portion of the tibial collateral ligament is firmly attached to the medial meniscus (*Atlas*, 5.69).

Lateral Aspect of Knee Joint (Fig. 5.32; *Atlas*, 5.63). On the **lateral aspect of the knee joint,** identify the **iliotibial tract.** It is about 2 to 3 cm wide. The tract is inserted into the anterior portion of the lateral tibial condyle (*Atlas*, 5.71B, 5.63, 5.64). Cut the biceps tendon close to its insertion into the head of the fibula (*Atlas*, 5.63). Subsequently, define the **fibular collateral ligament** of the knee. Notice that it does not blend with the underlying lateral meniscus (*Atlas*, 5.69). In fact, the space between fibular collateral ligament and lateral meniscus is wide enough so that the popliteus tendon can pass through it (*Atlas*, 5.68).

Anterior Aspect of Knee Joint (*Atlas*, 5.61, 5.65). On the **anterior aspect of the knee joint,** identify the **expansions of the vasti muscles** and the **ligamentum patellae.** Palpate the patella. Verify the existence of the **prepatellar bursa** just anterior to the patella. Detach the quadriceps tendon from the patella. Be careful *not* to damage the underlying synovial capsule of the knee joint (*Atlas*, 5.61, synovial capsule shown in blue). Make a transverse cut immediately superior to the patella through the synovial capsule into the joint cavity. With a blunt instrument, carefully explore the extent of the capsule. Note the superior recess of the joint cavity. This sac-like recess is the **suprapatellar or quadriceps bursa.**

Just superior to the quadriceps bursa, make a wide horseshoe-shaped section through the quadriceps from

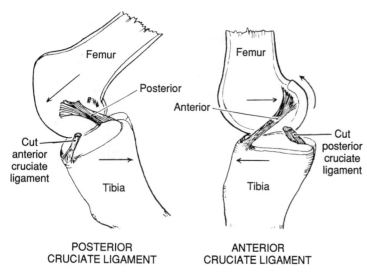

| POSTERIOR | ANTERIOR |
| CRUCIATE LIGAMENT | CRUCIATE LIGAMENT |

Figure 5.33. The posterior cruciate ligament prevents anterior displacement of the femur or posterior displacement of the tibia. The anterior cruciate ligament prevents posterior displacement of the femur and hyperextension.

epicondyle to epicondyle. Identify the quadriceps bursa. Note a layer of fat (fatpad) between bursa and femur.

Back of Knee Joint. Remove the major vessels and nerves of the popliteal fossa (*Atlas*, 5.55). Cut the semimembranosus and other hamstring muscles well superior to the knee joint. Free the plantaris and both heads of the gastrocnemius from the joint capsule. Then, remove these muscles from their bony origins (*Atlas*, 5.56). Cut through the fleshly fibers of the popliteus and remove this muscle (*Atlas*, 5.68). During this procedure, the synovial capsule will be opened posteriorly. Observe that the capsule extends inferior to the lateral meniscus (*Atlas*, 5.61).

Clear away the posterior aspect of the joint capsule (*Atlas*, 5.68). Remove any fat. Identify the **posterior cruciate ligament.** By means of transverse and vertical incisions, open the synovial cavity posterior to each femoral condyle. With a probe, explore the limits of the synovial cavity (*Atlas*, 5.68). Verify that the cruciate ligaments are located entirely *outside* the synovial capsule.

Interior of Knee Joint (*Atlas*, 5.58). Turn to the anterior aspect of the knee joint and open the synovial capsule widely with a transverse incision. Carry the incision around the sides of the knee.

During development, the medial and lateral halves of the knee joint were originally two independent joint cavities separated by the membranes of the **intercondylar septum.** This septum partially breaks down anterior to the anterior cruciate ligament. Examine the anterior part of the septum, the **infrapatellar synovial fold** (*Atlas*, 5.58). Posterior to the infrapatellar fold, the septum is complete. Here, the synovial membranes are reflected across both sides of the cruciate ligaments. Therefore, the cruciate ligaments are situated outside the synovial cavity (*Atlas*, 5.68). However, they lie inside the fibrous joint capsule.

Snip through the infrapatellar fold (*Atlas*, 5.58). Verify that the femur and tibia remain attached to each other by four ligaments (*Atlas*, 5.60A), the **two collateral liga-**ments and the **two cruciate ligaments.** Rotate the femur medially. Note that the **fibular collateral ligament** becomes taut and stops the movement. Sever it. Note that medial rotation of the femur is now free and results in untwisting of the cruciate ligaments.

Verify that the strong cruciate ligaments cross each other (*Atlas*, 5.60A). The **anterior cruciate ligament** attaches the femur to the tibia *anteriorly*. The **posterior cruciate ligament** attaches the femur to the tibia *posteriorly* (*Atlas*, 5.69, 5.71B). Study the functions of the cruciate ligaments (Fig. 5.33 or *Atlas*, 5.70). Extend the leg (knee joint) maximally. In this position, observe:

1. The articular surfaces of femur and tibia are in maximal contact.
2. The joint is "locked" in its most stable position.
3. The anterior cruciate ligament is taut and prohibits further extension.

Flex the leg (knee joint). Observe:

1. There is less contact between the articular surfaces.
2. Some rotation occurs in the knee joint (at the expense of its stability).
3. The posterior cruciate ligament prevents anterior displacement of the femur; i.e., it prevents the femur from sliding anteriorly off the "tibial plateau."
4. With the leg (knee joint) flexed to a right angle, the tibia cannot be pulled anteriorly; it is held back by the anterior cruciate ligament.

Cut the anterior cruciate ligament (*not* the posterior one!). Flex the leg to a right angle. Now, you will be able to pull the tibia anteriorly. This forward movement is an important clinical and diagnostic sign in cases of a ruptured anterior cruciate ligament (see later in this chapter).

Study the menisci or semilunar cartilages (*Atlas*, 5.69, 5.71B). Test the mobility of the menisci. The *C*-shaped **medial meniscus** is firmly attached to the tibia by the coronary ligament. Once again, examine its attachment to the tibial collateral ligament. The small *O*-shaped **lateral meniscus** is distinctly mobile. Remember, it has no attachments to the fibular collateral ligament.

The medial meniscus is injured about 6 to 7 times as often as the lateral meniscus. Why? The medial meniscus is firmly attached to the tibial collateral ligament and the underlying tibia (*Atlas*, 5.60, 5.69). It is virtually immobile. During forceful abduction of the leg, the tension exerted by the tibial collateral ligament can result in tearing of the medial meniscus. In contrast, the slightly mobile lateral meniscus is not attached to the fibular collateral ligament and, therefore, less likely to be torn.

Forced abduction and lateral rotation of the leg may result in the simultaneous rupture or damage of three structures: (a) tibial collateral ligament; (b) anterior cruciate ligament; and (c) medial meniscus. This injury is typical for football players. It has been named the "unhappy triad."

Once more, review the extensive collateral blood supply around the knee joint (*Atlas*, 5.40, 5.57). There are four named genicular branches (two superior branches and two inferior branches). In addition, there may be unnamed genicular branches that participate in the formation of the collateral vascular network around the knee. The vessels are closely applied to the skeletal plane. Note tiny nutrient foramina in the femur and in the tibia.

Study radiographs of the knee region (*Atlas*, 5.73). In addition, correlate your anatomical observations with a sagittal and coronal MRI (*Atlas*, 5.72).

Ankle Joint

Cut and reflect the structures crossing the anterior aspect of the ankle joint. However, leave the tibialis anterior tendon intact.

Medial Side of Ankle Joint (*Atlas*, 5.101). To display the medial aspect of the ankle joint, cut and reflect the flexor digitorum longus. Displace anteriorly (but do *not* cut) the tibialis posterior tendon. Now, clean and define the **medial or deltoid ligament**. It is a triangular ligament that attaches the medial malleolus to the tarsus. Note that the superficial fibers of this ligament are inserted into the whole length of the sustentaculum tali (*Atlas*, 5.120A). The most anterior fibers radiate toward the navicular bone. The deep portion of the ligament anchors the medial malleolus to the talus. This fact is best appreciated on coronal (vertical) section (*Atlas*, 5.126A).

Lateral Side of Ankle Joint (*Atlas*, 5.88). Identify the tendons of the peroneus longus and peroneus brevis. These tendons must be mobilized. Make sure that the superior and inferior peroneal retinacula are slit open. Displace anteriorly (but do *not* cut) the peroneus longus and peroneus brevis tendons. Clean and define the ligaments that hold the lateral malleolus of the fibula to the tarsus (*Atlas*, 5.121): the **calcaneofibular ligament** and the **anterior talofibular ligament**. At this time, also identify the strong **anterior inferior tibiofibular ligament**, one of the structures that hold the tibia and fibula together. The **posterior talofibular ligament** can be best appreciated on coronal section (*Atlas*, 5.126A). At this time, correlate your anatomical observations with a coronal MRI of the ankle joint (*Atlas*, 5.126B).

Plantarflex the foot. Incise transversely the **articular capsule of the ankle joint** (*Atlas*, 5.116, 5.117, 5.118, 5.119). Push the handle of the knife between body of talus

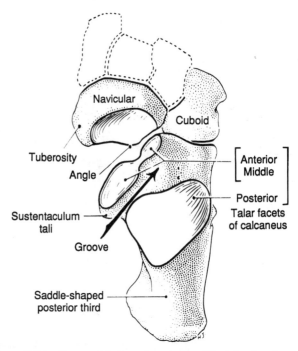

Figure 5.34. Bones of foot on dorsal view. The talus has been removed to show where inversion and eversion take place.

and tibia. To display the **articular surfaces**, sever the ligaments that connect the fibula to the talus and calcaneus: calcaneofibular ligament, anterior talofibular ligament, and posterior talofibular ligament, collectively also known as the **lateral ligament**. Dislocate the foot by swinging it medially. The **deltoid ligament** or medial ligament of the ankle, which remains intact, acts as a hinge. Study the articular surfaces (*Atlas*, 5.74, 5.83, 5.124).

Finally, study suitable radiographs of the ankle (*Atlas*, 5.123). Review pertinent magnetic resonance images (MRIs) of the region (*Atlas*, 5.126B).

Joints of Inversion and Eversion

Study the movements of inversion and eversion of the foot in suitable bony specimens (wired laboratory skele-

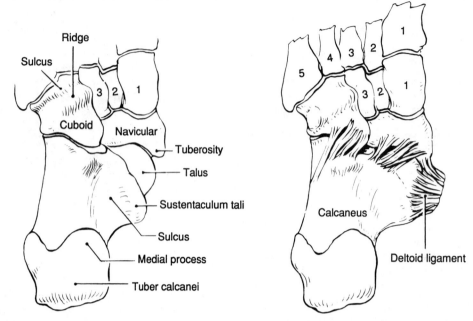

Figure 5.35. Bones of foot on plantar view. Plantar ligaments of joints of inversion and eversion.

tons can be damaged!). With one hand, immobilize the ankle joint, i.e., hold the talus tightly between tibia and fibula. With the other hand, invert and evert the foot. Observe the following:

1. The talus remains fixed in the ankle joint.
2. The entire foot rotates about the inferior and anterior surfaces of the talus.
3. This movement is augmented at the joint between calcaneus and cuboid.

Turn to the cadaver specimen. **Produce eversion** by pulling on the tendons of the peroneus longus and peroneus brevis. Follow the tendons to their insertions (*Atlas*, 5.88, 5.128). Produce inversion by pulling on the tendons of the tibialis anterior and tibialis posterior. Follow the tendons clearly to their insertions (*Atlas*, 5.128).

Study the complex articular interactions between the talus on the one hand, and the calcaneus and navicular on the other (*Atlas*, 5.83, 5.114, 5.120B, 5.122). The objective is to disarticulate the talus from the rest of the tarsus. Proceed as follows (*Atlas*, 5.116 to 5.121):

1. If not already done during dissection of the ankle, sever the ligaments that hold the lateral malleolus to the tarsus.

2. Cut the interosseous talocalcaneal ligament.
3. Cut the posterior part of the subtalar joint capsule.
4. Force the handle of the knife between the talus and calcaneus.
5. Swing the calcaneus and the foot medially. The deltoid ligament, which remains intact, acts as a hinge.

Identify the posterior talar facet of the calcaneus for the subtalar joint (Fig. 5.34; *Atlas*, 5.132B). Inspect the socket for the head of the talus. The articular components of this socket are formed by the **middle talar facet, anterior talar facet, and posterior articular surface of the navicular bone.** The floor of the socket is formed by the important **spring ligament** (*Atlas*, 5.132B). Force a probe or needle through the floor of the socket. Next, approach the probe and ligament from the sole of the foot (Fig. 5.35; *Atlas*, 5.128, 5.129). Identify the **spring ligament or plantar calcaneonavicular ligament.** Understand that this ligament and the tibialis posterior tendon are necessary for the support of the head of the talus. The socket for the head of the talus is of great importance to the integrity of the foot. The socket supports the "keystone" of the high medial arch. Finally, study a radiograph of the foot (*Atlas*, 5.123).

CHAPTER 6

THE UPPER LIMB

Introductory Remarks

The essential functional requirement of the upper limb is manual activity. Anatomically, the upper limb is divided into four segments:

1. **Shoulder,** the junction of arm and trunk;
2. **Arm** (brachium), the segment between shoulder and forearm;
3. **Forearm** (antebrachium), the segment between arm and hand;
4. **Hand** (manus).

It is advantageous to dissect the upper limb in the following sequence: first, the superficial veins and nerves and the deep investing fascia of the entire upper limb will be explored. Next, the muscles acting on the shoulder joint will be studied. If *The Thorax* (Chapter 1) has been covered previously, the muscles of the pectoral region have already been identified during dissection of the anterior chest wall. If *The Back* (Chapter 4) has already been explored, the superficial group of back muscles connecting the upper limb to the vertebral column has already been studied. If you are assigned *The Upper Limb* before dissection of *The Thorax* and *The Back*, the previously mentioned muscles of the shoulder region must as yet be dissected. Subsequently, the axilla and its contents as well as the brachial and anterior cubital regions will be explored. The flexor compartment of the forearm will be dissected and its contents will be followed into the palm of the hand. Finally, the extensor region of the forearm will be studied together with the dorsum of the hand.

Note: Remember that this manual is intended to guide you with the **dissection** of the human body. It is **not** the purpose of *Grant's Dissector* to provide you with a list of all muscles, their origins, insertions, and functions. However, you may find it advantageous to prepare or to copy such a list and to bring it to the laboratory for systematic review of all muscles of the upper limb you are held responsible for in your laboratory course.

Before you begin . . .

Do *not* dissect at this time. Realize that **superficial veins** and cutaneous nerves are contained in the **superficial fascia.** The first objective is to study these structures (superficial fascia; superficial veins; cutaneous nerves) of the entire upper limb as a whole. To accomplish this, the entire upper extremity will be skinned in an initial dissecting effort. The subcutaneous connective tissue and fat will be removed, leaving the more important superficial veins and nerves intact. Subsequently, the **deep fascia** will be demonstrated. The deep or investing fascia surrounds the various muscle compartments.

Skin Incisions

Refer to Figure 6.1. If *The Thorax* has been dissected previously, all skin incisions and skin reflections, as outlined in Figure 6.1A, have already been executed; if not, make the following skin incisions with the cadaver in the supine position:

1. From the jugular notch A along the clavicle and across the acromion B to point E, about 10 cm distal to the acromion;
2. From A to the xiphisternal junction C;
3. From C superiorly and along the anterior axillary fold to point E; avoid the nipple;
4. From C laterally until stopped by the table D;
5. Refer to Figure 6.1C; at the root of the arm, make a complete circular incision from E to E;
6. At the level of the wrist, make another circular incision from G to G;
7. Join the two circular incisions with a longitudinal one on the anterior aspect of the upper limb from E to G; make additional transverse incisions as necessary to speed up the skinning process; reflect the skin of the arm and forearm medially and laterally; then, remove it completely; do not damage the superficial veins and cutaneous nerves in the superficial fascia;

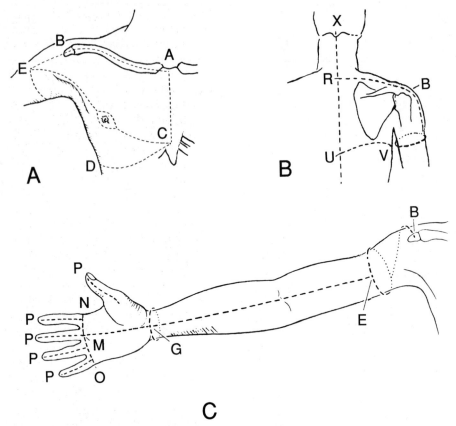

Figure 6.1. Skin incisions.

8. If the hand is tightly clenched, force it open and let your partner hold it open; make incisions in the middle of the palm from *G* to *M*, across the palm from *N* to *O*, and along the middle of all fingers to points *P*; remove the skin from the palmar and dorsal parts of the hand and finger; in peeling off the skin flaps from the fingers, proceed with intelligence and caution; note the thinness of the subcutaneous fat at the creases of the fingers; realize that there are digital nerves, vessels, and fibrous sheaths (*Atlas*, 6.88, 6.124); these structures must not be destroyed.

If *The Back* has been dissected previously, all skin incisions and skin reflections as outlined in Figure 6.1B have already been executed; if not, make the following skin incisions with the cadaver in prone position:

9. In the midline, make a vertical skin incision from the external occipital protuberance *X* via *R* to a point at the approximate level of the inferior angle of the scapula *U*;
10. Carry out a transverse incision from *U* to *V* at the level of the inferior scapular angle;
11. Make a transverse incision from *R* to *B* (superior to the scapula and to the tip of the acromion) and on to the circular incision at the root of the arm; reflect the skin laterally and remove it; check with your instructor.

Superficial Fascia, Veins, and Nerves

In the living, the superficial veins are conspicuous through the skin. They are most frequently used for drawing blood and injecting medications. In the cadaver, the superficial veins are empty and are not conspicuous through the skin. However, they can be easily demonstrated in the superficial fascia. The brachial plexus supplies the upper limb with many cutaneous nerves. At various levels, these cutaneous nerves pierce the deep fascia and reach the superficial fascia and skin.

The next objective is to remove the **superficial fascia** while leaving intact the deep fascia and the principal superficial veins and nerves. With the cadaver in the prone position, examine the structures contained in the superficial fascia of the **posterior aspect of the upper limb**.

On the dorsum of the hand, demonstrate a few tributaries to the **dorsal venous arch** (*Atlas*, 6.5B). Note **superficial dorsal veins**. Realize that the superficial veins of the hand drain into the **basilic vein** and the **cephalic vein**. These two structures will be followed proximally during dissection of the anterior aspect of the upper limb. The veins of the dorsum of the hand are often used for venipuncture and intravenous injection of fluids.

Continue to investigate the structures contained in the superficial fascia of the **posterior aspect of the upper**

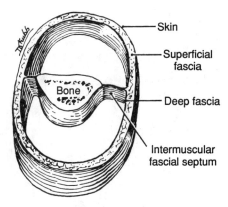

Figure 6.2. The two compartments of the arm.

limb. Familiarize yourself with the expected course of the **superficial nerves** and the cutaneous areas they innervate (*Atlas*, 6.6**B**): cutaneous branch of the axillary nerve; intercostobrachial nerve; posterior brachial cutaneous nerve; posterior antebrachial cutaneous nerve; medial antebrachial cutaneous nerve; lateral antebrachial cutaneous nerve. Pay special attention to the cutaneous nerve branches that supply the dorsum of the hand. Identify and trace to some extent the following two nerves:

1. At the radial aspect of the wrist, use a probe and pick up the **superficial branch of the radial nerve;**
2. At the ulnar aspect of the wrist, identify the **dorsal branch of the ulnar nerve.**

Next, turn the cadaver over and examine the structures contained in the **superficial fascia of the anterior aspect of the upper limb.** Focus your attention on the **superficial veins.** On the radial side of the wrist, use a probe and pick up the **cephalic vein** (*Atlas*, 6.5**A**). On the ulnar side of the wrist, identify the **basilic vein.** Follow these two main, superficial veins proximally (*Atlas*, 6.4). Verify the following:

1. Superiorly, the **cephalic vein** passes into the interval between the deltoid and pectoralis major muscles.
2. The **basilic vein** runs on the medial aspect of the forearm and arm. Before reaching the axilla superiorly, it pierces the deep fascia (*Atlas*, 6.4).
3. In the cubital fossa, the cephalic vein and the basilic vein communicate by means of the **median cubital vein.** (The veins in the region of the cubital fossa are prominent and easily accessible; therefore, they are commonly used for venipuncture).
4. With a probe, lift up various portions of the principal superficial veins. Note that they are connected to **perforating veins** that drain deeper structures (*Atlas*, 6.4, 6.5).

Continue to investigate the structures contained in the superficial fascia of the **anterior aspect of the upper limb.** Familiarize yourself with the expected course of the **superficial nerves** and the cutaneous areas they innervate (*At-las*, 6.6**A**): intercostobrachial nerve; medial brachial cutaneous nerve; medial antebrachial cutaneous nerve with ulnar and anterior branches; lateral antebrachial cutaneous nerve with anterior and posterior branches; various palmar cutaneous branches. (The nerves to the fingers will be explored later).

Deep Fascia. Next, remove all superficial fascia, leaving intact the deep fascia, and the principal superficial nerves and veins. Examine the **deep fascia** of the upper limb. The **deep fascia of the arm** is known as the **brachial fascia.** It is connected with the humerus by two fascial intermuscular septa, thus creating two fascial compartments for the muscles of the arm (Fig. 6.2). Superiorly, the brachial fascia is continuous with the deep fascia covering the pectoralis, the deltoid, and the latissimus dorsi muscles. Inferiorly, the brachial fascia is continuous with the **deep fascia of the forearm, the antebrachial fascia.** In the cubital fossa, the antebrachial fascia is connected to the biceps brachii muscle via a strong triangular band. This is the **bicipital aponeurosis** (*Atlas*, 6.57), which protects deeper structures in the cubital fossa. Positively palpate and identify this obliquely running structure in the cadaver and in your own cubital fossa. At the level of the wrist, the antebrachial fascia is thickened posteriorly and anteriorly to create strong transverse bands. The posterior band, the **extensor retinaculum,** retains the extensor tendons in their position (*Atlas*, 6.103). The anterior band, the **flexor retinaculum,** forms part of a tunnel that contains the flexor tendons (*Atlas*, 6.83). Study and review the deep fascia of the upper limb. Obviously, the deep fascia will have to be incised and removed in order to explore the deep structures of the upper limb.

Scapular and Deltoid Regions

General Remarks

If *The Back* (Chapter 4) has already been explored, the superficial group of back muscles connecting the upper limb to the vertebral column has already been studied. If you are assigned *The Upper Limb* before dissection of the back, the previously mentioned muscles of the shoulder region must, as yet, be dissected and studied. These muscles include the **trapezius, latissimus dorsi, the rhomboids, and the levator scapulae.** The latissimus dorsi acts directly on the arm, since it is inserted into the humerus. The trapezius, rhomboids, and levator scapulae act primarily on the scapula. Positional changes of the scapula are transferred to the humerus (since the scapula and the humerus articulate with each other; *Atlas*, 6.1). Review these previously mentioned muscles (Chapter 4, pp. 84–85).

Four muscles (supraspinatus, infraspinatus, teres major, teres minor) arise from the dorsal surface of the scapula and insert into the upper portion of the humerus. In order to have complete access to these muscles, the deltoid muscle must be detached from its scapular origin.

Bony Landmarks

Refer to a skeleton and study the following bony landmarks:

1. **Scapula** (*Atlas*, 6.1). The **spine** separates the dorsal surface of the scapula into **supraspinous fossa** and **infraspinous fossa.** At the lateral scapular border, the two spinous fossae are connected by the **great scapular notch.** Observe the **glenoid cavity** for the articulation with the head of the humerus. Above the glenoid cavity, note the **supraglenoid tubercle;** below it, observe the **infraglenoid tubercle.** Identify the **coracoid process.** Note the **suprascapular notch** incising the superior scapular border at the base of the coracoid process.
2. **Humerus** (*Atlas*, 6.1). Identify: **head,** articulating with the glenoid cavity; **greater tubercle,** located laterally; **lesser tubercle,** located anteriorly; **intertubercular sulcus or bicipital groove** between the two tubercles; **deltoid tuberosity** for insertion of the deltoid muscle.

Before you begin . . .

The deltoid muscle will be detached from its scapular origin and the course of its nerve and artery will be studied. Subsequently, the four muscles arising from the dorsal surface of the scapula (supraspinatus, infraspinatus, teres major, teres minor) will be dissected and their nerve and blood supplies will be demonstrated.

Dissection

With the cadaver prone, dissection will be easier if the arm is abducted about 45° and the shoulder is allowed to fall forward. Use a wooden block if necessary.

Define the borders of the **deltoid muscle.** Verify its origin from the lateral third of the clavicle (*Atlas*, 6.14), spine, and acromion of scapula (*Atlas*, 6.32, 6.33, 6.45**B**). With a scalpel, carefully detach the deltoid from the spine and the acromion of the scapula. Leave the muscle attached to the clavicle. Reflect the deltoid anteriorly. Observe the **axillary nerve** and the **posterior humeral circumflex artery** entering its deep surface (*Atlas*, 6.40). Dissect the nerve and vessels. Note the following:

1. The axillary nerve also supplies the teres minor (*Atlas*, 6.11**D**, 6.40).
2. The axillary nerve is a branch of the posterior cord of the brachial plexus (*Atlas*, 6.11**D**).
3. The posterior humeral circumflex artery is a branch of the axillary artery (*Atlas*, 6.7).

Push your fingers parallel to the axillary nerve and posterior humeral circumflex vessels into a space. This space is the **quadrangular space** (Fig. 6.3; *Atlas*, 6.40). Define the borders of the quadrangular space:

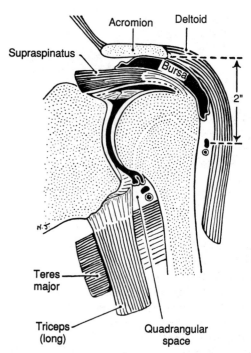

Figure 6.3. Shoulder region (coronal section). Quadrangular space.

1. Cranially, the capsule of the shoulder joint;
2. Laterally, the surgical neck of the humerus;
3. Medially, the long head of the triceps brachii;
4. Caudally, the upper border of the teres major.

Note the **long head of the triceps brachii** (*Atlas*, 6.40). Verify that it passes between teres minor and teres major and attaches to the infraglenoid tubercle. With your fingers, separate the **long and lateral heads of triceps.** Define the triangular interval between the two heads of the muscle inferior to the teres major. With a probe, explore the floor of the triangular interval: identify the humerus; observe the **radial nerve** and the **profunda brachii artery** within a broad groove directly on the humerus (*Atlas*, 6.40). Get into the habit of learning where vessels and nerves originate from and travel to. In this case, the profunda brachii artery is schematized in *Atlas*, 6.7. A scheme of the radial nerve with its origin and distribution is shown in *Atlas*, 6.11**D**.

Next, the **supraspinatus** and **infraspinatus muscles** must be explored. To clear the area, reflect the trapezius anteriorly (*Atlas*, 6.33). If dissection of the superficial back muscles has been done properly, the trapezius will remain attached only to the clavicle. Its nerve and blood supply should still be intact. Remove deep fascia from the supraspinatus and infraspinatus. Push your finger into the space bounded by the levator scapulae, superior border of the scapula, and anterior margin of reflected trapezius. Since this space is filled with loose fat, use scissors and forceps to remove it. Run your finger along the superior border of the scapula. Feel the ligament that bridges the suprascapular notch medial to the base of the coracoid

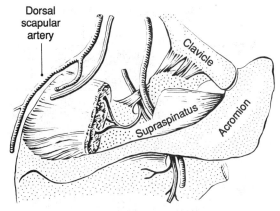

Figure 6.4. Supraspinatus muscle (section removed).

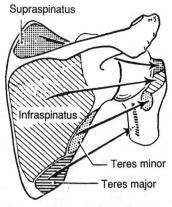

Figure 6.5. The supraspinatus, infraspinatus, and teres minor muscles insert into the greater tubercle of the humerus and contribute to the rotator cuff. The teres major muscle inserts into the crest of the lesser tubercle of the humerus.

process (*Atlas*, 6.33, 6.34, 6.35). This is the **suprascapular ligament.**

The next objective is to demonstrate the nerve and blood supply to the muscles occupying the supraspinous and infraspinous fossae. Vertically, cut across the supraspinatus muscle at the following location (Fig. 6.4; *Atlas*, 6.34): about 5 cm lateral to the superior angle of the scapula; that is, medial to the suprascapular notch and ligament. With the handle of the scalpel, free the lateral portion of the supraspinatus from its fossa. Reflect it laterally. Now, observe and clean the **suprascapular nerve and artery** (Fig. 6.4; *Atlas*, 6.34, 6.36). The nerve passes inferior to the suprascapular ligament whereas the artery passes superior to it. Realize that the nerve is derived from cervical segments (*Atlas*, 6.11D). The artery usually originates from the thyrocervical trunk (*Atlas*, 6.34).

Next, cut vertically across the **infraspinatus muscle**, about 5 cm lateral to the vertebral border of the scapula. Peel loose the lateral portion of the muscle. Reflect it laterally. Note the **suprascapular artery and nerve** reaching the muscle via the greater scapular notch (Fig. 6.4; *Atlas*, 6.34, 6.40).

Follow the **suprascapular artery and nerve** into the fossa bounded by the levator scapulae, the superior border of scapula, and the trapezius (*Atlas*, 6.33). Both nerve and artery are lateral to a small "rounded" muscle, the **posterior belly of the omohyoid**, which arises medial to the suprascapular notch. Deep within the fossa, find the **transverse cervical artery** (*Atlas*, 6.33). The transverse cervical artery is a branch of the thyrocervical trunk (*Atlas*, 6.34). It continues to the deep surface of the trapezius muscle where it supplies the middle third of this muscle.

> In 70% of the cases, there is a **dorsal scapular artery** that arises from the second or third part of the subclavian artery. The artery runs an independent course deep to the rhomboid layer of muscles to supply the rhomboids, the levator scapulae, and the serratus anterior. It also sends small branches to the dorsal and ventral surfaces of the scapula, providing anastomoses with the suprascapular and the subscapular arteries. When the dorsal scapular artery does *not* arise independently from the subclavian artery (in 30% of the cases), it is usually a branch of the transverse cervical artery (*Atlas*, 6.34). Regardless of its point of origin, the artery that runs deep to the rhomboid layer is called the **dorsal scapular artery.**

> The scapular region has an extensive collateral circulation (*Atlas*, 6.8). Its surgical importance becomes apparent during ligation (placement of thread or clamp) of an injured axillary or subclavian artery. Realize that the axillary artery may be ligated between the thyrocervical trunk and the subscapular artery. In this case, the direction of the blood flow in the subscapular artery becomes reversed, allowing arterial blood from anastomoses to reach the portion of the axillary artery distal to the ligature. Note that, in case of ligature, the subscapular artery receives its blood via several anastomoses with the suprascapular artery, transverse cervical artery, dorsal scapular artery, and some intercostal arteries (*Atlas*, 6.8). Ligation of the axillary artery distal to the subscapular artery interrupts the blood supply to the arm entirely and is intolerable.

Study the insertion of the four muscles arising from the dorsal surface of the scapula (Fig. 6.5). Verify that the tendons of the **supraspinatus, infraspinatus, and teres minor muscles** fuse with the capsule of the shoulder joint to form the major portion of the "rotator cuff" (*Atlas*, 6.37). These tendons insert into the **greater tubercle of the humerus.** Sometimes, the tendons of the infraspinatus and teres minor muscles are inseparable. The teres major is attached to the medial lip of the intertubercular sulcus of the humerus. Understand the principal actions of these four muscles (Fig. 6.5). The supraspinatus abducts the arm, infraspinatus and teres minor rotate the arm laterally, and the teres major rotates the arm medially. Realize and demonstrate that the supraspinatus tendon covers part of the capsule of the shoulder joint (*Atlas*, 6.35, 6.47).

> **Attrition of the supraspinatus tendon** (*Atlas*, 6.49) is a common finding among middle-aged persons. As the supraspinatus tendon degenerates and wears away, the underlying joint capsule is opened. Between the deltoid muscle and the acromion superiorly and the supraspinatus tendon inferiorly lies a bursa. This bursa (synovial sac) is the **subacromial bursa.** Attrition of the supraspinatus tendon ultimately leads to a wide-open communication between the shoulder joint and the subacromial bursa. The result is a "painful shoulder" (pathologically evidenced by a rupture of the rotator cuff of the shoulder joint with limitation of rotation of the arm).

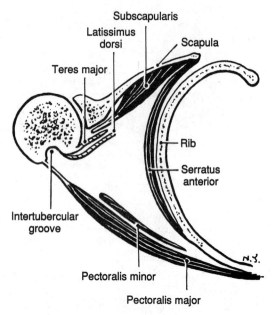

Figure 6.6. Walls of axilla (on transverse section).

Pectoral Region

The pectoral region (L., *pectus*, chest) covers the anterior and part of the lateral chest wall. The mammary gland is superficial. The muscles of the region comprise the pectoralis major, pectoralis minor, subclavius, and serratus anterior. The pectoralis major muscle is inserted into the humerus. The other muscles are inserted into the scapula and clavicle, which form part of the pectoral girdle (*Atlas*, 6.21, 6.29). If *The Thorax* (Chapter 1) has been covered previously, the mammary gland and the muscles of the pectoral region have already been identified during dissection of the anterior chest wall. For dissection instructions or review, please refer to Chapter 1, pp. 8–9. Dissect or review the following structures:

1. **Mammary gland** and its lymphatic drainage (p. 8);
2. **Pectoralis major** and related structures (deltopectoral triangle; clavipectoral fascia; cephalic vein; medial and lateral pectoral nerves, p. 9);
3. **Pectoralis minor** and **subclavius** (p. 9).

At this point, identify and study the **serratus anterior,** the 4th muscle of the pectoral region (*Atlas*, 6.28A). Note its extensive fleshy origin from the upper eight ribs. Realize that it is inserted into the whole length of the medial border of the scapula (*Atlas*, 6.28B). Identify the serratus anterior on a transverse section (Fig. 6.6). Review the components of the **pectoral girdle** (*Atlas*, 6.29). Finally, review the muscles acting on the scapula and study various **scapular movements** (*Atlas*, 6.31).

Axilla

General Remarks

The axilla is the region between the arm or brachium and the chest. Palpate your own axillary fossa and verify that it is a pyramidal space. The axillary fossa possesses an apex, a base, and four walls. The apex is bounded by the clavicle ventrally, the upper border of the scapula dorsally, and the 1st rib medially. The base of the pyramidal space is the skin and fascia of the armpit. The **four walls of the axilla** are (Fig. 6.6; *Atlas*, 6.18):

1. **Anterior wall**, the muscular anterior axillary fold;
2. **Posterior wall**; consists of muscles covering the ventral surface of the scapula;
3. **Medial wall**; consists of the upper portion of the thorax with overlying serratus anterior muscle;
4. **Lateral wall**; the narrow vertical groove of the humerus intervening between the converging anterior and posterior walls, i.e., the intertubercular sulcus.

The contents of the axilla are: axillary vessels and lymphatics, brachial plexus, and muscles (*Atlas*, 6.19).

Dissection of Axilla

Anterior Wall of Axilla. Review the **pectoralis major and pectoralis minor** (*Atlas*, 1.2, 6.14, 6.22). These muscles were discussed in detail with the dissection of the pectoral region. Reflect the pectoralis minor superiorly. Reflect the pectoralis major toward the arm. Abduct the arm to a right angle. Have your partner hold the limb in this position with the elbow raised off the table. This procedure relaxes the structures within the axilla.

Posterior Wall of Axilla (Fig. 6.6; *Atlas*, 6.17, 6.26). Identify and palpate the three muscles that form the posterior wall of the axilla: **latissimus dorsi** (responsible for producing the posterior axillary fold), **teres major**, and **subscapularis.** Do *not* clean these muscles at this time. This will be done after tracing nerves and blood vessel from the axillary contents.

Medial Wall of Axilla (Fig. 6.6; *Atlas*, 6.25). The medial wall is formed by the expansive and flat **serratus anterior** that covers the ribs and intercostal muscles. Identify the serratus. With your fingertips, follow it dorsally toward the medial margin of the scapula. Do *not* clean the muscle at this time so that its nerve and blood supply remain undisturbed.

Lateral Wall of Axilla (Fig. 6.6). This narrow wall is the **intertubercular sulcus** of the humerus. The sulcus is also called the **bicipital groove** since the tendon of the long head of biceps brachii lodges in it (*Atlas*, 6.19B).

Dissection of Contents of Axilla

Identify the following three muscles as part of the contents of the axilla (*Atlas*, 6.19B, 6.22):

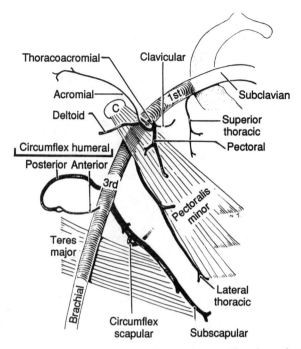

Figure 6.7. Axillary artery, its three parts, and its branches.

1. Tendinous **long head of biceps brachii;** it lies within the intertubercular sulcus; it arises from the supraglenoid tubercle of the scapula;
2. **Short head of biceps,** lying medial to the tendon of long head;
3. **Coracobrachialis,** the most medial of the muscles; observe that the coracobrachialis and short head of biceps are attached to the coracoid process of the scapula (*Atlas,* 6.22, 6.26).

Axillary Sheath (*Atlas,* 6.17, 6.19B). This sheath envelops the remaining contents of the axilla; i.e., the axillary artery, the axillary vein, and cords of the brachial plexus. If the axillary vein and its tributaries have already been removed, the axillary sheath must have been opened. If the axillary vein is still present, remove it and its tributaries so that the dissection field of the axilla can be clarified.

Axillary Artery and Its Branches (Fig. 6.7; *Atlas,* 6.7, 6.22, 6.25). The axillary artery is surrounded by the cords and branches of the brachial plexus. These nerves must *not* be destroyed. They should be retracted (*Atlas,* 6.25) during dissection of the axillary artery and its branches. Using scissors and forceps, clean the following structures:

1. **Axillary artery** (Fig. 6.7). This large artery begins at the lateral border of the 1st rib where it is continuous with the **subclavian artery.** The axillary artery ends at the inferior border of the teres major muscle. At this point, it continues distally as the **brachial artery.** Identify the three parts of the axillary artery (Fig. 6.7): the first part is located between the lateral border of the 1st rib and the superior border of the pectoralis minor; the second part lies deep to the pectoralis minor; the third part extends between the inferior border of the pectoralis minor and the inferior border of the teres major. Positively identify these three parts, which give rise to various arterial branches. Note, however, that there is considerable variation in the branching pattern of the axillary artery. If the pattern is different in your specimen, realize that the branches are named according to their distribution rather than their point of origin.

2. Branch of the **first part** of the axillary artery (Fig. 6.7): this single, small vessel is the **superior (or supreme) thoracic artery** that supplies part of the 1st and 2nd intercostal spaces (*Atlas,* 6.25).

3. Branches of the **second part** of the axillary artery (Fig. 6.7): these are the **thoracoacromial artery** and the **lateral thoracic artery** that arise deep to the pectoralis minor muscle. Identify the short wide **trunk of the thoracoacromial artery** at the superior border of the pectoralis minor muscle, and follow its branches (acromial; deltoid; pectoral; clavicular) to their respective fields of distribution (*Atlas,* 6.22). Next, identify the origin of the **lateral thoracic artery,** and follow it to the pectoral muscles. (In females of reproductive age, this vessel is relatively large since it also supplies the lateral portion of the mammary gland).

4. Branches of the **third part** of the axillary artery (Fig. 6.7): first, identify the largest branch of the axillary artery, the **subscapular artery.** Trace it along the lateral border of the subscapularis muscle (*Atlas,* 6.22). The vessel continues inferiorly as the thoracodorsal artery, which supplies the latissimus dorsi muscle. Note another branch of the subscapular artery, the circumflex scapular artery, which contributes to the rich anastomotic arterial network around the scapula (*Atlas,* 6.8, 6.22). Follow other branches of the subscapular artery to the following muscles (*Atlas,* 6.25): subscapularis, latissimus dorsi, and serratus anterior. Next, search for the **anterior and posterior humeral circumflex arteries.** Note that the larger vessel, the *posterior humeral circumflex artery,* passes through the quadrangular space together with the axillary nerve (*Atlas,* 6.40). Establish continuity of the vessel. With one finger, approach the quadrangular space from the axilla (Fig. 6.8; *Atlas,* 6.25, 6.26); with another finger, approach the quadrangular space from dorsally (*Atlas,* 6.40). Identify the posterior humeral circumflex artery as it passes through the quadrangular space. The artery is accompanied by the axillary nerve, which will be studied later in more detail.

Brachial Plexus (Fig. 6.9; *Atlas,* 6.22, 6.27). *Note:* only the infraclavicular part of the plexus will be dissected at this time. The supraclavicular part will be dissected with the neck. The axillary artery is surrounded by the **three cords** of the brachial plexus: lateral, medial, and posterior. First, identify the **lateral and medial cords** and their branches. Proceed in the following manner:

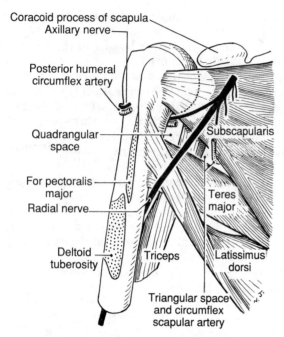

Figure 6.8. Posterior wall of axilla.

1. Identify the **musculocutaneous nerve.** It is the most lateral nerve of the plexus and enters the substance of coracobrachialis (*Atlas*, 6.26).
2. Trace the musculocutaneous nerve proximally to the **lateral cord** (Fig. 6.9).
3. Identify the other terminal branch of the lateral cord: this is the lateral root of the median nerve. Follow it distally and identify the **median nerve.**
4. Trace the medial root of the median nerve proximally to the **medial cord** (Fig. 6.9).
5. Identify the other terminal branches of the medial cord, the **ulnar nerve.**

Note that the three nerves (musculocutaneous; median; ulnar) describe the letter *M* anterior to the axillary artery (Fig. 6.9). The medial cord has a large collateral branch: the **medial cutaneous nerve of the forearm** (*Atlas*, 6.22). Follow the nerve distally to the point where it pierces the deep fascia (*Atlas*, 6.6A). Trace the pectoral nerves of the reflected pectoral muscles to their origins from lateral and medial cords (or divisions; *Atlas*, 6.11C, 6.19B).

With tape or a string, retract the axillary vessels and the M-shaped anterior nerves (*Atlas*, 6.25). This procedure exposes the **posterior cord** of the brachial plexus. Clean the posterior cord and dissect its branches (Fig. 6.8; *Atlas*, 6.26):

1. The **axillary nerve,** passing through the quadrangular space with the posterior humeral circumflex artery;
2. **Subscapular nerves** to subscapularis muscle; some nerve fibers continue distally to supply the teres major muscle;

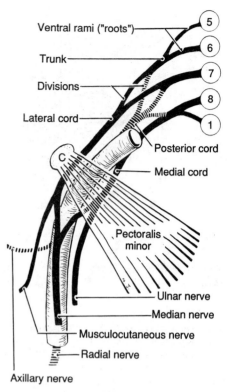

Figure 6.9. Brachial plexus.

3. The **nerve to the latissimus dorsi** and the **nerve to the subscapularis** run in the loose areolar or fatty tissue anterior to the subscapularis muscle; use probe and scissors to clean these nerves.

On the lateral axillary and thoracic wall, free the **nerve to the serratus anterior** (*Atlas*, 6.25, 6.26, 6.28A). Follow it proximally to the apex of the axilla. This nerve originates separately from lower cervical segments (*Atlas*, 6.11D).

Now, the contents of the axilla have been identified and dissected. Proceed by cleaning the surfaces of all muscles forming the walls of the axilla.

Examine the **contents of the axilla** with special reference to an important bony landmark: the **tip of the coracoid process.** Palpate this landmark. Verify (*Atlas*, 6.22):

1. The axillary sheath passes about 2 cm inferior to it.
2. All structures within the axillary sheath (artery; several nerves) may be easily severed here (stab wounds; piece of shrapnel).

Study the attachments of the **serratus anterior** (Fig. 6.6; *Atlas*, 6.28A). It is the essential protractor of the scapula (as when pushing). The muscle also abducts the arm above the horizontal plane. Paralysis of the serratus anterior will result in "winging" of the scapula and in inability to elevate the arm above the horizontal plane.

Identify the **subscapularis** muscle (*Atlas*, 6.26). Note that it fills the subscapular fossa (anterior aspect of scap-

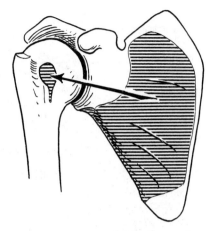

Figure 6.10. Attachments of the subscapularis muscle.

ula) and is inserted into the lesser tubercle of the humerus (Fig. 6.10; *Atlas*, 6.45A).

> The tendons of subscapularis, supraspinatus, infraspinatus, and the teres minor blend to form a continuous musculotendinous sheath. This sheath, which is intimately adherent to the underlying shoulder joint capsule, is called the rotator cuff (*Atlas*, 6.51, 6.52). Infraspinatus and teres minor *rotate* the arm laterally (Fig. 6.5), the subscapularis *rotates* the arm medially (Fig. 6.10), and the supraspinatus abducts (Fig. 6.5). Attrition of the rotator cuff may produce a "painful shoulder" (*Atlas*, 6.49).
>
> The attachment of muscle fibers or tendons to the capsule of the joint over which they pass is an anatomical principle that has functional as well as clinical implications. Look for other examples as you dissect and consider the implications in each case.

Review the essential anatomical features of the axilla. Examine additional cadavers in order to appreciate variations in the distribution of arteries and nerves. Study a transverse section through the axilla (*Atlas*, 6.19). Correlate your anatomical observations with a transverse magnetic resonance image (MRI) of the shoulder (*Atlas*, 6.20). Review the scapular movements (*Atlas*, 6.31).

Brachial and Anterior Cubital Regions

General Remarks

The muscles of the arm or brachium are contained in two fascial compartments (Figs. 6.2 and 6.11). The anterior compartment houses three muscles, their nerves, and vessels. The posterior compartment houses one extensor muscle, the triceps brachii, and its nerves and vessels (*Atlas*, 6.44). The cubital fossa (L., *cubitus*, elbow) is related to the anterior aspect of the elbow.

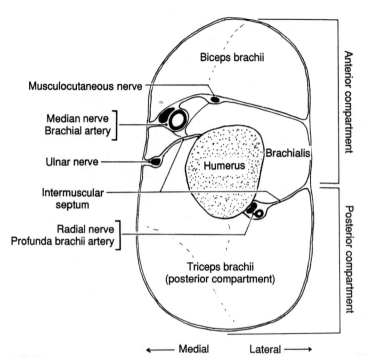

Figure 6.11. The two compartments of the arm. The anterior compartment contains flexor muscles, which are supplied by the musculocutaneous nerve. The posterior compartment contains an extensor muscle, the triceps brachii. It is innervated by the radial nerve.

Before you begin . . .

Within the cubital fossa, the positions of the brachial artery as well as the median and radial nerves will be investigated. Subsequently, the continuity of median, ulnar, and musculocutaneous nerves will be established. The brachial artery and its important collateral vessels will be demonstrated. Finally, the muscles in the two brachial compartments will be studied.

Dissection

Identify and define the **biceps brachii** (*Atlas* 6.57). In the cubital fossa, note the strong tendon of the biceps. From its medial side, the tendon gives off a strong triangular aponeurosis, the **bicipital aponeurosis** (lacertus fibrosis). It passes obliquely into the deep fascia covering the flexor muscles of the forearm. Note that the bicipital aponeurosis bridges and protects the **median nerve** and the **brachial artery**. Cut across the aponeurosis. Note the relative positions of bicipital tendon, brachial artery, and median nerve. Do not destroy the **lateral cutaneous nerve of the forearm** (the cutaneous branch of the musculocutaneous nerve). This nerve runs between biceps and brachialis, and reaches the cubital fossa lateral to the biceps tendon (*Atlas*, 6.55, 6.57).

On the lateral aspect (side of thumb) of the forearm, identify the **brachioradialis muscle** (*Atlas*, 6.57). With

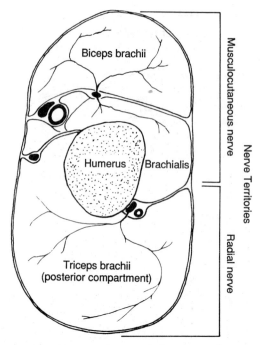

Figure 6.12. Nerve territories of the arm (brachial region).

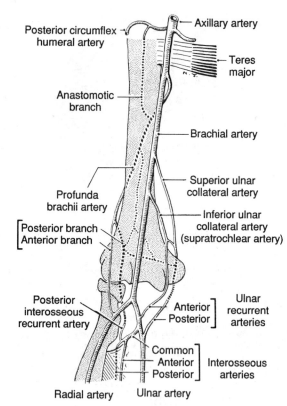

Figure 6.13. Brachial artery and branches. Anastomoses around the elbow.

your fingertips, explore the interval between brachioradialis, biceps, and brachialis (*Atlas*, 6.59). Deep in this interval, find the **radial nerve.**

Follow the **radial nerve** proximally. The next objective is to expose the nerve where it is covered by the lateral head of the triceps brachii (*Atlas*, 6.41). Proceed as follows: to have better access to the triceps, rotate the arm medially. Push a probe proximally along the course of the radial nerve. The probe lies between lateral head of triceps and humerus (*Atlas*, 6.41). Using the probe as a protective device to shield nerve and vessels, sever the lateral head of the triceps obliquely. Now, expose the **radial nerve** and the accompanying **profunda brachii artery.**

Establish the continuity of the radial nerve from the axilla to the elbow region. Observe that the radial nerve is in direct contact with the humerus (*Atlas*, 6.41). This area of contact is called the **groove for the radial nerve** or **the spiral groove** (*Atlas*, 6.1**B**; posterior view). In the area of this groove, the radial nerve can be easily injured during fracture of the humerus.

Realize that the **triceps brachii** lodges in the posterior compartment of the arm. Identify the **three heads of the triceps: long, lateral,** and **medial.** Observe that the triceps tendon inserts into the olecranon process of the ulna (*Atlas*, 6.41). Look for muscular branches of the radial nerve to the triceps. There is only one branch to the long head of the triceps (*Atlas*, 6.26). The other heads receive several branches.

Identify the **three muscles in the anterior compartment of the arm: coracobrachialis, brachialis,** and **biceps brachii** (*Atlas*, 6.26, 6.57, 6.59). Observe the tendon of the long head of biceps in the intertubercular sulcus (bicipital groove). Follow the tendon proximally, under the bridge of the transverse humeral ligament, and to the interior of the fibrous capsule of the shoulder joint (*Atlas*, 6.43**B**, 6.46).

Trace the **musculocutaneous nerve** distally through the coracobrachialis (*Atlas*, 6.26) and between biceps and brachialis (*Atlas*, 6.59). Sever the biceps about 5 cm proximal to the cubital region. Reflect the severed portions of the biceps. Now, the musculocutaneous nerve can be conveniently traced. Note its branches to the three muscles of the anterior brachial compartment (*Atlas*, 6.11A, 6.26). Follow the nerve distally where it becomes the **lateral cutaneous nerve of the forearm** (*Atlas*, 6.6A, 6.55).

Trace the **median nerve** from axilla to cubital fossa. Next, follow the **ulnar nerve** from the medial cord to the medial epicondyle of the humerus. Note that the nerve is applied to the posterior aspect of the medial epicondyle. There, palpate the nerve (*Atlas*, 6.41, 6.64, 6.66). Verify that the median and ulnar nerves do not supply any muscles in the arm (*Atlas*, 6.11A and **B**). Review the nerve territories of the brachial region (Fig. 6.12): the musculocutaneous nerve is responsible for the muscles in the anterior compartment. The radial nerve supplies the muscle of the posterior compartment, the triceps brachii.

The **brachial artery** is the continuation of the axillary artery. It begins at the inferior border of the teres major muscle. It ends at its bifurcation into the ulnar artery and radial artery (Fig. 6.13; *Atlas*, 6.7, 6.63). Verify that the brachial artery is palpable throughout the arm. It runs with the median nerve, which is the only important structure to cross it (*Atlas*, 6.43**B**). Identify (Fig. 6.13; *Atlas*, 6.63):

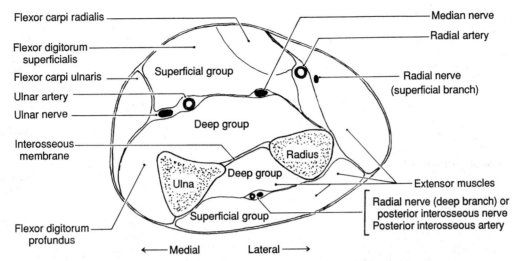

Figure 6.14. Schematic transverse section through the forearm.

1. **Profunda brachii artery;** it is highest in origin; review its course;
2. Several unnamed **muscular branches** (*Atlas*, 6.26, 6.43B);
3. **Superior and inferior ulnar collateral arteries** (*Atlas*, 6.43B, 6.63).

Understand the functionally and surgically important collateral circulation around the elbow joint (Fig. 6.13; *Atlas*, 6.63). The brachial artery may be tied off distal to the inferior ulnar collateral artery. Under these circumstances, sufficient blood reaches the ulnar and radial arteries via the existing anastomoses. Look for the superior ulnar collateral artery. This artery runs with the ulnar nerve posterior to the medial epicondyle where it anastomoses with the posterior ulnar recurrent artery (*Atlas*, 6.64, 6.66). The important anastomotic connections around the elbow are often difficult to demonstrate. Collateral circulation occurs between small vessels, often within muscles. Limit the time spent in pursuit of these anastomotic connections.

Always keep in mind that the brachial artery lies medial to the biceps and its tendon (*Atlas*, 6.57). At this location, palpate the arterial pulse in yourself and in your partner. Where should you place the stethoscope when taking blood pressure and listening to the pulsations of the brachial artery?

Flexor Region of Forearm

General Remarks

The flexor muscles of the forearm can be divided into a superficial and a deep group. Study a tranverse section through the middle of the forearm (Fig. 6.14; *Atlas*, 6.122A). Realize that the ulnar artery, ulnar nerve, and median nerve are located in an areolar septum. This septum separates the deep from the superficial flexors.

The superficial flexor muscles arise mainly on the medial side of the elbow from the medial epicondyle and its supracondylar ridge (*Atlas*, 6.77). The deep flexor muscles arise from radius and ulna. Their origin extends to the posterior border of the ulna. Thus, the posterior border of the ulna separates flexor region from extensor region (Fig. 6.14; *Atlas*, 6.122A).

In the living subject, verify the following:

1. Palpate the posterior border of the ulna throughout the forearm region. It lies subcutaneous and is not crossed by muscles or a motor nerve. Therefore, the posterior border of the ulna indicates a convenient "internervous line," where the surgeon may incise in order to reach deeper parts of the forearm.
2. Flex your fingers (make a fist). Palpate the contraction of superficial and deep flexors. Note that the active muscle group originates from the medial region of the elbow and around the medial aspect of the forearm as far as the posterior border of the ulna.

Bony Landmarks

Refer to a skeleton and study the following bony landmarks (Fig. 6.15; *Atlas*, 6.67, 6.69):

1. **Humerus.** The **medial epicondyle** and its medial supracondylar ridge give origin to the superficial flexor group; the **lateral epicondyle** and its lateral supracondylar ridge give origin to extensor muscles (*Atlas*, 6.45A); the **capitulum** for articulation with the radius; the **trochlea** for articulation with the ulna; the **olecranon fossa;**
2. **Radius.** The **head** for articulation with humerus; the **neck;** the **tuberosity** for biceps tendon; the **anterior**

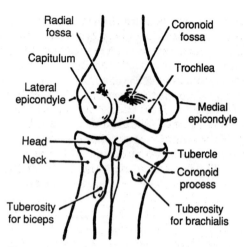

Figure 6.15. Bony parts of the elbow region.

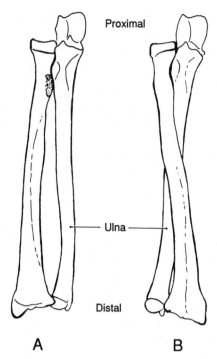

Figure 6.16. Anterior view of right ulna and radius; **A**, in supination; **B**, in pronation. Note proximal and distal radioulnar joints.

oblique line for origin of flexor digitorum superficialis; the **styloid process** (*Atlas*, 6.76C); the interosseous border for attachment of the important interosseous membrane between the radius and the ulna (*Atlas*, 6.76C);

3. **Ulna** (*Atlas*, 6.67). The **olecranon;** observe that it fits into the olecranon fossa of the humerus and thus limits hyperextension of the forearm; joint surface for articulation with trochlea of humerus; **head** at the distal extremity of the ulna (*Atlas*, 6.56); **interosseous border** for attachment of interosseous membrane;

4. It is essential to understand how the three bones (humerus; radius; ulna) articulate with each other. On the skeleton, examine the following:
    a. Joint between the capitulum of the humerus and the head of the radius (*Atlas*, 6.1, 6.69**B**);
    b. Joint between the ulna and the trochlea of the humerus (*Atlas*, 6.1, 6.69**A**);
    c. Proximal radioulnar joint, between the head of the radius and a corresponding notch on the proximal end of the ulna (Fig. 6.16; *Atlas*, 6.1);
    d. Distal radioulnar joint, between the head of the ulna and a corresponding notch on the lower end of the radius (Fig. 6.16; *Atlas*, 6.1);
    e. Observe the characteristic movements performed in the proximal and distal radioulnar joints (Fig. 6.16); in the position of supination (anatomical position), the radius and the ulna are parallel; in the position of pronation, the two bones cross each other;

5. On the palmar surface of the articulated hand, identify the pisiform bone (*Atlas*, 6.130A).

Before you begin . . .

At the level of the wrist, the relative positions of tendons, vessels, and nerves will be identified. After reflecting the superficial flexor group, the deep flexor group will be studied. The student should understand the relations of vessels, nerves, and muscles on transverse section (Fig. 6.14; *Atlas*, 6.122A).

Dissection

Remove the superficial and deep fasciae from the front of the forearm as far around as the posterior border of the ulna. Expose the superficial flexor muscles. Follow them distally to the wrist (*Atlas*, 6.79). Be careful. Do *not* destroy arteries and nerves. From the lateral to medial side, identify the following structures (*Atlas*, 6.79, 6.87): **radial artery,** tendon of **flexor carpi radialis, median nerve,** tendon of **palmaris longus** (absent in 10%), the four tendons of the **flexor digitorum superficialis** (sublimis), **ulnar artery, ulnar nerve,** and the tendon of **flexor carpi ulnaris.**

Palpate these structures in your own wrist (*Atlas*, 6.85, 6.86). Do you have a palmaris longus? Feel the pulse in the radial artery. Point to the site of the median nerve. Realize that this important nerve can be easily injured in the wrist region. Palpate the insertion of the flexor carpi ulnaris tendon into the pisiform bone, and through it to the pisohamate and pisocarpal ligaments (*Atlas*, 6.99). In reference to the pisiform bone, where do you expect to find the ulnar nerve and artery? (*Atlas*, 6.86).

Identify the **brachioradialis.** This muscle is a flexor of the elbow joint. Open the furrow medial to the brachioradialis. There, identify the **superficial branch of the radial nerve** (*Atlas*, 6.59). Follow the nerve proximally to the point where it arises from the radial nerve. Note that the **radial nerve** divides into its two end branches: **superficial branch** and **deep branch.** The deep branch and its relations will be examined later.

Pick up the **brachial artery.** Trace it to its subdivision into **ulnar and radial arteries** (*Atlas*, 6.81). Close to the origin of the radial artery, look for the radial recurrent artery. It is part of the anastomotic network around the elbow (*Atlas,* 6.63). Follow the radial artery inferiorly to the wrist. Look for muscular branches (*Atlas,* 6.81). Note: no motor nerve crosses the radial artery. Therefore, the course of the artery indicates a convenient "internervous line" where surgeons may incise to reach deeper parts of the forearm.

Pick up the **median nerve.** It supplies most muscles of the flexor region of the forearm (*Atlas,* 6.11A). Observe that these branches arise from the medial side of the median nerve (*Atlas,* 6.81, 6.83). Study a transverse section through the forearm (Fig. 6.14; *Atlas,* 6.122A). Correlate your anatomical observations with a transverse MRI of the forearm (*Atlas,* 6.122B). Understand that the median nerve runs in the plane between deep and superficial flexors. Therefore, in order to expose the median nerve, the superficial flexor muscles must be reflected. This is the next objective.

Cut the tendon of **palmaris longus** about 3 cm proximal to the wrist. Sever the **flexor carpi radialis** tendon about 5 cm proximal to the wrist. Reflect the muscles and tendons. Now, the **flexor digitorum superficialis** (sublimis) is fully exposed (*Atlas,* 6.81). Pull on its four tendons and observe that the middle phalanges of fingers 2 to 5 are flexed. Realize that the flexor digitorum superficialis is attached to the common flexor origin and to the anterior oblique line of the radius (*Atlas,* 6.77, 6.81). With scissors, carefully detach the superficialis from the radius. Reflect the muscle medially. Identify the **pronator teres.** Understand why it can pronate (*Atlas,* 6.77, 6.78A). Divide the muscle close to its insertion into the radius. Observe the **median nerve** clinging to the deep surface of the flexor digitorum superficialis. Free the nerve completely, and identify its muscular branches to palmaris longus, flexor carpi radialis, flexor digitorum superficialis, and pronator teres. Identify the ulnar nerve and follow it proximally to the elbow joint. Verify that the ulnar nerve sends a motor branch to the flexor carpi ulnaris (*Atlas,* 6.83, 6.84).

With the superficialis reflected, study the **ulnar artery** and its main branches (*Atlas,* 6.81, 6.83). First, establish the continuity of the ulnar artery from cubital fossa to wrist. Note that the vessel passes deep to the flexor digitorum superficialis to reach the ulnar (medial) side of the forearm. Refer to a diagram (*Atlas,* 6.7). Study the distribution of the **common interosseous artery.** Identify this vessel in the cadaver (*Atlas,* 6.76C, 6.83). The **anterior interosseous artery** descends on the anterior surface of the interosseous membrane. It gives off branches to the deep flexors and nutrient branches to the bones. Arterial twigs pierce the interosseous membrane to supply the extensors. The **posterior interosseous artery** reaches the posterior aspect of the forearm and the extensor muscles (*Atlas,* 6.122A). Identify the interosseous arteries (*Atlas.* 6.83).

Occasionally (in about 3% of cases), the ulnar artery arises high from the brachial artery. When it does so, it runs almost invariably superficial to the flexor muscles (*Atlas,* 6.58). The artery may be mistaken for a vein. If certain drugs are injected into this vessel, the result may be disastrous: gangrene with subsequent partial or total loss of the hand.

The ulnar artery is joined by the **ulnar nerve** (*Atlas,* 6.81, 6.83). Once more, follow the nerve proximally and observe that it passes deep to the junction of the two heads of the flexor carpi ulnaris. Note the motor branch to the flexor carpi ulnaris. Verify that the ulnar nerve lies in a groove between the olecranon and the medial epicondyle (*Atlas,* 6.64, 6.66). Here, the nerve is covered only by skin and fascia. In yourself, palpate the nerve. Understand the meaning of the popular term "funny bone."

Identify the **supinator muscle** (it belongs to the extensor group). The muscle arises mainly from the radial collateral ligament. It is inserted into the lateral aspect of the radius (*Atlas,* 6.77, 6.84). Verify that the **posterior interosseous nerve** (deep branch of radial nerve) pierces the supinator (*Atlas,* 6.59, 6.83). Subsequently, the nerve reaches the posterior aspect of the forearm to supply extensor muscles (*Atlas,* 6.114, 6.122A).

Study the **three deep flexor muscles of the forearm: flexor digitorum profundus, flexor pollicis longus, and pronator quadratus** (*Atlas,* 6.83, 6.84). Pull on the tendon of the profundus; observe the resulting flexion of the distal phalanges of digits 2 to 5. Pull on the tendon of the flexor pollicis longus; observe the resulting flexion of the distal phalanx of the 1st digit (thumb). The pronator quadratus runs transversely from ulna to radius in the inferior quarter of the forearm (*Atlas,* 6.78D, 6.99). Identify it.

Review the major arteries in the anterior forearm (*Atlas,* 6.7) and the nerve supply to the flexor muscles (*Atlas,* 6.11A and B). Note that the flexor digitorum profundus receives a dual supply from both the median nerve and the ulnar nerve. Review the layers of the anterior forearm muscles (*Atlas,* 6.78).

The next objective is to follow tendons, nerves, and arteries from the forearm into the palm of the hand.

Palm of the Hand

General Remarks

There are two superficial muscle masses in the hand: the **thenar group** forming the ball of the thumb, and the **hypothenar musculature** forming the ball of the little (5th) finger. In the middle of the palm is a thick fibrous sheet, the palmar aponeurosis (*Atlas,* 6.79). Deep to the palmar aponeurosis are the tendons of the deep and superficial digital flexors. These tendons reach the palm through the carpal tunnel. Deep in the palm is a series of small muscles.

The palm is supplied with blood by two arterial arches: the superficial arch is mainly derived from the ulnar artery and the deep arch from the radial artery (*Atlas,* 6.10, 6.96). The nerve supply of the palmar (or volar) aspect of the hand is derived from the median and ulnar nerves (*Atlas,* 6.11A and B).

Important Landmarks

Refer to an articulated skeleton of the hand. As a group, identify the **eight carpal bones** (Fig. 6.17). Distal to the

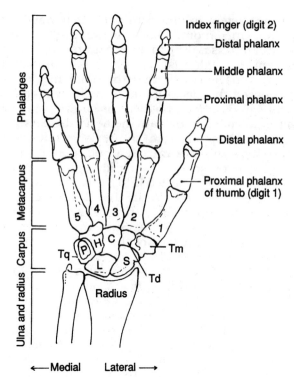

Figure 6.17. Important bony landmarks of the hand. The eight carpal bones include four distal bones (*H*, hamate; *C*, capitate; *Td*, trapezoid; *Tm*, trapezium) and four proximal bones (*Tq*, triquetrum; *P*, pisiform; *L*, lunate; *S*, scaphoid).

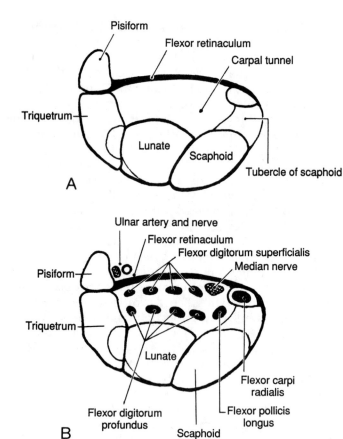

Figure 6.18. Transverse section through the carpal tunnel and its contents at the level of the proximal row of carpal bones. **A**, empty carpal tunnel; **B**, contents of carpal tunnel and related structures.

carpus (Gr. *karpos*, wrist) are the **five metacarpal bones.** Distal to the metacarpals are the **phalanges.** The thumb (digit 1) has only two phalanges: a proximal one and a distal one. Fingers 2 through 5 have three phalanges: proximal, middle, and distal (Fig. 6.17; *Atlas*, 6.130).

Be able to **identify the eight carpal bones** in the articulated skeleton (Fig. 6.17). Identify the **pisiform bone** and the **hook of the hamate** on the medial side of the carpus. On the lateral side of the carpus, identify the **tubercle of the scaphoid** and the **tubercle of the trapezium.** These bony landmarks on both sides of the carpus are bridged by a thick fibrous band, the **flexor retinaculum (transverse carpal ligament).** Between carpal bones and flexor retinaculum is an important space, the **carpal tunnel** (Fig. 6.18**A**; *Atlas*, 6.128). The carpal tunnel contains the median nerve and several tendons (*Atlas*, 6.126).

Realize that the **scaphoid** and **lunate** are supported by the radius (Fig. 6.17; *Atlas*, 6.139). By necessity, any transmission of force from hand to forearm or vice versa must pass through these two carpal bones. This is a fact of clinical significance. Study a radiograph of the hand (*Atlas*, 6.131).

Before you begin ...

The palmar aponeurosis and the flexor retinaculum will be examined. The ulnar nerve and artery will be traced into the palm. The carpal tunnel will be opened and its contents, the median nerve and the long flexor tendons, will

be followed into the palm and on to the digits. Subsequently, the long flexor muscles will be severed and reflected distally. This procedure will allow convenient access to the deep structures of the palm (muscles, deep palmar arch, and deep branch of ulnar nerve).

Dissection

Identify the **palmaris longus muscle** (*Atlas*, 6.80, 6.87). It is absent in about 14% of cases. Follow the palmaris longus tendon distally into the palm and into the palmar aponeurosis. Clean the **palmar aponeurosis** (*Atlas*, 6.79). Observe four longitudinal bands of aponeurosis, one to each finger.

> Nodular and fibrotic changes of the palmar aponeurosis may lead to a pulling down of one or more fingers via the longitudinal bands of the aponeurosis. This condition is known as Dupuytren's contracture.

Lateral to the palmar aponeurosis observe the thenar fascia enveloping the **thenar muscles.** The **palmaris**

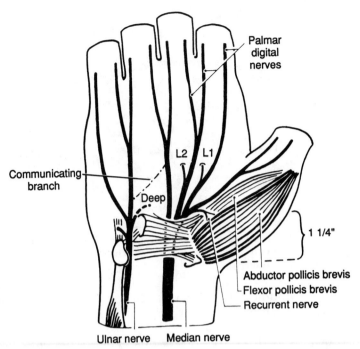

Palmar
digital
nerves

Communicating
branch

Deep

L2 L1

1 1/4"

Abductor pollicis brevis
Flexor pollicis brevis
Recurrent nerve

Ulnar nerve   Median nerve

Figure 6.19. Essential nerves of the hand: median and ulnar nerves (*L1* and *L2*, lumbrial branches of median nerve).

brevis muscle arises from the medial aspect of the aponeurosis (*Atlas*, 6.79, 6.88). Identify it.

Carefully remove the palmar aponeurosis. Do not damage nerves and blood vessels deep to it (*Atlas*, 6.88, 6.90). Detach the palmaris brevis from the palmar aponeurosis and reflect it medially. Now, the ulnar artery and nerve can be freely followed into the palm.

Study the arteries of the **superficial palmar arch** (*Atlas*, 6.7, 6.10, 6.96). Identify the pisiform bone and verify that the ulnar artery and nerve lie lateral to it (anatomical position). Follow the **ulnar artery** into the palm (*Atlas*, 6.90). Dissect the superficial palmar arch and the digital arteries springing from it. Subsequently, dissect the **ulnar nerve**. Clean its **superficial branch**, which supplies the 5th and the medial part of the 4th finger (Fig. 6.19; *Atlas*, 6.91, 6.92). The **deep branch of the ulnar nerve** disappears under cover of two of the hypothenar muscles (*Atlas*, 6.91). Identify its initial portion. Realize that it passes deep into the hand (*Atlas*, 6.99). Do not trace the deep branch of the ulnar nerve at this time.

Review the flexor retinaculum and its role in the formation of the carpal tunnel (Fig. 6.18). Identify the **flexor retinaculum** (*Atlas*, 6.84, 6.91, 6.93). Push a probe deep to the retinaculum through the **carpal tunnel**. With a scalpel, cut through the retinaculum down onto the probe. This procedure will prevent injury to the contents of the carpal tunnel. Examine the contents of the carpal tunnel. It consists of the median nerve and several digital flexor tendons (Fig. 6.18B). Examine the extent of the synovial tendon sheaths deep to the retinaculum (*Atlas*, 6.93). The synovial sheaths can be more clearly demonstrated if phenol or water is injected; check with your instructor.

Carefully dissect the **median nerve** and its branches (Fig. 6.19; *Atlas*, 6.92). Trace the small but important **recurrent branch of the median nerve** to the thenar muscles (*Atlas*, 6.90, 6.91). The only two other muscles supplied by the median nerve in the hand are the 1st and 2nd lumbricals. Attempt to locate these two small muscular branches (*Atlas*, 6.91). Subsequently, follow the **digital branches** of the median nerve to the first 3½ digits. Study the cutaneous nerve supply of hand and fingers. Be aware of variations. Consult a useful diagram (*Atlas*, 6.112, 6.113).

> The recurrent branch of the median nerve lies superficial (*Atlas*, 6.87). Therefore, it can be easily severed during "minor" cuts. If the nerve is injured, the thenar muscles are paralyzed and the thumb loses much of its usefulness. In the emergency room, never belittle superficial cuts over the thenar region. Always test the thenar muscles to make sure the important recurrent branch of the median nerve is intact.

Thenar muscles (Gr., *thenar*, hand). Examine the three thenar muscles (*Atlas*, 6.90, 6.91):

1. **Abductor pollicis brevis** (L. *pollex*, thumb; genitive, *pollicis*); raise the superficial muscle; sever it in the middle (*Atlas*, 6.91);
2. **Opponens pollicis**; deep to the severed abductor;
3. **Flexor pollicis brevis**; note the recurrent branch of the median nerve crossing over it;

Hypothenar muscles (*Atlas*, 6.90, 6.91). Identify:

1. **Abductor digiti quinti**, arising from the pisiform bone;
2. **Opponens digiti quinti**;
3. **Flexor digiti quinti**, sometimes absent.

Clean the **fibrous digital sheaths** of the tendons (Fig. 6.20; *Atlas*, 6.93, 6.94, 6.99). Understand that the fibrous digital sheath and the phalangeal bones together form an *osseofibrous digital tunnel*. In this tunnel, the long flexor tendons are housed (Figs. 6.20, 6.21; *Atlas*, 6.99, 6.124).

Turn your attention to the long flexor tendons that traverse the carpal tunnel. Realize that these tendons are surrounded by synovial sheaths (*Atlas*, 6.93). These sheaths are lubricating devices. There are two sets of synovial sheaths:

1. **Common synovial sheath** (sac) of the palm, within the carpal tunnel, and extending proximally and distally to it;
2. **Digital synovial sheaths**, within the osseofibrous digital tunnels; in most cases, the digital sheath of the little finger and thumb are connected to the common synovial sheath of the palm (*Atlas*, 6.93).

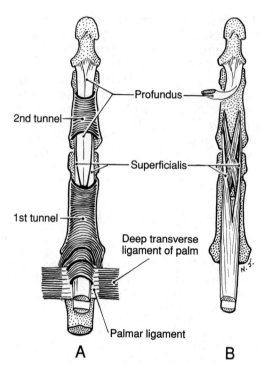

Figure 6.20. Long flexor tendons and their fibrous sheaths: **A**, fibrous digital flexor sheath showing the two osseofibrous tunnels; **B**, mode of insertion of the long digital flexors.

Frequently, bacterial infection involves the synovial sheaths (bacterial tenosynovitis). The constant movements of the tendons within the synovial sheaths further enhance the spread of infection. Understand that a minor infection of the 5th finger may spread along the flexor tendon sheath, involve the common synovial sheath in the palm, and finally reach the thumb.

A swelling of the common synovial sheath (as in the nonbacterial tenosynovitis) may encroach on the available space in the carpal tunnel. As a result, movements of the flexor tendons are interfered with and the median nerve may be compressed (carpal tunnel syndrome; pain and paresthesia of thumb, index finger, and middle finger; weakness of thenar muscles). With these clinical comments in mind, study again the contents of the carpal tunnel (Fig. 6.18B; *Atlas*, 6.126).

With your fingers, separate the **flexor digitorum superficialis** from the **profundus.** Cut across the fleshy part of the superficialis. Reflect the tendons distally. During this procedure, the common synovial sheath will be destroyed. In order to reflect the tendons even further, slit open the 1st osseofibrous tunnels of digits 2 through 5 (Fig. 6.20).

Now, the **flexor digitorum profundus** is exposed. Identify the four small **lumbrical muscles** originating from the profundus tendons (*Atlas*, 6.91, 6.93). Note that these muscles lie on the *radial* side of the corresponding digit. They insert into the dorsal or **extensor expansion** of the digits (*Atlas*, 6.100C and **D**). Thus, they flex the metacarpophalangeal joints and extend the interphalangeal joints. Know the nerve supply of the lumbricals (*Atlas*, 6.11A and **B**).

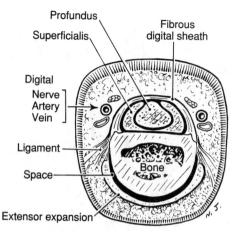

Figure 6.21. Transverse section of a finger. Note the osseofibrous digital tunnel with tendons in it. The digital nerves and vessels lie lateral to the tunnel.

On the middle digit, open the fibrous digital sheath. Study the interactions of the tendons of flexor digitorum superficialis and profundus (Fig. 6.20; *Atlas*, 6.85, 6.100C). Note that the profundus tendon pierces the superficialis tendon. Verify that the superficialis tendon acts on the middle phalanx, whereas the profundus tendon acts on the distal phalanx of fingers 2 through 5.

Now, identify the **flexor pollicis longus** (*Atlas*, 6.93, 6.95). Leave it intact. Follow the tendon proximally through the carpal tunnel into the forearm (*Atlas*, 6.84). Observe that it is supplied by a branch of the median nerve.

Cut across the fleshy fibers of the **flexor digitorum profundus.** Reflect its tendons and the associated lumbricals as far distally as possible. Now, the **pronator quadratus** is in full view, and the deep palmar space is exposed (*Atlas*, 6.99). This space is of surgical importance. Frequently, it is the site of infections that require surgical drainage.

Deep Structures in the Palm (*Atlas*, 6.95, 6.99). The first objective is to follow the deep branches of the ulnar nerve and artery deep into the palm. Detach the flexor digiti quinti from the flexor retinaculum (*Atlas*, 6.91). Push a probe parallel to the ulnar nerve and accompanying ulnar artery as they pierce the opponens digiti quinti. Carefully remove the muscle tissue in front of the nerve. Now, follow the **deep branch of the ulnar nerve** across the deep structures of the palm (*Atlas*, 6.99). Identify and clean the triangular **adductor pollicis** (*Atlas*, 6.95). This muscle draws the thumb toward the palm, a movement of considerable importance. Demonstrate the arteries of the **deep palmar arch** (*Atlas*, 6.95, 6.96).

Identify the *three palmar interossei* originating from the metacarpal bones of digits 2, 4, and 5 (*Atlas*, 6.99). Note that the palmar interossei are inserted into the bases of the proximal phalanges and into the dorsal expansions (*Atlas*, 6.100D). From the diagram in Figure 6.26, understand the actions of these muscles (Fig. 6.22; Atlas, 6.100A). They are adductors. They adduct the finger toward an imaginary line drawn through the long axis of the

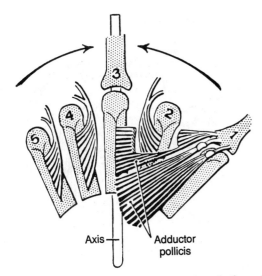

Figure 6.22. The three palmar interossei and the adductor pollicis.

middle finger. From the dissection, it is obvious that they are supplied by the ulnar nerve (*Atlas*, 6.99).

Review the movements of fingers and thumb. Define: flexion, extension, abduction, and adduction (Fig. 6.23). Which muscles are responsible for flexion? Which muscles are responsible for adduction of the fingers? Can you name the nerves that innervate the respective muscles? Review the motor branches of the median and ulnar nerves (*Atlas*, 6.11A and B).

Extensor Region of Forearm and Dorsum of Hand

General Remarks

The extensor muscles of the forearm can be divided into a superficial group and a deep group. The **superficial extensors** arise mainly on the lateral side of the elbow: from the lateral epicondyle, supracondylar ridge, and posterior border of the ulna (*Atlas*, 6.101, 6.102A and B). The tendons of these muscles reach across the posterior aspect of the wrist from side to side (*Atlas*, 6.103). They extend the carpus and the phalanges.

The **deep extensors** arise mainly from the ulna and the posterior aspect of the interosseous membrane (*Atlas*, 6.101, 6.102C). This deep layer is chiefly concerned with supination of the radius and reposition of the thumb into the anatomical position.

The extensors are supplied by the deep branch of the radial nerve, the posterior interosseous nerve (*Atlas*, 6.11D, 6.114). Nerve and vessels of the extensor compartment run in the plane dividing the superficial from the deep group (*Atlas*, 6.122A).

On the back of the hand, the bones are almost superficial. There are no fleshy extensor fibers here; accordingly, no motor nerve supply is required. The cutaneous nerve supply to the back of the hand is shared by the radial, ul-

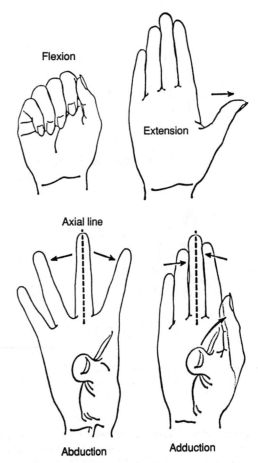

Figure 6.23. Movements of fingers and thumb.

nar, and median nerves (*Atlas*, 6.112). Variations in the pattern of the cutaneous nerve supply are common (*Atlas*, 6.113).

Before you begin . . .

First, the anatomical "snuff box" will be defined and studied. Next, the superficial posterior forearm muscles will be identified and their tendons will be followed distally. Subsequently, the deep (outcropping) extensor muscles will be studied.

Dissection

Anatomical "Snuff Box." Study its surface anatomy (*Atlas*, 6.117). Palpate it in a living person. Feel the pulsations of the radial artery within its boundaries. In the cadaver, define the tendons that constitute the boundaries of the anatomical snuff box (*Atlas*, 6.116B). The **abductor pollicis longus** and **extensor pollicis brevis** bound the snuff box anteriorly. The **extensor pollicis longus** bounds it posteriorly. These three tendons belong to muscles of the deep extensor group. Clean the tendons. Deep within the snuff box, find the **radial artery** (*Atlas*, 6.116B). Trace it distally to where it disappears between the two heads of

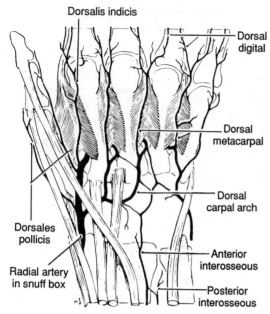

Figure 6.24. Dorsal interossei. Branches of radial artery on dorsum of hand.

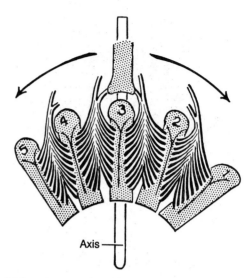

Figure 6.25. The four dorsal interossei. Abduction of fingers.

the **1st dorsal interosseous muscle.** Realize that small arteries exist on the dorsum of the hand, but do not dissect them (Fig. 6.24; *Atlas*, 6.104).

The deep fascia at the back of the wrist is thickened to form the **extensor retinaculum** (*Atlas*, 6.103). All tendons at the back of the wrist are enveloped in synovial sheaths; these extend distally and proximally to the extensor retinaculum (*Atlas*, 6.105).

Trace the three tendons bounding the anatomical snuff box proximally into the forearm. The fleshy bellies of the corresponding muscles crop out along a furrow that divides the extensors into a lateral and a medial group. Open this furrow as far as the lateral epicondyle (*Atlas*, 6.114). In doing this, it is necessary to split the intermuscular septum between **extensor carpi radialis brevis** and **extensor digitorum.**

Identify the **supinator,** which is wrapped around the upper third of the radius (*Atlas*, 6.114). Proceed as follows: on the anterior aspect of the forearm (*Atlas*, 6.83), identify the deep branch of the radial nerve as it traverses the supinator. Push a probe along the nerve through the substance of the muscle. Turn the upper limb and look for the tip of the probe on the posterior aspect of the forearm (*Atlas*, 6.114). After traversing the supinator muscle, the deep branch of the radial nerve becomes the **posterior interosseous nerve.** This nerve sends motor branches to the extensor muscles. Once more, establish the continuity of the posterior interosseous nerve with the radial nerve in front of the elbow joint.

Muscles of the superficial extensor group (*Atlas*, 6.114). Identify, clean, and study the following muscles:

1. Lateral to the outcropping of muscles of the anatomical snuff box find the **brachioradialis, extensor carpi radialis longus,** and **extensor carpi radialis brevis.**

2. Medial to the outcropping muscles of the anatomical snuff box find the **extensor digitorum, extensor digiti minimi,** and **extensor carpi ulnaris.**

Follow the flattened tendons of the **extensor digitorum** right to their insertions. Note their cross connections on the back of the hand (*Atlas*, 6.105, 6.107). Cut through the extensor retinaculum, thus freeing the tendons of the extensor digitorum. Retract the tendons medially.

Now, the five muscles of the **deep extensor group** can be studied in their entirety (*Atlas*, 6.114). These are: the three muscles bounding the snuff box (abductor pollicis longus; extensor pollicis brevis; extensor pollicis longus), the **supinator,** and the **extensor indicis** (i.e., the extensor for the 2nd or index finger).

Note that the tendons of the extensor muscles are contained in special tunnels between the bones of the forearm and the extensor retinaculum (*Atlas*, 6.106).

Check with your instructor whether or not you are required to dissect the **dorsal interossei muscles.** Note that these muscles occupy the intervals between the metacarpal bones (Fig. 6.24, *Atlas*, 6.103, 6.107). Remove the fascia covering the muscles. Follow the thin tendons of the dorsal interossei muscles into the extensor expansion (*Atlas*, 6.100C and D). Understand the action of the muscles (Fig. 6.25; *Atlas*, 6.100B). They abduct the fingers from an imaginary line drawn through the axis of the middle finger. The dorsal interossei are supplied by the ulnar nerve (*Atlas*, 6.11B, 6.99).

The four dorsal interossei abduct (*Atlas*, 6.100B). The three palmar interossei adduct (*Atlas*, 6.100A). All seven interossei are supplied by the ulnar nerve (*Atlas*, 6.11B). That means: if the ulnar nerve is paralyzed, abduction and adduction of the fingers is impossible.

Review the insertions of flexor and extensor tendons into metacarpal bones and phalanges (Fig. 6.26). Note that the strongest extensor tendons (extensor carpi radialis longus; extensor carpi radialis brevis; extensor carpi ulnaris) are inserted into the metacarpal bones (*Atlas*,

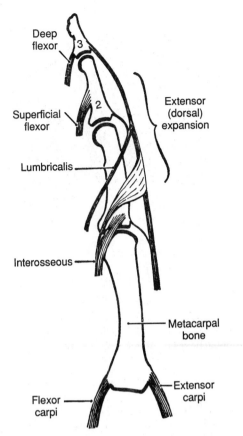

Figure 6.26. Insertions of tendons into metacarpal bone and phalanges of digit (lateral view).

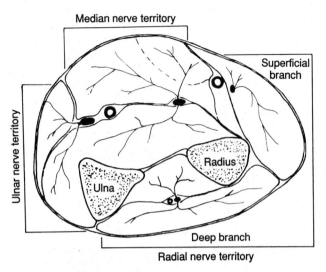

Figure 6.27. Nerve territories of the forearm.

6.101). These three extensors of the wrist are the strongest because they work synergistically with the flexors of the digits. Understand and test on yourself: the firmly grasping hand requires an extended wrist (*Atlas*, 6.120, 6.121). Review the extensor (dorsal) expansion of a finger (*Atlas*, 6.109).

Review the **nerve territories** of the forearm (Fig. 6.27; *Atlas*, 6.115). The **ulnar nerve** supplies the flexor carpi ulnaris and the ulnar half (medial half) of the flexor digitorum profundus. The **median nerve** innervates the superficial and deep flexor muscles. The **radial nerve** supplies its territory with a superficial branch and a deep branch (posterior interosseous nerve). Finally, review the motor nerve distribution to the entire upper limb (*Atlas*, 6.11).

Read an account of the lymphatic drainage of the upper limb. Lymph vessels from the radial side of the hand and forearm drain directly into the axillary nodes. Some lymph channels from the ulnar side of the hand and forearm may drain into the cubital lymph nodes (located at the medial side of the cubital fossa) and from there into axillary nodes. Lymphangitis (i.e., inflammation of lymph vessels, as a result of an infection of the hand, for example) is characterized by red streaks in the skin leading proximally toward the axilla.

Joints of the Upper Limb

General Remarks

It is advantageous to dissect the joints in only one upper limb. Keep the soft structures of the other limb intact for review purposes.

Refer to the articulated bones of the upper limb. Identify the following joints (*Atlas*, 6.1).

1. Sternoclavicular joint;
2. **Shoulder joint;**
3. **Elbow joint;**
4. Radioulnar joints (proximal, intermediate, distal);
5. **Wrist joint** (radiocarpal joint);
6. Joints of the digits.

If time is limited, dissect at least the following joints: **shoulder joint, elbow joint,** and **wrist joint.** If time permits, refer to the appendix regarding the dissection of smaller joints.

Shoulder Joint

Review the bony features pertinent to the **shoulder joint** (*Atlas*, 6.1). Remove the coracobrachialis, the short head of the biceps brachii, and the long head of the triceps. Clean the insertion of the subscapularis. Once again, observe that the tendons of the supraspinatus, infraspinatus, and teres minor muscles blend with the joint capsule (*Atlas*, 6.37). Cut these muscles.

The **fibrous capsule** is now completely exposed, except in front where the subscapularis remains intact. Verify that the capsule is attached just proximal to the glenoid

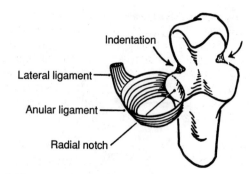

Figure 6.28. Anular ligament and radial notch of ulna form socket for head of radius.

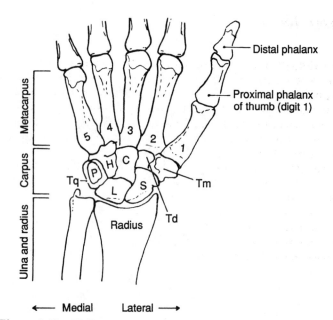

Figure 6.29. Wrist joint or radiocarpal joint is concerned with movements between radius and carpus. The eight carpal bones include four distal bones (*H*, hamate; *C*, capitate; *Td*, trapezoid; *Tm*, trapezium) and four proximal bones (*Tq*, triquetrum; *P*, pisiform; *L*, lunate; *S*, scaphoid).

cavity. On the humerus, it is attached to the anatomical neck (*Atlas*, 6.40, 6.47, 6.53).

Remove the posterior portion of the joint capsule (*Atlas*, 6.53). With a probe, explore the extent of the **synovial cavity** (*Atlas*, 6.46, 6.47). With a saw or a hammer and chisel, remove the head of the humerus. Now, identify the following structures (*Atlas*, 6.50, 6.53).

1. **Glenoid cavity;** around its margin, note a fibrocartilaginous rim, the **glenoid labrum;**
2. Three bands reinforcing the front of the joint capsule, the **glenohumeral ligaments;** they converge on the supraglenoid tubercle;
3. **Tendon of long head of biceps.**

Define and clean the strong **coracoacromial ligament** from the coracoid process to the acromion (*Atlas*, 6.46). This ligament, together with acromion and coracoid process, forms a continuous ligamentous and bony protection, the **coracoacromial arch.** It prevents upward displacement of the head of the humerus. Finally, study radiographic images of the shoulder (*Atlas*, 6.54).

Elbow Joint

Review the bony features of the elbow region (*Atlas*, 6.67). In the articulated skeleton, verify that the joint consists of three different portions:

1. The portion between the trochlea of the humerus and the trochlear notch of the ulna; it is a simple hinge joint (flexion and extension);
2. The portion between the capitulum of the humerus and the head of the radius; it is a gliding joint;
3. The portion between the circumference of the head of the radius and the radial notch of the ulna; rotation of the radius takes place here.

Turn to the cadaver. Remove the soft structures crossing the elbow joint. Dissect the brachialis off the capsule. Remove the triceps from the back of the thin capsule. Detach the tricipital aponeurosis from the olecranon. Re-

move the superficial flexor muscles of the forearm from the medial epicondyle.

On the medial side of the elbow joint, free the **ulnar collateral ligament** (*Atlas*, 6.75A). Observe that it consists of a strong anterior cord and a weaker posterior fan-like portion. Define the attachments of the ligament to humerus and ulna.

On the lateral side, detach the extensor muscles from their common tendon of origin. Remove the supinator. Expose the **radial collateral ligament** (*Atlas*, 6.75B). It fans out from the lateral epicondyle to the anular ligament of the radius.

The **anular ligament** encircles the head of the radius. It is in circumferential continuity with the radial notch of the ulna (Fig. 6.28; *Atlas*, 6.73). Note that the radius can freely rotate in the anular ligament. Place the hand in the pronated position (radius and ulna crossed). Now, pull on the remains of the biceps tendon, which is attached to the radial tuberosity. Note the strong supinating action of the biceps brachii.

Open the joint capsule anteriorly by making a transverse cut through the capsule between the ulnar and radial collateral ligaments. With a probe, explore the extent of the **synovial capsule** (*Atlas*, 6.72). Pass the probe (within the capsule) between the head of the radius and the anular ligament. Observe the smooth articular surfaces of the humerus, ulna, and radius. Notice the thin synovial fold and fatpads intervening between the head of the radius and the capitulum of the humerus. This fatpad may give radiologists a clue as to possible fractures in the elbow region. Review a transverse section through the elbow joint (*Atlas*, 6.74). Study radiographic images of the elbow region (*Atlas*, 6.68 through 6.71).

Wrist Joint

By definition, the **wrist joint or radiocarpal joint** is concerned with the movements between the **radius** and the **carpus.** Review the carpal bones (Fig. 6.29; *Atlas*, 6.130). Note that the distal end of the radius has two joint surfaces for two carpal bones. In the articulated skeleton, observe that the radius articulates with the **scaphoid** and **lunate** (*Atlas*, 6.138, 6.139).

Turn to the cadaver. Remove all soft structures crossing the wrist. On the anterior (palmar) aspect, observe a number of **radiocarpal ligaments** that hold radius and carpus together (*Atlas*, 6.133).

Force the hand backward (extend). Cut through the radiocarpal ligaments, and open the radiocarpal joint transversely (*Atlas*, 6.135). Leave the hand attached to the forearm by the dorsal part of the joint capsule.

Identify the smooth proximal surfaces of the **scaphoid, lunate, and triquetrum** (*Atlas*, 6.135). Study the corresponding articular surfaces of the radius and the articular disc. Verify that the **articular disc** holds the distal ends of the radius and the ulna firmly together. Understand that the articular disc forms part of the wrist joint. Note that it articulates with the triquetrum when adducted.

Correlate your anatomical observations with radiographs and magnetic resonance images (MRIs) of the hand and wrist (*Atlas*, 6.131, 6.132).

Perform the **principal movements** possible at the wrist joint: *flexion, adduction, extension,* and *abduction.* Carry out a *circumduction* by combining these movements in a consecutive fashion. Observe the articular surfaces during these movements.

CHAPTER 7

THE HEAD AND NECK

Front of Skull and Face

General Remarks

Developmentally, the facial muscles of expression and the muscles of the scalp originate from the right and left *2nd* branchial arches. The nerve associated with the 2nd arch is the **facial nerve or cranial nerve VII.** This nerve innervates all muscles derived from the second arch including the facial muscles of expression, muscles of the scalp and external ear, and the platysma. The facial muscles are subcutaneous. Most of their fibers are inserted into the skin. They not only express a variety of emotions, but also act as sphincters and dilators for orifices (mouth; nostrils; orbits).

The nerve of the *1st* branchial arch is the **trigeminal nerve or cranial nerve V.** It supplies the muscles of mastication which are derived from the first arch. However, the main part of the trigeminal nerve is sensory. Each of the three **divisions** of the trigeminal nerve (V^1, V^2, V^3) supplies an area of skin in the facial region (Fig. 7.1; *Atlas*, 7.8). In general, these areas of skin may be mapped out by drawing two lines: (a) from the nose across the lateral angle of the eye; and (b) from the corner of the mouth to a point about midway between eye and ear. The central V-shaped region (forehead, eyes, nose) is supplied by the **1st or ophthalmic division** of the trigeminal nerve (V^1). The intermediate area (cheek) is that of the **2nd or maxillary division** (V^2). The lower part of the face (mandibular region) is supplied with sensory fibers from the **3rd or mandibular division** (V^3).

Bony Landmarks

Warning: Handle the skull with great care. Never hold a skull by placing your fingers into the orbital cavities. Their medial walls are paper thin. They are very easily broken.

Orientation: Anatomists have agreed to examine skulls in the following position: The lower margins of the orbital apertures and the

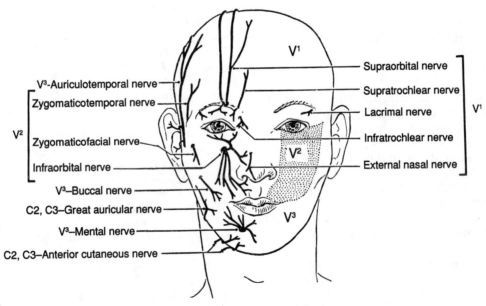

Figure 7.1. Sensory nerves of the face.

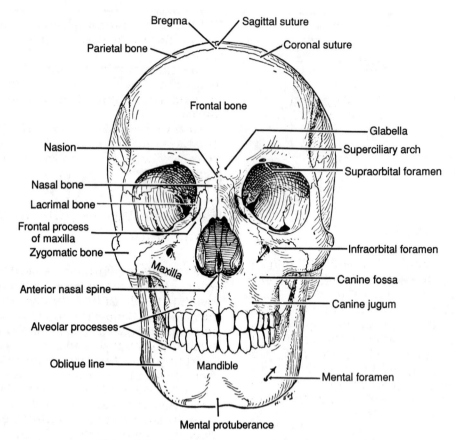

Figure 7.2. Skull on anterior view (norma frontalis).

upper margins of the external acoustic (auditory) canals lie on a horizontal plane. This position approximates very closely the anatomical position.

Skull on Frontal View (Norma Frontalis).   Examine the front of a skull. Identify the following landmarks (Fig. 7.2; *Atlas*, 7.1):

1. **Frontal bone;**
2. **Maxilla;** it has a *frontal process* that joins the frontal bone;
3. **Zygomatic bone;**
4. **Mandible;**
5. **Anterior nasal aperture** (piriform aperture); define its borders: two *nasal bones* superiorly; two *maxillae* laterally and inferiorly; *anterior nasal spine* of maxilla positioned inferiorly in the median plane;
6. **Nasion,** the depression at the root of the nose;
7. **Superciliary arch** (ridge);
8. **Glabella,** the smooth eminence above the nasion and between the superciliary arches;
9. **Entrance to the orbit;** each of three bones (frontal; maxillary; zygomatic) forms approximately one-third of the orbital margin;
10. **Lacrimal bone;** positioned at the anterior part of the medial orbital wall; together with the frontal process of the maxilla, it forms the **lacrimal fossa** (*Atlas*, 7.43); the lacrimal fossa is continuous inferiorly with

the **nasolacrimal canal;** gently push a flexible wire through the canal into the nasal cavity;
11. **Teeth** (*Atlas*, 7.91B, 7.94); if fully developed, the adult has 32 permanent teeth, 16 in the upper jaw (maxilla), and 16 in the lower jaw (mandible); the roots of the teeth are embedded in the **alveolar processes.**

Briefly familiarize yourself with the primary or deciduous teeth (temporary; milk teeth). At the end of the 2nd year, there are normally 20 teeth, 10 in each jaw (*Atlas*, 7.96, 7.97).

Lateral Aspect of Skull (Norma Lateralis).   Examine the lateral aspect of the skull. The following bony landmarks are of immediate interest (*Atlas*, 7.2):

1. **Mandible;** identify its **body, ramus, angle,** and **posterior border;** the condylar process consists of the constricted **neck** and the **articular condyle or head;**
2. **Temporomandibular joint (TMJ),** between head of mandible and a fossa on the temporal bone;
3. **External auditory meatus** (canal), which is part of the temporal bone;
4. **Zygomatic arch;** it is formed by two bony processes, the zygoma of the temporal bone and the temporal process of the zygomatic bone; note the suture line in the anterior third of the arch;
5. **Coronal suture;** it separates the frontal from the parietal bones.

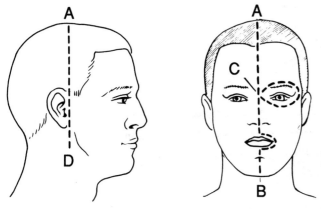

Figure 7.3. Skin incisions.

Correlate the bony landmarks of the skull with appropriate radiographs. Realize that the radiographic images of several bony structures may be superimposed. For example, in a lateral view (*Atlas*, 7.3**B**), right and left structures are more or less superimposed, depending on the accuracy of positioning and the direction of the x-ray beam. In the posteroanterior (PA) view (*Atlas*, 7.3**A**), images of the posterior skull are superimposed with facial images. As you make progress and learn more about the bony details of the skull, refer back to these radiographs for correlation.

Before You Begin . . .

After reflection of the skin, the muscles of the face will be exposed. Branches of the facial nerve that are motor to these muscles will be identified as they emerge from the substance of the parotid gland. Two important sphincter muscles will receive particular attention: the orbicularis oris (mouth), and the orbicularis oculi (eye). The essential nerves responsible for the sensory supply of the facial skin will be exposed. Finally, the lacrimal apparatus will be explored.

Skin Incisions

Make the following skin incisions (Fig. 7.3):

1. In the midline, from vertex to chin (*A* to *B*); encircle the mouth at the margin of the lips.
2. Start at the nasion (*C*), widely encircle the orbital margins, and return to the nasion.
3. Make other incisions from the vertex, anterior to the ear, inferiorly to a point just posterior to the angle of the mandible (*A* to *D*).

First, reflect the skin between eyebrows and vertex. Notice that the skin is closely adherent to the thick and tough subcutaneous fascia. Leave this fascia intact; nerves and vessels run in it. Do *not* reflect the **frontalis muscle** (*Atlas*,

7.10). If the skin is raised without difficulty, you are probably in the areolar space deep to the frontalis and its aponeurosis.

The skin of the face is thin. There may be a considerable amount of subcutaneous fat. Reflect the skin carefully. Do not damage the underlying pale and inconspicuous facial muscles.

Observe the thin and loose skin of the eyelids. Remove the skin at the margins of the eyelids. Reflect the skin of the face inferior and parallel to the inferior border of the mandible.

Facial Nerve, Vessels, and Related Structures

The **platysma** (*Atlas*, 8.1) reaches as far inferiorly as the 2nd rib. Demonstrate the superior attachment of the muscle sheet to the inferior border of the mandible. Subsequently, cut the posterior part of the platysma along the inferior border of the mandible, and reflect it toward the angle of the mouth.

Identify the rhomboid **masseter muscle** that extends from the zygomatic arch to the ramus of the mandible (*Atlas*, 7.10). About 2.0 to 2.5 cm inferior to the zygomatic arch, the **parotid duct** crosses the lateral aspect of the masseter muscle (Fig. 7.4; *Atlas*, 7.10, 7.12). Identify the duct. It is empty, collapsed, and flattened like a piece of narrow white tape. Follow the parotid duct to the anterior border of the masseter. Here, the duct turns at a right angle to pierce the buccinator, the muscle of the cheek. Superior to the duct, find the **transverse facial artery** and the *zygomatic branch* of the **facial nerve** (*Atlas*, 7.10). Preserve the nerve. The artery, unless injected, is often difficult to trace.

The **parotid duct** opens into the oral cavity opposite the upper 2nd molar tooth. Usually, the opening is marked by a slight elevation of buccal mucosa, the **parotid papilla**. Palpate your own right or left parotid papilla with your tongue or your finger. Inspect the papilla in a fellow student. Realize that the parotid duct and the papilla transmit the saliva secreted by the parotid gland.

Facial Nerve (Fig. 7.4; *Atlas*, 7.12, 7.13). After its emergence at the base of the skull, the facial nerve turns anteriorly and traverses the substances of the parotid gland. Within the gland, the nerve divides into various branches that radiate to the facial muscles of expression. To find these nerve branches, proceed by following the parotid duct posteriorly to the point where it emerges from the **parotid gland.** This point is about 5 to 7 mm anterior to the posterior border of the mandible. Then raise the anterior border of the gland from the masseteric fascia. Find the white, flattened branches of the facial nerve issuing from the substance of the gland. Note that they run deep. They are separated from the masseter only by its fascia. Trace the nerve branches to the muscles they supply. The highest of these radiating branches, the *temporal branch*, crosses the zygomatic bone. The lowest branch, the *cervi-*

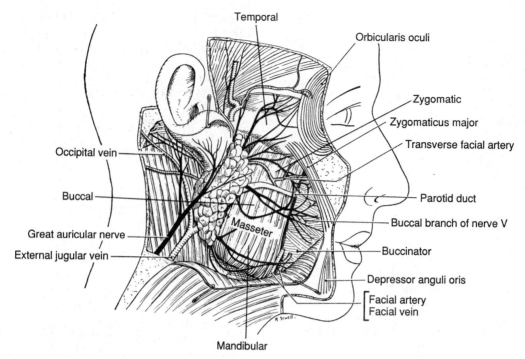

Figure 7.4. Dissection of the lateral aspect of the face.

cal branch, runs below the angle of the mandible. This branch sends twigs to the platysma (*Atlas*, 9.12B).

Define the free, anterior border of the **masseter** in its entire length. Anterior to the masseter is an extensive **buccal fatpad** (*Atlas*, 7.6). Remove this buccal fatpad in order to expose the underlying **buccinator muscle** (*Atlas* 7.12). Once again, verify that the **parotid duct** pierces the buccinator. Notice that two different nerves enter the substance of the buccinator:

1. The *buccal branch* of the **facial nerve**; it runs *lateral* to the masseter to supply the buccinator with motor fibers.
2. The **buccal branch of the trigeminal nerve (V³)**; it runs *medial* to the masseter. Observe its twigs (*Atlas*, 7.6, 7.12). The nerve does *not* supply the buccinator muscle. It merely pierces the muscle to send sensory fibers to the buccal mucosa of the vestibule of the mouth. (The buccal nerve also sends a small branch to the skin of the cheek (*Atlas*, 7.8)). This cutaneous branch was destroyed during the skinning process.

Facial Artery and Vein (*Atlas*, 7.10, 7.11). On yourself, palpate the pulse of the **facial artery**. This vessel crosses the mandible at the anterior border of the masseter. The accompanying **facial vein** lies posterior to the artery. Find these vessels in the cadaver. Trace the facial artery to the medial angle of the eye. In its course, the artery crosses successively the mandible, buccinator, and maxilla. Follow the vein to the medial angle of the eye.

Muscles of the Mouth

There are numerous muscles that alter the shape of the mouth and lips. Define the more important muscles (Fig. 7.5; *Atlas*, 7.6):

1. **Depressor anguli oris** (depresses corner of mouth; aided by the posterior fibers of the platysma);
2. **Zygomaticus major**, descending from zygomatic bone to corner of mouth (draws angle of mouth superiorly and posteriorly);
3. **Levator labii superioris**, descending from infraorbital margin to upper lip (elevates upper lip).
4. **Orbicularis oris**, the important sphincter muscle of the mouth. Demonstrate the circular arrangement of its muscle fibers. Realize that the orbicularis oris intimately blends with the fibers of the other muscles of the mouth. If time permits, demonstrate additional muscles of facial expression (*Atlas*, 7.6).

Clean the surface of the **buccinator** (*Atlas*, 7.62). Define its superior and inferior attachments to the outer surfaces of the alveolar processes of maxilla and mandible (*Atlas*, 7.63, 8.54, 8.55). Note that the buccinator fibers blend with the orbicularis oris.

With a probe, loosen the tissue deep to the levator labii superioris. Carefully cut horizontally through the muscle close to the infraorbital margin. Reflect the muscle inferior and thus expose the **infraorbital nerve** (*Atlas*, 7.6). Trace some of its branches to the inferior eyelid, side of the nose, and upper lip.

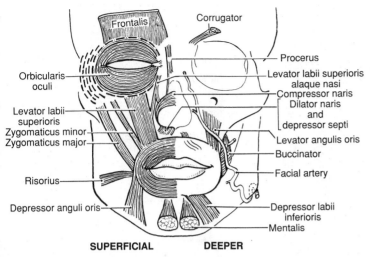

Figure 7.5. Muscles of the face.

Labels in figure: Frontalis, Corrugator, Procerus, Orbicularis oculi, Levator labii superioris alaque nasi, Compressor naris, Dilator naris and depressor septi, Levator labii superioris, Levator anguli oris, Zygomaticus minor, Buccinator, Zygomaticus major, Facial artery, Risorius, Depressor anguli oris, Depressor labii inferioris, Mentalis

SUPERFICIAL   DEEPER

Study the infraorbital foramen and canal in the skull. Pass a wire through the foramen into the canal. For purposes of local anesthesia, the infraorbital nerve is often infiltrated at the level of the foramen or in the canal. In the cadaver, palpate the foramen and push a probe through it.

Lower Lip, External Nose, and External Ear

Lower Lip. Make a midline incision through the entire thickness of the lower lip. Parallel to this incision, make a second vertical incision inferiorly from the angle of the mouth (do this on one side of the body only). Reflect the quadrangular piece of lip inferiorly. Cut through the mucous membrane along the line of its reflection from lips to gums. Dissect the mucous membrane from the underlying muscle fibers up to the red line of the lip.

Observe the small **labial glands** immediately deep to the mucous membrane. At the red line of the lip, see the **inferior labial artery** (the cut end of the artery may, of course, be seen in the cut edge of the flap). This artery is a branch of the facial artery. The nerve fibers that ascend in the flap are branches of the **mental nerve.** Now, strip the flap from the bone and locate the **mental foramen.** It is located approximately 3 cm from the median plane. Observe that the mental nerve traverses the foramen (*Atlas*, 7.6).

> The mental nerve is a branch of the inferior alveolar nerve (*Atlas*, 9.11A). The inferior alveolar nerve runs within the substance of the mandible. Dentists frequently anesthetize the inferior alveolar nerve and, therefore, also the mental nerve. The resulting local anesthesia of the mental nerve involves the region of the chin and the lower lip on the concerned side.

External Nose. The nose is held in shape by the **nasal cartilages** that consist of hyaline cartilage (Fig. 7.6; *Atlas*, 7.100). Palpate the inferior borders of the two nasal bones.

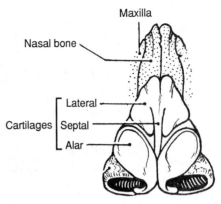

Figure 7.6. Framework of the external nose (anterior view).

Labels in figure: Maxilla, Nasal bone, Cartilages — Lateral, Septal, Alar

Adjacent to these bony borders, identify the paired **lateral nasal cartilages.** They are not independent structures, but merely triangular expansions of the large **septal cartilage.** This median, unpaired septal cartilage extends between the right and left nasal cavities. It forms the anterior part of the nasal septum (*Atlas*, 7.102B).

On each side of the septal cartilage is an **alar cartilage** (Fig. 7.6; *Atlas*, 7.100). These U-shaped cartilages are responsible for the formation of the nares (nostrils). Make a small midline incision at the tip of the nose. Separate the two alar cartilages from the septal cartilage. Follow the free inferior edge of the septal cartilage to the anterior nasal spine (*Atlas*, 7.102B).

External Ear (*Atlas*, 7.135). The external ear consists of the **auricle** and the **external acoustic meatus** (external ear canal). Examine the **auricle** and identify the following parts: *helix*, the prominent rim; *antihelix*, the curved prominence anterior to the helix; *tragus*, usually showing hairs on its medial surface; *lobule*, the characteristic shape of the auricle maintained by a single piece of elastic cartilage. There is no cartilage in the lobule.

You may not have enough time for a detailed dissection of the auricle, its cartilage, and its six tiny intrinsic muscles. Palpate the auricular cartilage on yourself. By palpation, verify that the cartilage is continuous with the cartilage of the external acoustic meatus.

Inspection of Eye and Eyelids

Inspect or palpate the living eye. Your own eye can be examined with the aid of a mirror. Identify the following structures (*Atlas*, 7.45):

1. **Palpebral commissures,** uniting the eyelids medially and laterally;
2. **Palpebral rima or fissure,** the opening between the lids;
3. **Medial and lateral angles (canthi)** of the fissure;
4. **Cornea,** the transparent anterior 1/6 of the outer coat of the eyeball;
5. **Sclera,** the whitish, opaque, posterior 5/6 of the outer coat of the eyeball;

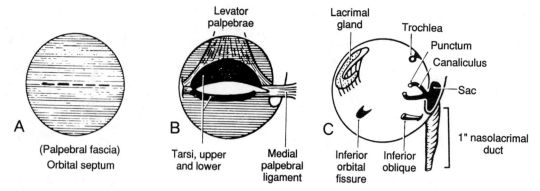

Figure 7.7. *A*, orbital septum; *B*, tarsi, ligaments, and levator palpebrae; *C*, the four corners of the orbital margin and the lacrimal apparatus (schematic).

6. **Iris,** the varied colored diaphragm seen through the cornea;
7. **Pupil,** the aperture in the center of the iris;
8. **Conjunctival sac,** the potential space between the eyeball and the eyelids (*Atlas,* 7.52);
9. **Conjunctiva,** the membrane lining the sac;
10. **Fornices** (L., *fornix,* arch; one fornix; two fornices), the regions of conjunctival reflection from the eyelid to the eyeball;
11. **Medial palpebral ligament,** a fibrous band deep to the medial commissure. It becomes conspicuous and palpable when the skin at the lateral commissure is pulled laterally (Fig. 7.7; *Atlas,* 7.6, 7.7).

Inspect the **margins of the eyelids** (*Atlas,* 7.45). The margins are flat and thick. They carry double or triple irregular rows of **eyelashes or cilia.** Observe the lack of cilia close to the medial angle of the eye. Posterior to the cilia are the pinpoint orifices of the **tarsal glands.** Examine the inner surfaces of the eyelids. Note yellowish streaks shining through the conjunctiva. These are the tarsal glands (*Atlas,* 7.52, 7.53).

Inspect the medial palpebral commissure (medial canthus). Here, the upper and lower lids are separated by a triangular space, the **lacus lacrimalis** (L., *lacus,* lake; *lacrima,* tear; "lake of tears"). The lacus contains a small reddish prominence, the **caruncula.** Focus your attention on the area where the base of the triangular lacus lacrimalis meets the eyelids. Here, on both eyelids, find a small elevation, the **lacrimal papilla.** Each papilla has a minute orifice, the **lacrimal punctum.** It is the opening of the **lacrimal canaliculus** that drains lacrimal fluid into the **lacrimal sac** (Fig. 7.7).

Dissection of Orbital Region

Dissect the circularly disposed fibers of the **orbicularis oculi** (Fig. 7.5; *Atlas,* 7.6, 7.9). Note that this sphincteric muscle consists of two parts: (a) a thick *orbital portion,* which surrounds the orbital margin and is responsible for the tight closure of the eye (*Atlas,* 7.9) and (b) a thin, pale *palpebral portion,* which is contained in the eyelids and is involved in the usual blinking of the eye. The orbicularis

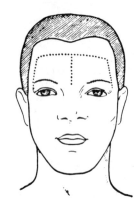

Figure 7.8. Muscle flaps to be reflected.

oculi originates from the medial part of the bony orbital margin and from the medial palpebral ligament. Raise the lateral part of the muscle and reflect it medially. Raise the thin palpebral portion off the underlying tarsus, and also turn it medially. Examine the **medial palpebral ligament** (Fig. 7.7; *Atlas,* 7.6). Its lower border is free. Fibers of the orbicularis oculi arise from its upper border.

The next objective is to reflect part of the frontalis muscle and to expose the supraorbital nerve. Proceed as follows (Fig. 7.8): from the nasion to a point 3 cm above the glabella, make a midline incision through *all* layers of the scalp right down to the bone. Subsequently, make three incisions, two parallel and one horizontal, as outlined in Figure 7.8. Reflect the quadrangular flap inferiorly.

In the flap, identify the following structures (*Atlas,* 7.6):

1. **Frontalis muscle,** interlacing with the orbicularis oculi;
2. **Supraorbital nerve (V[1]) and vessels.** These emerge from the **supraorbital foramen** (or notch).

Turn the flap inferiorly as far as the supraorbital margin and the medial palpebral ligament. Then, remove the flap entirely.

Now, examine the **orbital septum** (palpebral fascia). It is an oval membranous sheet that is attached to the margin of the orbit (Fig. 7.7A and **B**; *Atlas,* 7.6, 7.52). It is continuous with the periorbita (the periosteum of the orbital cavity).

Examine the tarsi (*Atlas*, 7.52, 7.53). Each **tarsus** is a condensed thickening of the orbital septum, designed to stiffen the eyelid. Evert the larger superior lid and study its free margin. Note the cilia. With the handle of the scalpel, stroke the posterior surface of the upper lid firmly toward its margin. This action will extrude secretions from the **tarsal glands.**

> There are about 20 to 30 **tarsal or Meibomian glands** in each tarsus. These are sebaceous glands that secrete an oily substance onto the free margin of the eyelids. This lipid prevents an overflow of lacrimal fluid under normal conditions.
>
> If the duct of a tarsal gland becomes obstructed, a cyst will develop. This is a **chalazion.** Understand that a chalazion will be located between tarsal plate and conjunctiva (*Atlas*, 7.53). The chalazion must he distinguished from a **hordeolum** (sty), which involves an inflammation of a small sebaceous gland around the follicle of a cilium.

Cut through the orbital septum in its superior lateral quadrant close to the orbital margin. Pass a probe through the incision. Keep the probe close to the bony orbital roof and free the **lacrimal gland** (*Atlas*, 7.6). Attempt to find some of the 6 to 10 ducts that connect the gland to the fornix of the upper part of the conjunctival sac (Fig. 7.7C; *Atlas*, 7.50).

The next objective is to study the structures that collect and drain the lacrimal fluid. Once again, refer to the bony skull and identify the **lacrimal fossa** for the **lacrimal sac** (*Atlas*, 7.43). Observe the *anterior crest* of the fossa. Understand that the **medial palpebral ligament** is attached to this crest. Consequently, the lacrimal sac lies just posterior to the ligament (Fig. 7.7; *Atlas*, 7.6). Turn to the cadaver. With a probe, puncture the lacrimal sac just below and posterior to the medial palpebral ligament. Explore the extent of the sac (*Atlas*, 7.44). Use a stiff wire or a thin probe and push the instrument downward within the sac. The instrument will traverse the **nasolacrimal duct** and enter the inferior meatus of the nose. Looking through the nostril on the corresponding side, you may or may not be able to see the tip of the probe (depending on the configuration of the nasal structures in each particular specimen).

Understand that the normal flow of lacrimal fluid is obliquely across the eye, from the ductules of the lacrimal gland, i.e., the lateral portion of the superior fornix to the medial angle (Fig. 7.7C). Excessive tear production and drainage via the nasolacrimal duct into the nose will induce the characteristic sniffing during crying.

Sensory Nerves of the Face

Review the sensory nerves of the face that are derived from the three divisions of the trigeminal nerve (Fig. 7.1; *Atlas*, 7.6, 7.8):

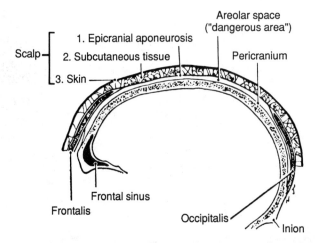

Figure 7.9. Sagittal section of the skull cap and overlying tissues.

1. **Supraorbital nerve,** a branch of the ophthalmic division (V^1);
2. **Infraorbital nerve,** a branch of the maxillary division, (V^2);
3. **Mental nerve,** a branch of the mandibular division, (V^3).

Note that the skin of the nose is supplied by the **external nasal nerve,** a branch of V^1. There are several smaller branches of the trigeminal nerve (*lacrimal; infratrochlear; zygomaticofacial; zygomaticotemporal*). Do not dissect these twigs. The auriculotemporal nerve (V^3) will be dissected later.

Scalp

General Remarks

The scalp is the covering of the cranial vault. It consists of three layers that are firmly bound together (Fig. 7.9; *Atlas*, 7.15):

1. **Skin,** usually covered with hair;
2. **Superficial fascia** (subcutaneous tissue), which is exceedingly tough and dense; vessels and nerves run in it;
3. **Muscular layer,** consisting of the **frontalis** anteriorly and the **occipitalis** posteriorly; the two muscles are united by a broad aponeurosis, the **galea aponeurotica or epicranial aponeurosis.**

The bones of the cranial vault are intimately covered with **pericranium** or periosteum. The pericranium is separated from the three layers of the scalp by a very **loose areolar tissue.** This loose areolar layer permits the frontalis and occipitalis muscles to produce a limited amount of movement.

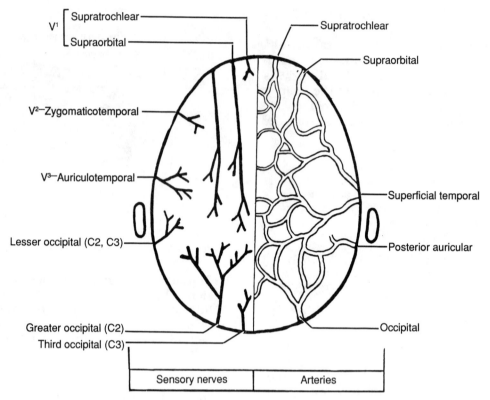

Figure 7.10. Sensory nerves and arteries of the scalp.

Blood vessels and sensory nerves reach the scalp from all around its periphery. These structures are contained in the exceedingly tough superficial fascia. You may not have time for the dissection of nerves and vessels in the scalp region. However, be aware of the fact that a rich nerve and blood supply exists (Fig. 7.10; *Atlas*, 7.14).

> The loose areolar layer between the scalp and the pericranium is of clinical importance. Once an infection has reached the loose layer, it can spread readily in it. Therefore, this layer has been called the "dangerous area" (Fig. 7.9; *Atlas*, 8.84). From the "dangerous area," the infection is easily carried along veins that traverse the bony vault. As a result, the infection may spread to the substance of the bones, to venous channels within the cranial cavity or to the brain. The physician must be aware of this fact and its anatomical basis.

Bony Landmarks

Refer to a skull and identify the following pertinent landmarks (*Atlas*, 7.1, 7.2):

1. **Nasion,** the depression at the root of the nose;
2. **Frontal bone;**
3. **Vertex,** the highest point on the calvaria or skull cap;
4. **Parietal bones;**

5. **Occipital bone;** note the **external occipital protuberance or inion;**
6. **Temporal bone with mastoid process;**
7. **Zygomatic arch,** jointly formed by processes of the temporal and zygomatic bones.

Skin Incisions

Make the following skin incisions (Fig. 7.11):

1. In the midline, from nasion (*A*) to vertex (*B*), and on to the external occipital protuberance (*C*);
2. On the right and left sides, from vertex to a point just above and in front of the ear (*B* to *D*);
3. On the right and left sides, from external occipital protuberance transversely to the mastoid process (*C* to *E*).

Dissection

Reflect the four flaps of scalp inferiorly. Do this by working in the loose areolar space ("dangerous area") with your fingers or the handle of the scalpel. On the side of the skull, reflect the scalp from the underlying **temporalis fascia,** which covers the temporalis muscle (*Atlas*, 7.62). At the level of the zygomatic arch and at the superior nuchal line, the loose areolar layer is closely adherent to bone (that means, infections of the scalp cannot readily spread beyond these areas).

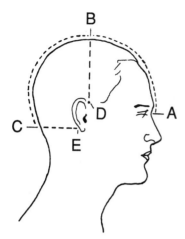

Figure 7.11. Skin incisions.

Realize that nerves and vessels are contained within the flaps of scalp. The **occipitalis muscle** is contained in the posterior flap. The anterior flap contains the **frontalis.** Examine the **galea aponeurotica,** which unites these two muscles (Fig. 7.9).

Next, observe the **pericranium** that intimately covers the skull cap. With a sharp instrument, scrape off the pericranium superior to the attachment of the temporalis fascia. Do not remove the temporalis fascia. Now, the **suture lines** separating the individual bones can be seen. In the cadaver and the bony skull, identify the following (*Atlas,* 7.2):

1. **Coronal suture,** separating the large unpaired frontal bone from the two parietal bones;
2. **Lambdoid suture,** separating the unpaired occipital bone from the two parietal bones;
3. **Sagittal suture,** separating the two parietal bones (*Atlas,* 7.31);
4. **Lambda,** the point where sagittal and lambdoid sutures meet;
5. **Bregma,** the point where sagittal and coronal sutures meet;

In the skull, identify the large unpaired frontal bone. Note the remains of the metopic or frontal suture extending a short distance superiorly from the nasion (*Atlas,* 7.1A). In about 2% of the population, the frontal bone of the adult is paired, as is normally the case in infants up to 2 years of age (*Atlas,* 7.4A). In the mentioned adult cases, the persisting frontal or metopic suture is of radiological importance. It must not be mistaken for a fracture line.

Interior of Skull

Removal of Skull Cap (Calvaria)

Refer to the bony skull. Remove the calvaria. Note that the bones of the roof of the skull consist of three parts: a compact *outer lamina*; a compact and very hard *inner lamina*; the *diploe*, a layer of spongy bone that is sandwiched in between the outer and inner laminae. The diploe contains diploic veins (*Atlas,* 7.16). Observe that there is no diploe in the temporal region where the bones are covered with the thick and fleshy temporalis muscle.

Return to the cadaver specimen. Pull the anterior half of the scalp well over the face and the posterior half well over the nuchal region. With a sharp scalpel, incise the temporalis fascia along the temporal lines (*Atlas,* 7.2B), i.e., incise it in a semicircular fashion along the superior and posterior margins of the temporalis muscle. Now, insert the handle of the scalpel between muscle and bones. Lift off the temporalis muscle. Reflect it inferiorly to the level of the zygomatic arch. Scrape the bones clean.

Place an elastic rubber band or a string around the circumference of the skull. Anteriorly, the band must be at least 2 cm above the supraorbital margin. Posteriorly, place the rubber band about 2 cm above the inion (external occipital protuberance). Use the band as a guide and encircle the calvaria with a pencil line.

With a saw, cut through the external lamina along the pencil line. During the sawing, turn the body alternately on the back or the face. Moist red bone indicates that the saw is well within the diploe. Be particularly careful on the sides where the bones are thin. If you saw through the inner table, you are liable to damage the underlying dura mater or even the brain. Therefore, break the inner table by repeatedly inserting a chisel into the saw cut and by striking the chisel gently with a mallet. Continue with this procedure until the calvaria can be pried loose. Remove the calvaria by gently detaching it from the dura mater. Use your fingers, the handle of a scalpel, or a pair of forceps. Do not use more force than necessary. Violent pulling will frequently result in tearing of the dura and in damage to the brain.

In 6% of all female specimens, the frontal bone is of unusual thickness. This condition is known as "hyperostosis frontalis."

Removal of Wedge of Occipital Bone

At this stage, the removal of a large wedge-shaped area of the occipital bone offers many advantages: The brain and its coverings can be more easily examined in situ. The superior sagittal and the transverse sinuses can be demonstrated in situ. After removal of the cerebellum, the brain stem and the cranial nerves emerging from it can be studied in situ. Finally, the removal of the brain is greatly facilitated.

Turn to the bony skull. Examine the landmarks pertinent to the removal of the bony wedge:

1. **Mastoid process;**
2. **Foramen magnum;**
3. **External occipital protuberance or inion;**
4. Examine the *internal surface* of the **occipital bone** (*Atlas,* 7.23, 7.35): **groove for superior sagittal sinus;**

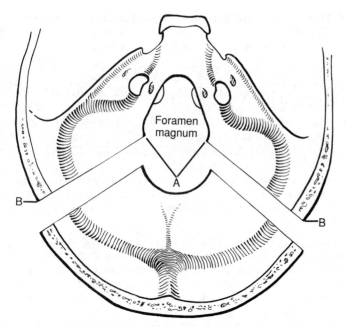

Figure 7.12. Large wedge removed from the occipital bone.

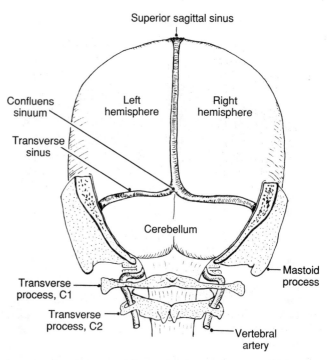

Figure 7.13. Calvaria and large wedge of the occipital bone removed. Dura mater and venous sinuses in posterior view (schematic).

grooves for right and left transverse sinuses; two fossae for cerebellum, inferior to the grooves for the transverse sinuses; **two fossae for the occipital poles** of the cerebral hemispheres, superior to the grooves for the transverse sinuses.

On the right and left side of the skull, identify two reference points. Identify (*A*) the lateral margin of the foramen magnum and (*B*) the point where the cut edge of the skull intersects with the lambdoid suture (suture between occipital and parietal bone). On the right and left sides, connect points (*A*) and (*B*) with pencil lines. You have now demarcated the wedge that is to be removed in the cadaver (Fig. 7.12).

Turn to the cadaver, which must be in the prone position (face down). Briefly review the suboccipital region (Chapter 4; *Atlas*, 4.56, 4.57). Detach all muscles from the occipital bone. Clearly identify the interval between **occipital bone** and **atlas** (C1).

Preserve the **vertebral arteries.** Using fine scissors, carefully incise the **posterior atlanto-occipital membrane** transversely from vertebral artery to vertebral artery.

Scrape the occipital bone clean of muscle remains and pericranium. With pencil lines, mark the bony wedge between points *A* and *B* as explained previously. Cut along these lines with a small saw (Hey's saw). As in the removal of the calvaria, do not cut through the inner compact layer of bone. Loosen the bony wedge with chisel and mallet. Carefully pry it loose from the moistened dura mater. Protect the vertebral arteries. Remove the wedge (Fig. 7.13).

Examine the inner surface of the removed bony wedge (*Atlas*, 7.23, 7.35). Verify that the two **cerebellar fossae** were in contact with the dura mater overlying the **cerebellum.** Demonstrate that the **grooves for the transverse sinuses** were in contact with these venous channels.

Meninges of Brain

The brain is covered with three membranes, the meninges (Gr., *meninx*, membrane). These are (Fig. 7.14; *Atlas*, 7.15):

1. **Dura mater,** the outer tough membrane;
2. **Arachnoid,** the intermediate membrane with spider-web-like processes toward the pia mater;
3. **Pia mater,** a soft delicate membrane that is closely applied to the brain tissue.

The *dura mater* (L., *dura*, hard) is also known as *pachymeninx* (Gr., *pachys*, thick). The two soft membranes, *arachnoid* and *pia mater*, are also collectively called *leptomeninx* (Gr., *leptos*, thin; delicate). The meninges of the brain are continuous with those covering the spinal cord (Chapter 4).

Dura mater (*Atlas*, 7.18). It consists of two layers:

1. A rough, outer layer; it was adherent to the cranial bones where it formed an endocranium (periosteal covering for the bone);
2. A smooth inner layer.

The two dural layers are indistinguishable except where they separate to enclose the venous sinuses.

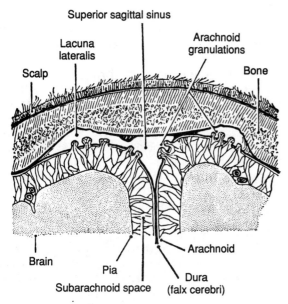

Superior sagittal sinus

Lacuna
lateralis

Arachnoid
granulations

Scalp

Bone

Brain

Pia

Arachnoid

Subarachnoid space

Dura
(falx cerebri)

Figure 7.14. Coronal section through the superior sagittal sinus and related structures.

Examine the rough, outer layer of the dura mater that covers the cerebral and cerebellar hemispheres. In the outer dural layer, observe the branches of the important **middle meningeal artery** (*Atlas*, 7.18). This vessel supplies the dura mater. The bulk of blood, however, reaches the adjacent cranial bones. Examine the internal surface of the removed calvaria. Note the distinct grooves for the branches of the middle meningeal artery. In the immediate vicinity of these grooves, observe numerous, tiny nutrient foramina leading to the substance of the bones. The use of a magnifying glass is helpful!

> The **middle meningeal artery** is of great clinical importance. If it is torn in a head injury, blood will quickly accumulate between the bony skull and dura mater (epidural hematoma). The expanding hematoma may exert fatal pressure on the brain unless it is promptly recognized and surgically treated. Surgeons must be aware of the course of the middle meningeal artery and its projection on the surface of the cranium (*Atlas*, 7.17). In the interior of a skull, examine the **groove for the middle meningeal artery**. Note that its **anterior branch** crosses the area of the **pterion** (*Atlas*, 7.23, 7.35, 7.153). Identify the pterion on the outside of a skull (*Atlas*, 7.2A). Fractures through this area are likely to result in tearing of the middle meningeal artery with the consequence of epidural hematoma.

In certain areas, the two layers of dura split to enclose the venous sinuses. Identify the **superior sagittal sinus** and the right and left **transverse sinuses** (Fig. 7.13). With scissors, slit these sinuses open. Examine closely the superior sagittal sinus, and verify that:

1. It increases in caliber as it passes posteriorly (direction of venous blood flow);
2. It is triangular on transverse section (Fig. 7.14);

3. It has lateral expansions, the **lacunae laterales** (Fig. 7.14).

In relation to the superior sagittal sinus and its lacunae, observe numerous cauliflower-like masses, the **arachnoid granulations** (Fig. 7.14; *Atlas*, 7.18).

> The **arachnoid granulations** are projections of the subarachnoid space filled with **cerebrospinal fluid (CSF)**. The CSF is constantly produced by the choroid plexuses in the ventricular system of the brain. To avoid undue and harmful pressure, any excess of CSF must be removed. This is accomplished by the arachnoid granulations. They empty the CSF into the venous sinuses by diffusion.
> The arachnoid granulations are responsible for small shallow depressions on the inner aspect of the calvaria. Examine the removed calvaria. Note these depressions, the *foveolae granulares*, in the vicinity of the sulcus for the superior sagittal sinus.

On both sides, **reflect the dura mater** from the cerebral and cerebellar hemispheres in the following manner:

1. Make an incision through the dura corresponding to the coronal suture. Be very careful not to injure the underlying arachnoid: With a forceps, produce a small fold of dura, nick it, and insert the scissors.
2. Cut the dura parallel to the superior sagittal and transverse sinuses. Stay about 2 cm clear of the venous channels. Now, expose the cerebral hemispheres by reflecting the dural flaps inferiorly. Note the smooth inner surface of the dura.
3. Cut the dura just inferiorly to the transverse sinuses. Then, cut it along the margins of the removed bony wedge. You may enlarge the exposed area by carefully resecting the posterior arch of the atlas. Remove the dura, but leave a small, sickle-shaped dural fold between the two cerebellar hemispheres. This is the **falx cerebelli** (*Atlas*, 7.19).

Now, with the dura mater reflected, the arachnoid is widely exposed. Realize that there is an extensive potential space between the dura mater and the delicate membrane of the arachnoid.

> As a complication of head injury, bleeding into the potential space between the dura mater and the arachnoid may occur. This hemorrhage is called a **subdural hematoma**. Because the potential space is only limited by the falx cerebri and the tentorium cerebelli, a subdural hemorrhage may spread thinly and widely over a hemisphere. The subdural hematoma, which is venous in origin, is a serious and insidious complication of head injuries. It must be distinguished from the epidural hematoma.

Arachnoid (Gr., *arachne*, spider; referring to the fine spiderweb-like processes between arachnoid membrane and pia). The arachnoid is a thin, nonvascular mem-

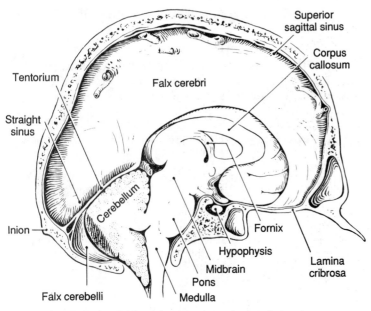

Tentorium · Falx cerebri · Superior sagittal sinus · Corpus callosum · Straight sinus · Fornix · Hypophysis · Midbrain · Lamina cribrosa · Inion · Cerebellum · Pons · Medulla · Falx cerebelli

Figure 7.15. Folds of dura mater and related structures.

brane that surrounds the brain loosely (Fig. 7.14; *Atlas*, 7.15). The **subarachnoid space** is a real space that contains cerebrospinal fluid. In the living, this fluid-filled space acts as an effective shock absorber. In the embalmed cadaver, the CSF is absent. Restore it artificially over a limited area of the cerebral hemisphere; use a syringe with a fine needle. Puncture the arachnoid membrane obliquely. Inject 5 to 10 cc of fluid (colored or plain water) into the subarachnoid space. An effective fluid cushion is being formed that covers several gyri and sulci. Note that the arachnoid smoothly covers all gaps and fissures of the brain surface.

Substantial intervals between pia and arachnoid are known as cisternae. Find the largest of these, the **cisterna cerebellomedullaris (cisterna magna)**. It is the enlarged subarachnoid space between the caudal part of the cerebellar hemispheres and the medulla oblongata. In the patient, the cisterna cerebellomedullaris can be tapped by a needle inserted through the posterior atlanto-occipital membrane.

Pia Mater (L., *pius*, tender; faithful). On part of one cerebral hemisphere, remove the arachnoid. Identify the pia. It is a delicate membrane that follows (faithfully) the brain tissue in between all sulci and fissures. The pia carries the blood vessels that supply the brain (Fig. 7.14, *Atlas*, 7.15). Observe the **cerebral veins** that empty into the superior sagittal sinus.

Exposure of Brain Stem and 4th Ventricle

It is desirable to maintain the structural integrity of the brain so that it can be used for future detailed studies (courses in neuroanatomy or the neurosciences). If it is

not necessary to preserve the brain, follow special directions from your instructors. Only half of the cerebellum will be sacrificed to expose the brain stem and the 4th ventricle.

The objective is to expose the brain stem and the cranial nerves emerging from it, as depicted in *Atlas*, 7.33. The cerebellum covers the brain stem posteriorly (Fig. 7.15; *Atlas*, 8.84). Remove the *right half* of the cerebellum in the following manner: with a scalpel, carefully split the narrow median portion (vermis) of the cerebellum in the midsagittal plane. Start just inferior to the confluens of the sinuses (Fig. 7.13) and just to the right of the falx cerebelli. Avoid cutting into the medulla. Next, make a parasagittal cut about 5 mm lateral to the midsagittal incision. Remove the narrow slice of cerebellar tissue. Gently force the two cerebellar hemispheres apart to obtain a partial view of the 4th ventricle. Remove several more thin slices of cerebellum. Finally, cut through the attachments of the right cerebellar hemisphere to the brain stem and remove the remains of the right half of the cerebellum. The right half of the brain stem and of the 4th ventricle is now exposed.

On the right side only, identify the following important structures (*Atlas*, 7.33):

1. **Vertebral artery,** entering the cranial cavity through the foramen magnum;
2. **Trochlear nerve (IV);** it is the most delicate of the cranial nerves; see it just caudal to the colliculi of the midbrain (also compare to a different view; *Atlas*, 7.36).
3. **Trigeminal nerve (V);** it is the largest of the cranial nerves emerging from the brain stem (*Atlas*, 7.33);
4. **Facial nerve (VII)** and **vestibulocochlear nerve (acoustic nerve; VIII)**, taking a common course toward the internal acoustic meatus;
5. Three cranial nerves that converge on the **jugular foramen: glossopharyngeal nerve (IX), vagus nerve (X), and accessory nerve (XI).**

Folds of Dura Mater

The *inner layer* of dura mater forms inwardly projecting folds that serve as incomplete partitions of the cranial cavity. Three of these folds will be examined now: **tentorium cerebelli, falx cerebelli, and falx cerebri** (Fig. 7.15; *Atlas*, 7.19).

Tentorium Cerebelli (L., *tentorium*, tent). In the cadaver, examine the inferior surface of the tentorium where the right cerebellar hemisphere was removed. Verify that it separates the cerebellar lobe from the corresponding occipital pole of the cerebral hemisphere. In fact, in the anatomical position, the tentorium supports the weight of the occipital poles. Observe the *posterior convex border* of the tentorium. It encloses the transverse sinuses. Review its attachments to the inner surface of the occipital bone along the grooves for the transverse sinuses. The *anterior and medial borders* of the tentorium are free and concave and form the tentorial notch that surrounds the midbrain (*Atlas*, 7.37).

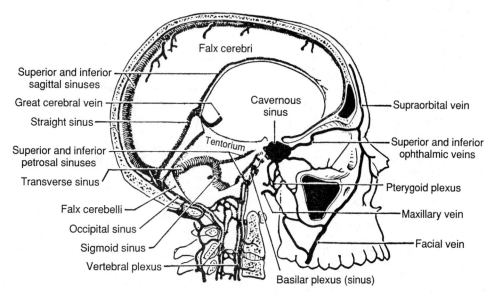

Figure 7.16. Folds of dura mater and venous sinuses.

Falx Cerebelli (L. *falx*, sickle). It is small. Observe its anterior free border that projects between the cerebellar hemispheres in the median plane (Fig. 7.15; *Atlas*, 7.19).

Falx Cerebri. This large, sickle-shaped membrane lies in the midsagittal plane between the two cerebral hemispheres (Figs. 7.14 to 7.16; *Atlas*, 7.19). Anteriorly, it is attached to the *crista galli* of the ethmoid bone. Posteriorly, it is fused with the tentorium cerebelli. The superior convex border encloses the **superior sagittal sinus** (Figs. 7.14, 7.16). Review its attachments to the inner surface of the calvaria, along the groove for the superior sagittal sinus. On the right and left sides, cut the **cerebral veins** that empty into the superior sagittal sinus. Free the falx cerebri. Gently pull the cerebral hemispheres apart and observe the free inferior border of the falx. It lies above the *corpus callosum* of the brain (Fig. 7.15).

The inferior concave border of the falx cerebri encloses the **inferior sagittal sinus** (Fig. 7.16, *Atlas*, 7.20). This sinus joins the great cerebral vein (of Galen) to form the **straight sinus**. The straight sinus runs obliquely between the falx cerebri and the tentorium cerebelli. Find the straight sinus as it empties into the **confluens of the sinuses** (Fig. 7.13). Push a thin probe from the confluens of the sinuses (confluens sinuum) into the straight sinus.

Review the folds of dura mater and obtain a clear concept of their arrangements. These dural folds will be detached during removal of the brain from the cranial cavity.

Removal of Brain

All attachments of the brain to the cranium must be freed. With the cadaver in the prone position (face down), transect the following structures (*Atlas*, 7.33):

1. The **spinal cord** at the level of the atlas (C1);
2. Both **vertebral arteries,** anywhere between the foramen magnum and the transverse processes of the atlas;

3. On the right side, where the cerebellum has been removed, cut with fine scissors the following **cranial nerves** close to the brain stem: **IV, V, and VII through XI.** Reflect cranial nerves **X and XI** posteriorly, and expose the fiber bundles of the **hypoglossal nerve (XII).** Sever this nerve.

Which structures must still be severed to completely mobilize the brain? Cranial nerves I, II, III, and VI on the right side; all cranial nerves on the left side; blood vessels; attachments of dural folds.

At this stage, it is necessary that you familiarize yourself with **relevant bony landmarks** and certain soft structures. In the bony skull, identify the following (*Atlas*, 7.23, 7.35):

1. **Crista galli;** a triangular plate of the ethmoid bone projecting into the interior of the skull in the median plane;
2. **Cribriform plate** (L., *cribrum*, sieve); a plate on either side of the crista galli; its numerous foramina transmit the filaments of the olfactory nerve; the olfactory bulb rests on the cribriform plate;
3. **Optic foramen** (canal); a round opening traversed by the optic nerve and the ophthalmic artery; view this foramen from the orbital cavity (*Atlas*, 7.1, 7.43);
4. **Groove for the internal carotid artery;** just inferior to the optic canal (*Atlas*, 7.35);
5. **Petrous portion of the temporal bone** (*Atlas*, 7.23, 7.35); note its sharp **superior margin;** the tentorium cerebelli is attached here; the margin also contains a small groove for the superior petrosal sinus.

In preparation for further dissection, examine the base of a brain (demonstration specimen) and identify the following **pertinent soft structures** (*Atlas*, 7.22):

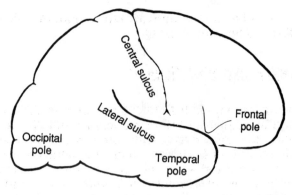

Figure 7.17. Lateral aspect of the right cerebral hemisphere (schematic).

1. **Olfactory bulbs and tracts** (cranial "nerve" **I**);
2. Right and left **optic nerves** (cranial "nerve" **II**); they unite to form the optic chiasma;
3. **Infundibulum,** just posterior to the optic chiasma; essentially, it is the stalk of the hypophysis cerebri (pituitary); the gland must be severed from its stalk during removal of the brain;
4. Right and left **internal carotid arteries,** lying in their grooves just inferior to the optic nerves (*Atlas,* 7.36, 7.40);
5. **Oculomotor nerve (III),** just cranial to the pons (*Atlas,* 7.22);
6. **Abducent nerve (VI),** just caudal to the pons.

Procedure. Turn the cadaver into the supine position (face up). Ask your partner to support the brain posteriorly with one or two hands. Gently separate the frontal poles of the cerebral hemispheres. Cut the **falx cerebri** close to the **crista galli** (*Atlas,* 7.19). Pull the falx superiorly and posteriorly.

Gently lift up the frontal poles. To both sides of the crista galli, note the **olfactory bulbs and tracts.** Dislodge the bulbs from the cribriform plates. Accomplish this with the aid of forceps and probe. Elevate the brain further until you see the **infundibulum** just posterior to the **optic chiasma.** Cut across the infundibulum. Next sever the **optic nerves** and the two **internal carotid arteries** close to the optic foramina. Lift up the brain further. Identify the two **oculomotor nerves** and cut them.

With a scalpel, **detach the tentorium cerebelli** on both sides. Start the cut at the free border of the tentorial notch. Carry the cut posteriorly, close to the **superior margin of the petrous bone.** Complete the detachment by cutting all the way to the free margin of the excised occipital wedge. Ask your partner to support the weight of the brain.

Next, identify and cut the two **abducent nerves.** Subsequently, sever the remaining cranial nerves on the *left side* (IV, V, VII through XII). Pull the brain gently posteriorly, and remove it from the cranial cavity.

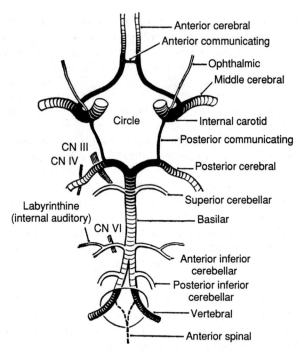

Figure 7.18. Two vertebral and two internal carotid arteries supply the brain. These arteries join to form an arterial circle (of Willis).

Gross Examination of the Brain

Examine the **cerebral hemispheres** and identify the following (Fig. 7.17; *Atlas,* 7.29, 7.30):

1. **Frontal pole;**
2. **Temporal pole;**
3. **Occipital pole;**
4. **Lateral sulcus** (lateral cerebral fissure; fissure of Sylvius);
5. **Central sulcus** (fissure of Rolando);
6. **Frontal lobe,** the largest of the lobes; it is bounded posteriorly by the central sulcus, inferiorly by the lateral sulcus;

Refer to a skull and identify the **three cranial fossae:** *anterior, middle, and posterior* (see Fig. 7.19). By placing the brain back into the cranial cavity, verify the following:

1. The frontal pole is located in the anterior cranial fossa.
2. The temporal pole fits into the middle cranial fossa.
3. The occipital pole is located in the posterior cranial fossa (above the grooves for the transverse sinuses).

Examine the base of the brain. Note that it is covered with arachnoid. Remove the arachnoid. Note the arteries at the base of the brain (Fig. 7.18; *Atlas,* 7.24, 7.25). The two vertebral and the two internal carotid arteries supply the brain. These arteries join to form the **cerebral arterial circle** (of Willis). Verify the following:

1. The right and left **posterior inferior cerebellar arteries** arise from the respective **vertebral arteries.** The right and left vertebral arteries join to form the **basilar artery.**
2. The **basilar artery** gives off several branches: anterior inferior cerebellar, superior cerebellar, and posterior cerebral. Note the **oculomotor nerve** (III) emerging between **posterior cerebral artery** and **superior cerebellar artery** (*Atlas*, 7.24).
3. After giving off the ophthalmic artery, each **internal carotid artery** terminates by dividing into a **middle cerebral artery** and an **anterior cerebral artery.**
4. The **arterial circle** (Fig. 7.18; *Atlas*, 7.25) is completed by communicating arteries. Anteriorly, the two anterior cerebral arteries are united by the unpaired and very short **anterior communicating artery.** Posteriorly, the **posterior communicating arteries** connect the internal carotid arteries with the posterior cerebral arteries.

Note that the flat *medial surfaces* of the cerebral hemispheres are supplied by the anterior and posterior cerebral arteries (*Atlas*, 7.26B). Specifically, the **anterior cerebral artery** supplies the anterior and superior aspects of the medial surface. The **posterior cerebral artery** supplies the posterior aspect of the medial surface and the inferior surface of the hemisphere.

Follow the large **middle cerebral artery** through the lateral sulcus. Gently widen the sulcus by retracting the gyri, which bound it superiorly and inferiorly. This procedure will expose the **insula.** Note that the insula is supplied by branches of the middle cerebral artery. Follow the artery on to the convex aspect of the hemisphere. Note that the superolateral surface of the cerebral hemisphere is predominantly supplied by branches of the middle cerebral artery (*Atlas*, 7.26A). Correlate the course of these dissected vessels with a carotid arteriogram (*Atlas*, 7.27). Also study a vertebral arteriogram (*Atlas*, 7.28).

> If time permits, examine more closely the middle cerebral artery within the lateral cerebral fissure. Note several small but important branches that supply the corpus striatum and the internal capsule. These branches are also known as "arteries of cerebral apoplexy" since they are frequently involved in apoplexy (stroke).

At the base of the brain (*Atlas*, 7.22), identify **cranial nerves I through XII.** After completion of your studies, moisten the brain with embalming fluid and store it in an airtight plastic bag. Detailed studies of the brain must be conducted in a separate neuroanatomy course.

The Three Cranial Fossae

The interior of the base of the skull can be divided into three parts, each forming a fossa: anterior, middle, and posterior. The anterior and posterior cranial fossae will be discussed first. The middle cranial fossa, which lies between the other fossae and which is anatomically more complex, will be studied last.

Anterior Cranial Fossa

Refer to the bony skull. Note that the interior of the base of the skull is subdivided into three fossae: anterior, middle, and posterior (Fig. 7.19). The **anterior cranial fossa** is sharply marked off from the middle cranial fossa by three concave crests: the sharp posterior borders of the **right and left lesser wings of the sphenoid bone,** and the **anterior margin of the optic (chiasmatic) groove** (Fig. 7.20; *Atlas*, 7.35).

Identify the three bones that participate in the formation of the anterior cranial fossa: **sphenoid bone;** crista galli and cribriform plate of **ethmoid bone;** orbital plates of **frontal bone,** forming the roofs of the orbital cavities.

Recall the topographic relations of soft structures and bony landmarks. The olfactory bulbs rest on the cribriform plates. The falx cerebri is attached to the triangular crista galli. The frontal poles of the cerebral hemispheres rest on the orbital plates of the frontal bone.

Posterior Cranial Fossa

Refer to the bony skull and the cadaver specimen. Realize that the **posterior cranial fossa** is the largest and the deepest of the three fossae (Fig. 7.19). It is separated from the middle fossa by the dorsum sellae and the superior borders (margins) of the right and left petrous bones.

The posterior cranial fossa is dominated by the enormous unpaired **foramen magnum,** which is oval in shape (Fig. 7.19; *Atlas*, 7.35). At the level of this foramen, the medulla oblongata becomes continuous with the spinal cord. The inclining bony surface anterior to the foramen magnum is the clivus. It is topographically related to the pons and to the medulla oblongata (*Atlas*, 8.84). The fossae for the cerebellum and the occipital poles of the cerebral hemispheres were examined earlier.

In the bony skull, identify the following openings (*Atlas*, 7.35).

1. **Hypoglossal canal** for cranial nerve XII;
2. **Jugular foramen,** which transmits cranial nerves IX, X, XI, and the sigmoid sinus;
3. **Internal acoustic meatus** for cranial nerves VII and VIII.

Turn to the cadaver. Identify the **stumps of cranial nerves VII through XII** and follow them to their respective foramina (Figs. 7.21, 7.23). Note the large **trigeminal nerve (V)** as it curves superior to the most medial part of the superior margin of the petrous bone. The nerve passes inferior to the attached margin of the tentorium into the middle cranial fossa to enter the trigeminal cave.

Slit open the **transverse sinus** (*Atlas*, 7.23). After leaving the tentorium, the transverse sinus becomes the sig-

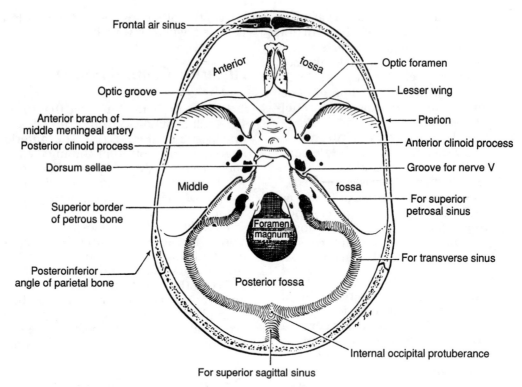

Figure 7.19. Interior of the base of the skull: the three cranial fossae.

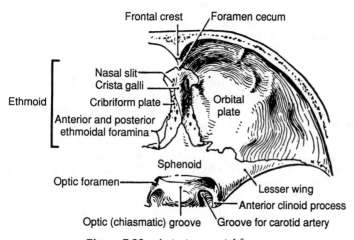

Figure 7.20. Anterior cranial fossa.

moid sinus. Open the sigmoid sinus. Verify that it leads to the jugular foramen. Slit open the **superior petrosal sinus.** Note that it runs in the attachment of the tentorium cerebelli to the superior margin of the petrous bone. This small sinus connects the large cavernous sinus with the transverse sinus. Finally, identify the stump of the **abducent nerve** (VI). It pierces the dura within the posterior cranial fossa.

Middle Cranial Fossa

In the bony skull, identify the **middle cranial fossa** (Fig. 7.19). Note that the main part of the fossa is composed of

two bones, the **sphenoid bone** and the **temporal bone.** On each side, the greater wing of the sphenoid contains a crescent of foramina (*Atlas,* 7.38). Identify the following important openings:

1. **Superior orbital fissure,** which transmits cranial nerves III, IV, V^1, VI, sympathetic nerve fibers, and the superior ophthalmic vein;
2. **Foramen rotundum** for cranial nerve V^2;
3. **Foramen ovale** for nerve V^3;
4. **Foramen spinosum** for the middle meningeal vessels; the **groove for the middle meningeal artery** leads from it.

In addition, identify the following pertinent bony landmarks in the middle cranial fossa (*Atlas,* 7.35):

5. **Hypophyseal fossa** for the hypophysis cerebri (pituitary gland);
6. **Optic groove** (chiasmatic sulcus), leading on each side to the optic canal;
7. **Optic canal,** for the optic nerve and ophthalmic artery;
8. **Dorsum sellae;**
9. **Foramen lacerum,** situated between hypophyseal fossa and apex of petrous bone;
10. **Carotid groove** for the internal carotid artery.

Recall that the middle cranial fossae are occupied by the temporal poles and lobes of the cerebral hemispheres.

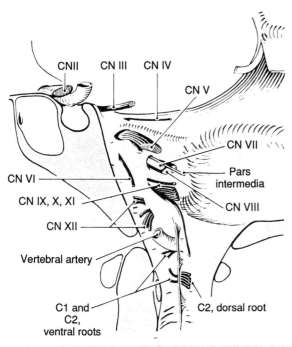

Figure 7.21. Stumps of nerves and vessels.

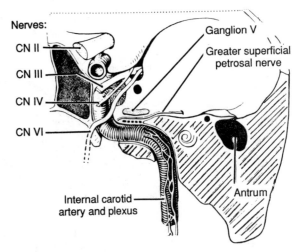

Figure 7.22. The internal carotid artery and its relations.

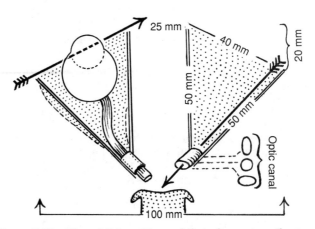

Figure 7.23. The orbital cavities and their dimensions (horizontal section).

Identify the optic nerve, which traverses the optic canal. During removal of the brain, the **hypophysis cerebri** (pituitary gland) was severed from its stalk. This small but important master gland lies beneath a circular dural fold, which covers the hypophyseal fossa (*Atlas*, 7.23). This fold is the **diaphragma sellae**. With a probe, define the circular aperture of the diaphragma sellae. Enlarge the opening and scoop out the pituitary gland.

Certain soft structures of the middle cranial fossa lie between *two layers of dura*. Therefore, the dura must be split to expose these structures: cavernous sinus; internal carotid artery; cranial nerves III, IV, V, and VI.

If not already done, slit open the **superior petrosal sinus** (*Atlas*, 7.23). Carry the cut anteromedially into the **cavernous sinus**. The sinus is large and important (*Atlas*, 7.20). Study a coronal section through the cavernous sinus (*Atlas*, 7.41). Realize that the sinus is actually traversed by the internal carotid artery and by cranial nerves.

These relations (*Atlas*, 7.41) are of clinical significance. In fractures of the base of the skull, the **internal carotid artery** may rupture within the **cavernous sinus**. As a result, an **arteriovenous fistula** (shunt) occurs. There is an abnormal reflux of blood from the cavernous sinus into the ophthalmic veins, which normally drain the contents of the orbital cavity. As a result, the eye is protruded, engorged, and is pulsating in synchrony with the radial pulse (pulsating exophthalmos).

During injuries or infections of the cavernous sinus, the cranial nerves traversing it may also be affected.

Pick up the **abducent nerve (VI)** in the posterior cranial fossa (*Atlas*, 7.23). Slit open the dura. Follow the nerve into the **cavernous sinus**. Trace the **oculomotor nerve (III)** anteriorly by slitting the dura. Identify a portion of **internal carotid artery** within the cavernous sinus.

Pick up the **trigeminal nerve (V)** where it crosses the superior border of the petrous bone (*Atlas*, 7.23). Here, the nerve lies in a 1-cm long cave that is lined with arachnoid. Slit open the roof of the cave. In doing so you will necessarily cut across the superior petrosal sinus. Remove the dura from the greater wing of the sphenoid to expose the **trigeminal ganglion** and the **three trigeminal divisions** (*Atlas*, 7.36). Trace the **mandibular division (V^3)** to the foramen ovale. Follow the **maxillary division (V^2)** to the foramen rotundum. Trace the small **ophthalmic division (V^1)** toward the superior orbital fissure.

Clean the **internal carotid artery** and demonstrate its sinuous course. Note its close relations to cranial nerves III, IV, and VI (Fig. 7.22; *Atlas*, 7.37, 7.40).

The **middle meningeal vessels** are embedded in the outer layer of the dura mater. Follow these vessels to the foramen spinosum (*Atlas*, 7.23).

If you have time, look for a very small branch of the facial nerve, the **greater petrosal nerve**. It carries important parasympathetic fibers to the pterygopalatine ganglion (*Atlas*, 9.12). The nerve lies extradurally. Therefore, remove the moistened dura in the vicinity of

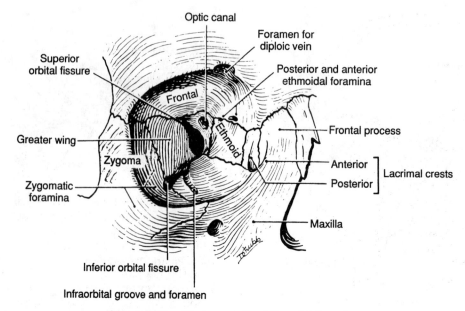

Figure 7.24. The bony walls of the orbital cavity.

the foramen lacerum. Be sure the dura is moist. If it is dry, it will break. The fine nerve may be seen running from the hiatus for the greater petrosal nerve in the petrous bone to the foramen lacerum (*Atlas*, 7.36, 7.37). After traversing this foramen, the nerve enters the pterygoid canal.

The tiny **lesser petrosal nerve** carries parasympathetic fibers to the otic ganglion (*Atlas*, 9.14**B** and **C**). The nerve runs lateral to the greater petrosal nerve to the foramen ovale or to a tiny foramen just posterior to the foramen ovale (*Atlas*, 7.36).

Read an account of the dural sinuses and review them in the cadaver (Fig. 7.16; *Atlas*, 7.20). Correlate your anatomical observations with a venogram of the sinuses (*Atlas*, 7.21). Study an outline of the cranial nerves (*Atlas*, 8.2). In the bony skull, review the openings (foramina; fissures) through which the cranial nerves pass.

Orbit and Contents

General Remarks

The two orbits are deep bony sockets for the eyeballs and their related structures (muscles; nerves; vessels). Certain vessels and nerves traverse the orbit in close contact with its roof or floor to reach the scalp or face.

Each orbit is pyramidal in shape (Fig. 7.23). It has four walls. The orbital margin is at the base. The apex is at the optic canal. The medial walls are parallel and about 25 mm apart. The lateral walls are at right angles to each other.

The eyeball is about 25 mm long; i.e., it is half as long as the orbit. It occupies the anterior half of the orbit (Fig. 7.23). The posterior half of the orbit is largely filled with muscles and loose fatty tissue.

Bony Landmarks

Refer to a skull and verify that a number of different bones participate in the formation of the **orbital cavity** (Fig. 7.24; *Atlas*, 7.43):

1. **Maxillary bone;**
2. **Zygomatic bone;**
3. **Frontal bone;**
4. **Lacrimal bone;**
5. **Ethmoid bone;**
6. **Sphenoid bone.**

In addition, observe the following details:

7. **Optic canal,** at the junction of the lesser wing and body of the sphenoid bone;
8. **Superior orbital fissure,** positioned between the greater and the lesser wings of the sphenoid;
9. **Inferior orbital fissure,** a gap between the maxilla and the greater wing of the sphenoid;
10. **Infraorbital groove,** continuous with the infraorbital canal and continuing anteriorly to the infraorbital foramen;
11. **Anterior and posterior ethmoidal foramina,** on the medial wall of the cavity (a passageway for small nerves between the orbit and the anterior cranial fossa (*Atlas*, 7.43);
12. The **lateral wall of the orbit** is stout and strong;
13. Understand that an object pushed through the **roof of the orbit** will enter the anterior cranial fossa (Fig. 7.25).
14. An object pushed through the **floor of the orbit** will enter the large maxillary sinus (Fig. 7.25);

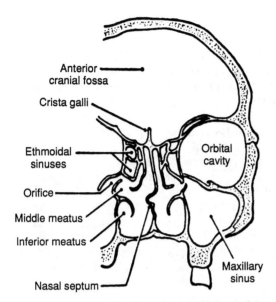

Anterior cranial fossa

Crista galli

Ethmoidal sinuses

Orbital cavity

Orifice

Middle meatus

Inferior meatus

Nasal septum

Maxillary sinus

Figure 7.25. Coronal section of the skull at the level of the orbits.

15. An object pushed through the paper-thin **medial wall** of the orbital cavity, the **lamina papyracea** of the ethmoid bone, will enter the ethmoidal sinuses of the nasal cavity (Fig. 7.25);

16. Explore this realistic possibility: a sharp object (pencil, nail, or a bullet) entering the orbit in an anteroposterior direction will traverse the superior orbital fissure and enter the middle cranial fossa. The physician will be confronted with such penetrating injuries; he or she must understand which anatomical substrates have been injured.

The bones of the orbital cavity are lined with periosteum called **periorbita.** At the optic canal and the superior orbital fissure, the periorbita is continuous with the dura mater of the cranial cavity.

Before you begin . . .

It is recommended that the right orbital cavity be approached superiorly (from above) through its roof. The orbital plate of the frontal bone must be removed. This procedure will reveal nerves, vessels, and muscles that are in contact with the roof of the orbit. The extraocular muscles will be studied. Two muscles will be divided and reflected to expose various important nerves and vessels located in the posterior half of the cavity. It will be seen that the optic canal transmits the optic nerve and the ophthalmic artery. The ophthalmic vein and nerves III, IV, V^1, and VI will be followed through the superior orbital fissure.

In contrast, the left orbital cavity should be dissected by using the anterior (or surgical) approach. General knowledge of the topographic anatomy in the orbit is a prerequisite for this most useful exercise. Eventually, the dissection is concluded with the enucleation of the right eyeball. Subsequently, the interior of the removed eye may be dissected.

Dissection

Special Technique. In most cases, the eyeball is partially collapsed. Distend it by injecting preservative fluid or glycerine into it with a fine needle attached to a syringe. Insert the needle very obliquely through the transparent cornea in front of the pupil. This precedure will make the dissection of the orbital contents easier.

Right Orbit, Superior Approach

In the cranial cavity, incise the moistened dura mater along the posterior sharp margin of the lesser wing of the sphenoid and along the lateral margin of the cribriform plate. Now, strip the dura from the anterior cranial fossa (roof of the orbital cavity).

With a chisel or another suitable metal instrument, break the center of the roof of the orbit. With bone forceps, nibble away the whole roof piece by piece:

Anteriorly, the bone is hollow. The exposed spaces belong to the **frontal sinus** (*Atlas,* 7.46A). Note its mucosal lining. Remove the roof of the orbit as far anteriorly as possible, but leave the superior orbital margin intact.

Medially, the roof may also be hollow. Here, the **anterior and posterior ethmoidal cells** will be exposed. Understand that the ethmoidal cells have a tendency to invade the adjacent frontal bone. Observe the mucosal lining of these cells (*Atlas,* 7.46A). At this stage, identify the tough membrane just inferior to the removed roof of the orbit. This is the **periorbita** that envelops the contents of the orbital cavity.

Posteriorly and laterally, the lesser wing of the sphenoid must be removed. This procedure will expose the **superior orbital fissure** and the optic canal. Push a probe between the bony roof and the periorbita posteriorly through the superior orbital fissure. With the probe still in a guiding position, remove the lesser wing of the sphenoid, which forms the upper margin of the superior orbital fissure. Next, with the aid of a probe, carefully break away the roof and the lateral wall of the **optic canal** (*Atlas,* 7.46B). Finally, remove the anterior clinoid process. Shell it out of the investing dura with a pair of forceps.

Next, incise the **periorbita** transversely near the anterior margin of the orbit. Make a second incision in an anteroposterior direction, but only as far posterior as the periorbita is free. Reflect or remove the flaps. Now, the most superior parts of the orbital contents are exposed (*Atlas,* 7.46A).

Locate the intracranial stump of the delicate **trochlear nerve** (*Atlas,* 7.36). Carefully follow it anteriorly. Observe the nerve along the lateral wall of the cavernous sinus and lateral to the internal carotid artery. In the superior orbital fissure, the nerve is in intimate contact with the **frontal nerve.** Separate the nerves with a delicate instrument, such as fine sharp-sharp scissors. Follow the trochlear nerve to the superior border of the **superior oblique muscle** in the orbit (*Atlas,* 7.36, 7.46A).

Trace the **frontal nerve** from the 1st trigeminal division through the superior orbital fissure (*Atlas,* 7.36). In the

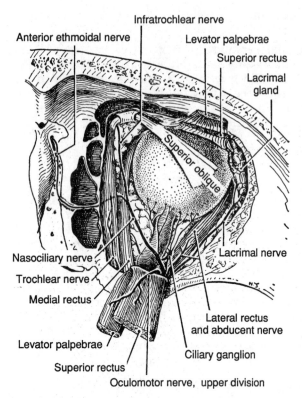

Anterior ethmoidal nerve
Infratrochlear nerve
Levator palpebrae
Superior rectus
Lacrimal gland
Superior oblique
Nasociliary nerve
Trochlear nerve
Medial rectus
Lacrimal nerve
Levator palpebrae
Superior rectus
Lateral rectus and abducent nerve
Ciliary ganglion
Oculomotor nerve, upper division

Figure 7.26. Dissection of the orbital cavity (superior approach).

orbit, trace the nerve anteriorly to its division into the small **supratrochlear nerve** and the larger **supraorbital nerve.** Push a probe through the supraorbital notch or foramen, and establish the continuity of the nerves onto the forehead and scalp region (*Atlas*, 7.6, 7.8). At this stage, you may extend the dissection field. If you wish to do so, carefully remove the part of the frontal bone that forms the superior orbital margin. This procedure completely exposes the upper eyelid and the **levator palpebrae superioris** (*Atlas*, 7.52, 7.53).

The delicate **lacrimal nerve** (*Atlas*, 7.36) enters the superior orbital fissure lateral to the frontal nerve. In the orbit (*Atlas*, 7.46A), trace the nerve anteriorly to the **lacrimal gland.** Arteries accompany the frontal and lacrimal nerves.

With forceps, pick out fine lobules of loose fatty tissue and expose the surface of the most superiorly positioned muscle, the **levator palpebrae** (*Atlas*, 7.46A, 7.52, 7.53). Examine this muscle. Gently pull on it. Verify that it raises the upper eyelid. Understand that various layers of the muscle are inserted into different parts of the lid (*Atlas*, 7.53). Cut the muscle as far anteriorly as possible and reflect it posteriorly (*Atlas*, 7.46A). Now, the underlying **superior rectus** lies exposed. Clean it. Note that the muscle is attached to the eyeball by a tendinous expansion (*Atlas*, 7.47A). Cut the superior rectus close to the eyeball and reflect it posteriorly. Note that a branch of the **oculomotor nerve (III)** reaches its deep surface (Fig. 7.26; *Atlas*, 7.46A). Examine the **superior oblique** muscle and trace it forward to its pulley, the **trochlea** (Atlas, 7.46B). Note that the tendon of the muscle bends at an acute angle and

passes to its insertion into the lateral and posterior portion of the eyeball.

At this stage, the **origin of the four recti muscles** must be considered. They arise from a tough tendinous ring or cuff, the **anulus tendineus** (*Atlas*, 7.51). This fibrous ring surrounds the optic canal and its contents. In addition, the ring partially includes the superior orbital fissure. The two heads of the **lateral rectus** are attached to the ring. The narrow interval overlying the superior orbital fissure, encircled by the fibrous ring and bounded by the heads of the lateral rectus, is of strategic importance. Several structures pass through this gap: **nasociliary nerve, abducent nerve, oculomotor nerve,** and **ophthalmic vein.**

In the dissection field, identify the **lateral rectus** and its superior head. Gently push a probe through the interval between the two heads of the muscle. Carefully sever the superior head and the anulus tendineus. Now, all structures passing through the narrow interval can be studied (*Atlas*, 7.46A).

Nasociliary Nerve (Fig. 7.26; *Atlas*, 7.46A and **B**). It is a branch of the 1st trigeminal division (V^1). Follow it into the orbit. As the nerve crosses the optic nerve, it gives off two or three delicate **long ciliary nerves** to the posterior part of the eyeball. Subsequently, the nasociliary nerve runs obliquely toward the medial wall of the orbit, at the level between the superior oblique and the medial rectus. To clarify the dissection field, pick out the numerous tiny lobules of loose fatty tissue that fill the interval between muscles, nerves, and vessels.

A small branch of the nasociliary nerve, the **anterior ethmoidal nerve,** passes through the anterior ethmoidal foramen (*Atlas*, 7.43, 7.46A). The nerve enters the cranial cavity, runs lateral to the cribriform plate, and enters the ethmoid bone to reach the nasal cavity (*Atlas*, 7.46B). It supplies part of the mucous membrane in the nasal cavity. Finally, it sends a terminal twig to the tip of the nose as the **external nasal nerve** (*Atlas*, 7.8).

Abducent Nerve (VI). Once again, follow it through the cavernous sinus and lateral to the internal carotid artery to the superior orbital fissure (*Atlas*, 7.36). In the orbital cavity (Fig. 7.26; *Atlas*, 7.46B), find the nerve applied to the medial surface of the lateral rectus.

Oculomotor Nerve (III). In the cranial cavity, identify the nerve where it pierces the dura between the anterior and posterior clinoid processes (*Atlas*, 7.37). Follow it to the superior orbital fissure. Here it divides into two divisions. Identify the **superior division,** which supplies the reflected levator palpebrae superioris and the superior rectus (Fig. 7.26; *Atlas*, 7.46A). The **inferior division** supplies the **medial rectus, inferior rectus,** and **inferior oblique** (*Atlas*, 7.46B, 7.51). Identify the **ciliary ganglion,** which receives parasympathetic fibers from the inferior division of the oculomotor nerve (III). This parasympathetic ganglion is only 1 to 2 mm in diameter. Find it lateral to the optic nerve, about 1 cm anterior to the apex of the orbit (*Atlas*, 7.46, 7.50). Delicate short ciliary nerves connect the ganglion to the posterior portion of the eyeball. Understand the functional importance of the ciliary ganglion and the ciliary nerve (*Atlas*, 9.5).

Look for the **superior ophthalmic vein** (Fig. 7.16; *Atlas*, 7.20, 7.60). At the medial angle of the eye, this vein anastomoses with tributaries of the facial vein. In the orbit, the superior ophthalmic vein and its tributaries accompany the ophthalmic artery. Identify the vein on the basis of two facts: (a) it passes through the superior orbital fissure, and (b) it drains into the cavernous sinus.

The anastomoses between facial vein and ophthalmic veins (*Atlas*, 7.20, 7.60) are of clinical importance. Infections (boils) of the nasal cavity, upper lip, cheeks, and forehead region may spread along venous channels into the ophthalmic veins and on into the cavernous sinus. The resulting **cavernous sinus thrombosis** is a most dangerous complication.

Optic Nerve (*Atlas*, 7.46B).   If not already done, open the roof of the optic canal. The optic "nerve" is actually a brain tract. Therefore, it is surrounded with the three meningeal layers: dura, arachnoid, and pia (*Atlas*, 7.57). Pass a thin probe underneath the external (dural) sheath and slit it open. Cut across the optic nerve inside the sheath. Lift up the nerve. Examine the cut surface of the nerve, and identify a dark spot at the center. This is the sectioned **central artery of the retina** (*Atlas*, 7.51).

Ophthalmic Artery (*Atlas*, 7.59).   Identify the artery where it arises from the internal carotid artery. In the optic canal, the vessel lies inferior and lateral to the optic nerve. With the tip of a probe, elevate the optic nerve slightly and observe the ophthalmic artery. Follow the artery into the orbital cavity. Note that it curves superior to the optic nerve and, subsequently, reaches the medial wall of the orbit. Observe the fine **ciliary arteries** to the eyeball. If time permits, examine other branches of the ophthalmic artery (*Atlas*, 7.59).

The **central artery of the retina** was already seen on the sectioned surface of the optic nerve. The artery enters the nerve about 13 mm posterior to the eyeball (*Atlas*, 7.59), runs in the center of the nerve (*Atlas*, 7.51), pierces the sclera, and reaches the retina (*Atlas*, 7.57). Its occlusion leads to instant and total blindness of the concerned eye.

Remove the optic nerve and its sheath. Now, the muscles at the floor of the orbital cavity can be observed (*Atlas*, 7.46B). Identify the **inferior rectus**. Raise the posterior pole of the eyeball, and observe the insertion of the **inferior oblique** into the sclera (*Atlas*, 7.47B). Identify and study the **medial rectus**. Review the distribution of the superior and inferior divisions of the oculomotor nerve (*Atlas*, 9.5).

Review the insertion of the extraocular muscles (*Atlas*, 7.47, 7.49): the four **recti** muscles are inserted by thin, wide tendons into the scleral coat near the cornea. The two **oblique** muscles are also inserted by thin wide tendons; but they are attached to the sclera of the posterior half of the eyeball.

Students particularly interested in the orbit and its contents should consider an additional or alternative procedure: the *lateral approach*. This useful approach was devised by Professor Laurenson. It allows an excellent exploration of the orbital contents. Refer to *Atlas*, 7.50.

Left Orbit from Facial Aspect (Surgical Approach)

Review the extent of the conjunctival sac (*Atlas*, 7.52). Verify that the conjunctiva is firmly adherent to the cornea, but loosely attached to the sclera (*Atlas*, 7.47A). With a sharp scalpel, make a complete circular incision through the conjunctiva, about 6 to 8 mm from the sclerocorneal junction. Push a probe through the incision, and find at least one of the recti muscles.

In order to facilitate the dissection, remove both eyelids and the orbital septum. Compare your field of dissection with *Atlas* 7.44 (the *Atlas* depicts the right orbit; you are dissecting the left one).

Examine three corners of the orbit (Fig. 7.7C). Notice:

1. Superior lateral: the lacrimal gland;
2. Superior medial: the trochlea for the superior oblique;
3. Inferior medial: the lacrimal sac; the origin of inferior oblique.

Observe the insertion of the **four recti muscles**. Study the insertions of the **superior and inferior obliques**. Notice that the obliques pass *inferior* to the corresponding recti (*Atlas*, 7.44).

Enucleation of Eyeball.   With a probe, hook up each rectus tendon and cut across it. Cut all four recti. Adduct the eyeball (turn medially) and pull it anteriorly. Insert a cutting instrument (preferably long, curved scissors) into the orbit from the lateral side. Cut the optic nerve. Now, pull the eyeball anteriorly and sever the two oblique muscles. Remove the eyeball. Keep it moist, and store it in a small plastic bag.

Study the socket (Fig. 7.27; *Atlas* 7.51). Remove the loose fatty tissue from the posterior portion of the orbital cavity. Pick up the nerve to the inferior oblique and follow it posteriorly as far as possible. Trace the **four recti** to their origin from the **anulus tendineus**. Identify the structures that pass between the two heads of the lateral rectus: **nerve VI, inferior and superior divisions of nerve III, and nasociliary nerve.**

Once more, observe the superficial origins of the cranial nerves at the base of the brain (*Atlas*, 9.1). Review the distribution of the optic nerve (*Atlas*, 9.4). Study an account of cranial nerves III, IV, and VI (*Atlas*, 9.5 through 9.7). Review the course of the ophthalmic nerve (*Atlas*, 9.9).

Dissection of the Human Eyeball

In most cases, the removed human eyeball is not well preserved enough to warrant its dissection. If the eye is in

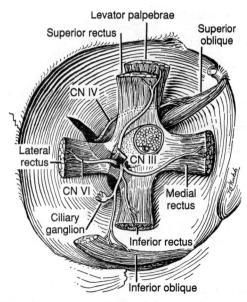

Figure 7.27. The anulus tendineus. Stumps of extrinsic ocular muscles. Distribution of cranial nerves III, IV, and VI.

acceptable condition, cut it into two halves along a sagittal plane. Use a sharp scalpel (new blade!). Carefully remove the remains of the vitreous body. Gently wash it out, if necessary. Note the following essential features (*Atlas*, 7.57):

1. **External or fibrous coat**, consisting of **sclera** (posterior 5/6) and **cornea** (anterior 1/6); the cornea is more convex than the sclera.
2. **Middle or vascular coat**, consisting of **choroid, ciliary body, and iris**; blood vessels and the ciliary nerves are contained in this coat.
3. **Internal or retinal coat**; in the cadaver, the retina is gray and partially detached. In well-preserved specimens, you may find the macula. Identify the region where the optic nerve and retinal vessels enter or leave. This is the **optic papilla or disc**.
4. Two of the **four refractive media** are still present: **cornea** and **lens**. The now empty space between the cornea and the lens is normally filled with **aqueous humor**. The jelly-like **vitreous body** has been removed earlier.

The principal gross anatomical structures of the eye can be conveniently examined in the large and fresh eye of the bull. If a detailed dissection of the eye is on your agenda, refer to the *Appendix*.

Posterior Triangle of Neck

General Remarks

The **boundaries** of the posterior triangle of the neck are (Fig. 7.28; *Atlas*, 8.2):

1. Anteriorly, the posterior border of the **sternocleidomastoid muscle;**
2. Posteriorly, the anterior border of the **trapezius;**
3. Inferiorly, the middle third of the **clavicle.**

The posterior triangle has a **fascial roof** of deep fascia that stretches between the two muscles forming its boundaries. This fascia splits to envelop the trapezius and the sternocleidomastoid. Superficial veins lie superficial to the fascial roof. The roof is pierced by cutaneous nerves.

The **floor** of the triangle is formed by a series of muscles that are covered with a thin, firm layer of fascia.

The **contents** of the posterior triangle consist largely of nerves and vessels connecting the neck region with the upper limb.

Before you begin . . .

Following reflection of the skin and a portion of the platysma, the posterior triangle will be fully exposed. First, the accessory nerve, an important guiding structure for dissection, must be identified (Fig. 7.28; *Atlas*, 8.2). Subsequently, a number of sensory nerves radiating from the posterior border of the sternocleidomastoid muscle will be dissected. At the base of the triangle, tributaries of the external jugular vein and branches of the thyrocervical trunk will be observed. Dissection in this area will be greatly facilitated by partial resection of the clavicle.

Finally, the fascia forming the floor of the triangle will be removed and the underlying muscles will be exposed. The important brachial plexus will be followed from the neck into the axilla.

Skin Incisions

If not already done, make an incision along the clavicle from its medial end to a point 3 cm beyond the acromion (*The Upper Limb*, Chapter 6, Fig. 6.1).

Refer to Figure 7.29. Make an incision from the base of the mastoid process to the medial end of the clavicle (*E* to *F*). Reflect the skin posteriorly. Subsequently, remove the triangular flap along the anterior border of the trapezius. Anteriorly, reflect the skin overlying the sternocleidomastoid muscle.

Superficial Structures and Contents of Triangle

The posteroinferior portion of the **platysma** covers the basal part of the triangle. The platysma passes over the whole length of the clavicle (*Atlas*, 1.2, 8.1). The **supraclavicular nerves**, which cling to the deep surface of the platysma, also cross the clavicle. Reflect the platysma upward. Do not injure the supraclavicular nerves.

Find the **accessory nerve** (Fig. 7.28; *Atlas*, 8.9). Its approximate course is marked by a line connecting two

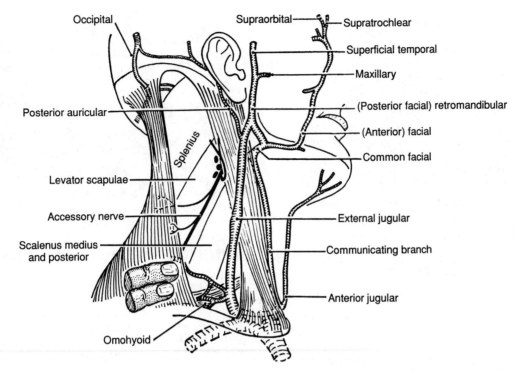

Figure 7.28. The posterior triangle of the neck showing superficial veins and the accessory nerve (cranial nerve XI).

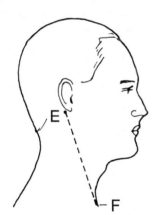

Figure 7.29. Skin incisions.

In addition to cranial nerve XI and the lesser occipital nerve (C2, C3), three other nerves radiate from the posterior border of the sternocleidomastoid (*Atlas*, 8.4A):

1. **Great auricular nerve** (C2, C3). Together with the external jugular vein, it ascends vertically on the surface of the sternocleidomastoid. The nerve supplies the back of the auricle and a cutaneous area extending from the angle of the mandible to the mastoid process.
2. **Transverse cervical nerve** (C2, C3). Follow it transversely across the middle of the sternocleidomastoid. It supplies the skin of the anterior triangle of the neck.
3. **Supraclavicular nerves** (C3, C4). Note *medial, intermediate,* and *lateral* branches.

External Jugular Vein (*Atlas*, 8.4A). This vein runs superficially from an area posterior to the angle of the mandible to a point about 3 cm superior to the clavicle. At this point, the vein pierces the roof of the posterior triangle. Clean the vein and follow it through the fascia. Then, remove the remains of the fascial roof.

Resection of Middle Portion of Clavicle. With a small saw, cut through the clavicle at two points (*Atlas*, 8.4C and **D**): (a) laterally, close to the anterior attachments of the trapezius and deltoid muscles; and (b) close to the medial end of the clavicle. Detach the clavicular head of the sternocleidomastoid as far as necessary. Remove the middle portion of the clavicle. Observe the slender **subclavius muscle,** then remove it. Now, the structures at the base of the posterior triangle can be displayed.

Next, examine the slender **omohyoid muscle** (*Atlas*, 8.2). Its inferior (posterior) and superior bellies are sepa-

points: (a) a point slightly superior to the middle of the posterior border of the sternocleidomastoid; and (b) a point about 5 cm superior to the clavicle at the anterior border of the trapezius. Incise the roof of the triangle along the course indicated. Spread the tissue with scissors along the expected course of the accessory nerve (XI). Find the nerve and free it from its surrounding tissue. Be aware of the function of nerve XI (*Atlas*, 9.16).

Find the **lesser occipital nerve** (*Atlas*, 8.4A). It emerges from the posterior border of the sternocleidomastoid in close proximity to cranial nerve XI. Trace the lesser occipital nerve superiorly along or near the posterior border of the sternocleidomastoid. The nerve supplies the scalp (*Atlas*, 7.14). At the apex of the posterior triangle, search for the occipital artery (*Atlas*, 8.4A).

rated by an intertendon (*Atlas*, 8.20, 8.23). This intertendon is held down to the clavicle by a fibrous expansion. Note this fibrous band (omohyoid fascia) deep to the clavicular attachment of the sternocleidomastoid. Remove the omohyoid fascia, thereby exposing the blood vessels at the base of the posterior triangle.

Blood Vessels (*Atlas*, 8.4**C** and **D**).   Follow the external jugular vein through the omohyoid fascia to the subclavian vein. Note the **suprascapular vein** that runs posterior to the clavicle. Note the **transverse cervical artery** running about 2 to 3 cm superior to the clavicle and deep to the omohyoid (*Atlas*, 8.4**D**). This artery heads toward the levator scapulae. The **suprascapular artery** takes a retroclavicular course to reach the suprascapular notch. Review the origin and destination of the two arteries (*Atlas*, 8.46). Note that both arteries pass anterior to the scalenus anterior. Variations in the origin of the transverse cervical and suprascapular arteries are common. In over 50% of the cases, one of the arteries does not arise from the thyrocervical trunk.

Structures Deep to Floor of Triangle

Now, after securing the contents of the posterior triangle, the **fascial floor** of the triangle (fascial carpet) can be removed (*Atlas*, 8.4**B** and **C**). Expose the underlying muscles: **splenius capitis, levator scapulae,** and the **three scaleni: scalenus posterior, scalenus medius,** and **scalenus anterior.**

Define the **scalenus anterior** and the **scalenus medius.** Clean the muscles. Observe the following (*Atlas*, 8.4**D**):

1. The two muscles are inserted into **rib 1.**
2. An elongated triangular space is formed by the two muscles and rib 1. This is the **interscalene triangle.** Through this interval pass two important structures: the **subclavian artery** and the **brachial plexus.**
3. The **subclavian vein** passes anterior to the scalenus anterior.
4. The **transverse cervical artery** and **suprascapular artery** commonly cross anterior to the scalenus anterior.
5. The **phrenic nerve** (C3, C4, C5) descends vertically across the surface of the scalenus anterior toward the thorax. The nerve is intimately applied to the muscle; therefore, nerve and muscle are crossed anteriorly by the three vessels: transverse cervical artery, suprascapular artery, and subclavian vein.
6. The scalenus medius is pierced by motor nerves to the rhomboids (C5) and to the serratus anterior (C5, C6).

If not already done, clean the **axillary artery** and the **brachial plexus** at the level of the scaleni. Review the brachial plexus, its rami, trunks, and divisions (*Atlas*, 6.27).

The **interscalene triangle** becomes of clinical significance when it is too narrow and, therefore, compresses the structures passing through it. Anatomical variations such as additional muscular slips, an accessory cervical rib, or exostosis on the 1st rib may narrow the available interval. As a result, the subclavian artery and/or the brachial plexus may be compressed. This compression may lead to ischemia and to disturbances in nerve function in the upper limb.

The supraclavicular nerves and the phrenic nerve have essentially the same segmental origin, C3 and C4. This fact explains the phenomenon of "referred pain" in pleurisy. Irritation of the phrenic nerve in the diaphragmatic region may produce pain sensations in the cutaneous area supplied by the supraclavicular nerves (shoulder; clavicular region).

Anterior Triangle of Neck

General Remarks

The **boundaries** of the anterior triangle of the neck are (*Atlas*, 8.2):

1. Anteriorly, the median line of the neck;
2. Posteriorly, the anterior border of the sternocleidomastoid;
3. Superiorly, the inferior of the mandible.

The anterior triangle is further subdivided into smaller triangles: *muscular, carotid, submandibular,* and *submental.*

Study a **transverse section through the neck** (*Atlas*, 8.43, 8.44). The anterior part of the neck may be regarded as a "cervical cavity." It is bounded by walls:

1. Posteriorly, by the cervical vertebrae;
2. Posterolaterally, by the scaleni;
3. Laterally, by the sternocleidomastoid;
4. Anteriorly, by the strap-like infrahyoid muscles.

The "cervical cavity" houses the **cervical viscera,** which lie in the median plane (*Atlas*, 8.43):

1. Superior part of digestive tract: **pharynx** and **esophagus;**
2. Superior part of respiratory tract: **larynx** and **trachea;**
3. **Thyroid gland,** anterior to the tube-like digestive and respiratory tracts.

The big vessels and nerves lie to each side of the cervical viscera. **Three major structures, carotid artery, internal jugular vein,** and **vagus nerve,** are wrapped together in the fascial carotid sheath.

Arterial Supply (*Atlas*, 8.12).   The **common carotid artery** bifurcates into the internal and external carotid arteries. The **external carotid artery** supplies almost all structures of the head and neck outside the cranial cavity. The **internal carotid artery** supplies the structures within the cranial and orbital cavities. The **vertebral arteries,** which ascend in the neck through the foramina transversaria, enter the cranial cavity through the foramen magnum to contribute to the cerebral arterial circle. A branch of the subclavian artery, the **thyrocervical trunk,** supplies the lower part of the neck.

Exposure of Anterior Triangle

Make a skin incision in the midline from the tip of the chin to the suprasternal notch. Remove entirely the skin from the front of the neck.

Once again, observe the fibers of the **platysma** (*Atlas,* 8.1A). Reflect and remove it. Review the cutaneous nerve to the region of the anterior triangle, the **transverse cervical nerve** (*Atlas,* 8.4A).

Superficial Veins (Fig. 7.28; *Atlas,* 8.9). Expect to *find variations* in the venous pattern. Review the course of the **external jugular vein.** Trace the facial vein along the lower border of the mandible to a point where it is joined by the anterior division of the **retromandibular vein.** The facial vein continues for a short distance and drains into the internal jugular vein deep to the sternocleidomastoid muscle. Follow the facial vein. If present, find the small **anterior jugular vein.** On occasion, this vein is connected to the facial vein by a **communicating branch.** Clean the deep fascia within the confines of the anterior triangle.

Bony and Cartilaginous Landmarks

Study bony and cartilaginous **landmarks** that will be used as reference structures (*Atlas,* 8.71, 8.73):

1. **Hyoid bone,** at the angle between floor of mouth and superior end of neck; palpate your own hyoid bone; distinguish **body, greater horn,** and **lesser horn;**
2. **Thyroid cartilage,** the large cartilage of the larynx; in the midline, note and palpate the **laryngeal prominence** (Adam's apple);
3. **Thyrohyoid membrane,** stretching between thyroid cartilage and hyoid bone;
4. **Cricoid cartilage,** inferior to thyroid cartilage and superior to the 1st tracheal ring; it lies at the level of C6;
5. **Cricothyroid membrane,** stretching between cricoid and thyroid cartilages; the cricothyroid muscles unite the two cartilages more laterally;
6. **Trachea;** note its 1st, 2nd, and 3rd rings.

Muscular Triangle

The **muscular triangle** is separated from the carotid triangle by the superior belly of the omohyoid (*Atlas,* 8.2). On each side of the median line are four ribbon-like muscles

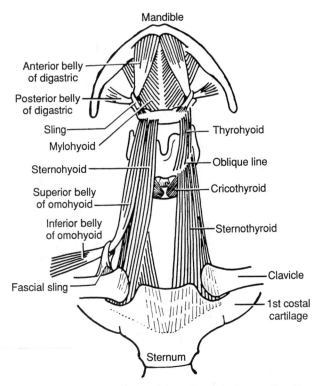

Figure 7.30. The muscles bounding the anterior median line of the neck and a diagram of the infrahyoid muscles.

that descend from the hyoid bone or the thyroid cartilage. These are the **infrahyoid muscles** (Fig. 7.30; *Atlas,* 8.33). Their names are descriptive of their attachments. In a *superficial plane,* identify the superior belly of the **omohyoid** and the **sternohyoid.** *Deep* to these two muscles are the **sternothyroid** and the short **thyrohyoid.** The muscles are supplied by nerve branches from C1 to C3 via the **ansa cervicalis** (*Atlas,* 8.19). These nerves to the infrahyoid muscles will be identified later.

Widen the gap in the midline between the right and left infrahyoids by gently pulling the muscles laterally. Now, palpate and identify (*Atlas,* 8.36): **laryngeal prominence, cricoid cartilage, cricothyroid membrane, 1st tracheal ring,** and **isthmus of thyroid gland.**

Tracheotomy (tracheostomy) is the formation of an opening into the trachea. As an emergency operation, it must be rapidly performed in cases with sudden obstruction of the vital airways (aspiration of foreign body; edema of larynx; paralysis of vocal cords). A superior (high) tracheotomy is performed superior to the level of the isthmus of the thyroid gland. An inferior (low) tracheotomy is done inferior to the isthmus.

The simplest and most rapid access to the airway inferior to the vocal cords may be created by opening the cricothyroid membrane (cricothyrotomy). It is often used prior to tracheotomy in certain emergency respiratory obstructions. Perform this important emergency procedure in the cadaver. Palpate the thyroid and cricoid cartilages and the membrane stretching between them. Then, incise the membrane transversely.

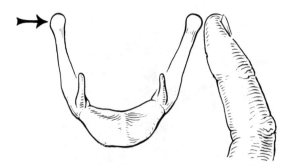

Figure 7.31. Steady the tip of one horn of the hyoid bone while palpating the other.

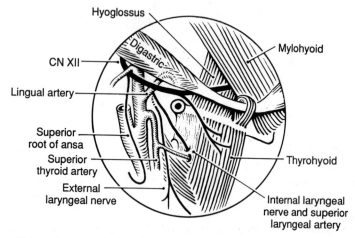

Figure 7.32. The tip of the greater horn of the hyoid bone is the reference point for many structures: nerves, arteries, and muscles.

Carotid Triangle

The **carotid triangle** is bounded by the superior belly of the omohyoid, the posterior belly of the digastric, and the anterior border of the sternocleidomastoid. The **common carotid artery** ascends through the triangle. The pulse of the common carotid artery can be palpated and auscultated within the boundaries of this triangular space.

Nerves in the Carotid Triangle (*Atlas*, 8.20). The first objective is to find the **accessory nerve (XI)** as it enters the sternocleidomastoid muscle. Transect the sternocleidomastoid muscle about 5 cm superior to its insertion into sternum and clavicle. Free and clean the upper portion of the sternocleidomastoid from its surrounding fascia. Do not damage the nerves that radiate from the posterior border of the muscle into the posterior triangle. Note the arterial branches that enter the muscle; then cut them. Find the **accessory nerve** where it enters the *deep surface* of the sternocleidomastoid: about 5 cm inferior to the tip of the mastoid process and about 2 cm posterior to the anterior border of the muscle (*Atlas*, 8.23). Trace the accessory nerve superiorly as far as possible. The nerve may cross the internal jugular vein anteriorly or posteriorly. The nerve and the vein pass through the same opening, the jugular foramen. Review cranial nerve XI (*Atlas*, 9.16).

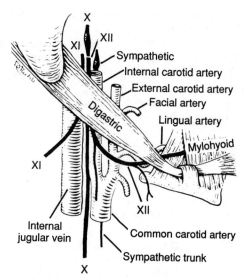

Figure 7.33. The posterior belly of the digastric muscle and structures deep to it.

To allow better access to deeper structures, cut the **facial vein** where it empties into the internal jugular vein.

The **tip of the greater horn of the hyoid bone** is an important reference point for many structures. The greater horn on one side is palpable only when the greater horn of the opposite side is steadied. Palpate the greater horn on the side of the dissection with one index finger while you press against the greater horn of the opposite side with your other index finger (Fig. 7.31).

The next objective is to find the **hypoglossal nerve (XII)**. It is the motor nerve to the tongue; therefore, it courses anteriorly. Palpate and locate the tip of the greater horn of the hyoid bone. Then, pick up the large, flat hypoglossal nerve just superior to the tip (Fig. 7.32; *Atlas*, 8.21, 8.23). At this point, nerve fibers belonging to spinal cord segments C1 and C2 and adhering to the hypoglossal nerve leave the nerve to supply the thyrohyoid muscle (*Atlas*, 9.17B and C). Follow this slender branch across the tip of the greater horn to the lateral border of the thyrohyoid muscle.

Trace the **hypoglossal nerve** anteriorly and proximally. Verify that the posterior belly of the digastric muscle lies lateral to the nerve (Fig. 7.33; *Atlas*, 8.20). Retract the posterior belly of the digastric and demonstrate the course of the hypoglossal nerve. Proximally, study the relationship of the nerve to the occipital artery (*Atlas*, 8.23). Note that a branch of the occipital artery, the muscular branch to the sternocleidomastoid, hooks over the nerve. At this point, find the **superior root of the ansa cervicalis** that is closely adherent to nerve XII (Fig. 7.32; *Atlas*, 8.21, 8.23). Study the components of the **ansa cervicalis** (*Atlas*, 8.19). The *superior root* (descendens hypoglossi) is mainly composed of fibers from C1 that adhere to and run with the hypoglossal nerve. The *inferior root* of the ansa (descendens cervicalis; C2, C3) descends from the more superior neck region to join the superior root. Thus, a loop or ansa is formed. Dissect the ansa. Trace nerve branches from it to the **infrahyoid muscles** (*Atlas*, 8.23).

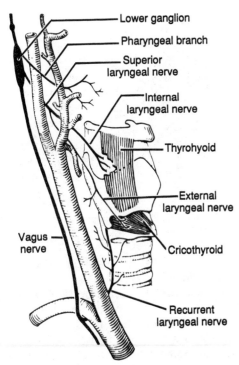

Figure 7.34. Laryngeal branches of the right vagus nerve (cranial nerve X).

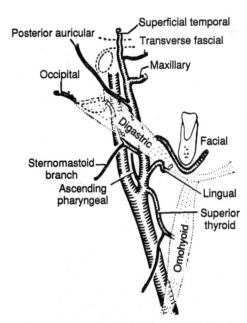

Figure 7.35. Arteries in the carotid triangle.

The next objective is to find the **vagus (X)** nerve and one of its branches. The vagus lies in the carotid sheath, in the posterior angle between the internal jugular vein and the great arterial trunk. Pull the internal jugular vein and nerve XI laterally; pull the carotid arteries and nerve XII medially. This will expose the vagus nerve (Fig. 7.33). Free the vagus and trace it inferiorly.

Now, find the **superior laryngeal nerve** and its major branch, the **internal laryngeal nerve** (Fig. 7.34; *Atlas*, 8.38A, 8.39). Proceed as follows: relax the anatomical structures of the neck by flexing the head (bending it anteriorly). With scissors, sever the omohyoid and the sternohyoid close to the hyoid bone. Reflect the muscles inferiorly. Next, carefully sever the exposed thyrohyoid muscle close to the hyoid bone; reflect it inferiorly. Now, the **thyrohyoid membrane** lies exposed. Identify this membrane that extends between the thyroid cartilage and the hyoid bone. Palpate these two topographic landmarks. The internal laryngeal nerve pierces the thyrohyoid membrane just inferior to the greater horn of the hyoid bone to supply the superior portion of the larynx with sensory fibers.

Find the **external laryngeal nerve** that supplies the cricothyroid muscle and the adjacent part of the inferior constrictor (Fig. 7.34; *Atlas* 8.48). Proceed as follows: trace the internal laryngeal nerve proximally to a point where it is crossed by the internal carotid artery. Here, find the external laryngeal nerve. Trace the delicate nerve inferiorly. Carefully sever the sternothyroid muscle from the oblique line of the thyroid cartilage. Raise the muscle. Find the external laryngeal nerve deep to it. Trace the nerve to the cricothyroid muscle.

Arteries in the Carotid Triangle (Fig. 7.35; *Atlas*, 8.12). The arteries in this triangle are: (a) parts of the common, internal, and external carotid arteries; and (b) the stems of most of the six collateral branches of the external carotid artery.

Remove the **carotid sheath.** Be aware of the relationship of internal jugular vein and common carotid artery (*Atlas*, 8.40). Note that the internal jugular vein lies in close lateral contact with the **common carotid artery** and the **internal carotid artery.** These two arteries have *no collateral branches* in the neck. The **external carotid artery,** which lies anteromedial to the internal carotid artery, gives off several branches before reaching the posterior belly of the digastric. Identify these branches (Fig. 7.35; *Atlas*, 8.14):

1. **Superior thyroid artery.** Identify its origin just inferior and posterior to the tip of the greater horn of the hyoid bone (Fig. 7.32). The artery descends to the superior pole of the thyroid gland. Identify one of its branches, the **superior laryngeal artery.** This artery pierces the thyrohyoid membrane together with the internal laryngeal nerve (*Atlas*, 8.39).
2. **Lingual artery.** Identify its origin just posterior to the tip of the greater horn of the hyoid bone (Fig. 7.32). Expect to find variations (*Atlas*, 8.22).
3. **Facial artery.** It arises just superior to the lingual artery. In 20% of all cases, the lingual and facial arteries have a common stem. Expect to find variations.
4. **Occipital artery.** It gives off a muscular branch to the sternocleidomastoid muscle.
5. **Ascending pharyngeal artery.** Usually, it is the first branch to arise from the external carotid artery close to the carotid bifurcation. It is often difficult to find.

Clean the **bifurcation of the common carotid artery.**
Notice the dilation of the superior end of the common carotid and the beginning of the internal carotid. Here, the
walls of the artery are thinner, less muscular, and more
elastic. This dilated region is the **carotid sinus.** The wall of
this sinus contains pressoreceptors that respond to
changes in blood pressure (*Atlas*, 9.15). Compare the
gross anatomical features of the dissected vessels with a
carotid arteriogram (*Atlas*, 8.13).

If time permits, look for the carotid body (*Atlas*, 9.14**B**
and **D**). It is a small mass of tissue, darker, and more firm
than fat, located on the medial aspect in the crotch of the
carotid bifurcation. The carotid body responds to changes
in the chemical composition of the blood. Cranial nerves
IX and X supply the carotid body and sinus.

Veins in the Anterior Triangle (*Atlas*, 8.10). Identify
the following tributaries to the **internal jugular vein: common facial vein; lingual vein;** and **superior thyroid vein,**
which accompanies the respective artery. To clarify the
dissection field, remove the tributaries of the internal jugular vein.

Submandibular Triangle

The **submandibular or digastric triangle** (*Atlas*, 8.2) is
bounded by:

1. Inferior border of mandible;
2. Anterior belly of digastric;
3. Posterior belly of digastric.

In the bony skull, identify the following relevant
landmarks:

1. In the **temporal bone,** examine (*Atlas*, 7.2A): the **mastoid process** and **styloid process;** in many skulls, the
   long and sharp styloid process is broken off;
2. Examine the inner aspect of a **mandible** (*Atlas*, 7.71**B**)
   and identify: **digastric fossa** for the attachment of the
   anterior belly of the digastric; **mylohyoid line,** for the
   attachment of the mylohyoid; **submandibular fossa,**
   inferior to the mylohyoid line; **mylohyoid groove,** in
   which the nerves and vessels to the mylohyoid and the
   anterior belly of the digastric run.

Part of the submandibular salivary gland and some
lymph nodes fill the submandibular triangle (*Atlas*, 8.18).
The **submandibular gland** is wrapped around the free posterior border of the mylohyoid like the letter U on its side.
The deep part of the gland and its duct (*Atlas*, 7.78**B**) must
not be disturbed. The superficial part of the gland, lying
within the boundaries of the submandibular triangle, may
be severed and removed. Proceed as follows: clamp a hemostat or a forceps to the gland. Pull the gland medially. Free
the superficial part of the gland from its surrounding fascia. Separate the **facial artery** and vein from the gland.
Note blood vessels supplying the glandular tissue. Now,

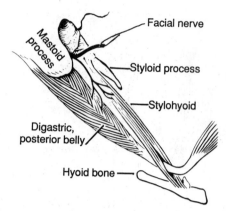

Figure 7.36. The stylohyoid muscle is perforated by the intermediate tendon of the digastric muscle.

cut through the gland at the posterior border of the
mylohyoid and remove it.

Now, the **anterior and posterior bellies of the digastric**
can be well defined. Note that the two bellies are connected
to each other by an intermediate tendon (Fig. 7.36; *Atlas*,
8.20, 8.21, 8.25**A**). This tendon is held to the body and the
greater horn of the hyoid bone by a fibrous sling. Note that
the intermediate tendon perforates a slender, round muscle, the **stylohyoid** (Fig. 7.36). Verify that the posterior
belly of the digastric arises from the medial aspect of the
mastoid process. The anterior belly arises from the digastric fossa of the mandible.

Trace the **hypoglossal nerve (XII)** into the submandibular triangle (*Atlas*, 8.23, 8.25**A**, 8.26). Observe that the
nerve disappears under cover of the mylohyoid muscle.

Pull the anterior belly of the digastric medially to expose
the **mylohyoid nerve,** a branch of V³ (*Atlas*, 8.25**A**). Observe that the nerve is sheltered by the lower border of the
mandible. Its more distal portion is closely applied to the
mylohyoid. One of its branches reaches the anterior belly
of the digastric (the posterior belly of the digastric and the
stylohyoid muscles are supplied by a branch of cranial
nerve VII; *Atlas*, 7.65, 9.12**B**).

Submental Triangle

The **boundaries** of the submental (suprahyoid) triangle
are (Fig. 7.30; *Atlas*, 8.2, 8.34):

1. Inferiorly, the body of the **hyoid bone;**
2. Laterally, the right and left **anterior bellies of the digastric muscles.**

The **floor** of the triangle is formed by the two **mylohyoid
muscles.** These muscles arise from the mandible and are
inserted into the body of the hyoid bone. The fibers of the
right and left muscles meet in a median fibrous raphe.

Clean the anterior bellies of the digastrics. Occasionally, these anterior bellies are fused and, therefore, may
hide the underlying mylohyoid muscle. If this is the case,

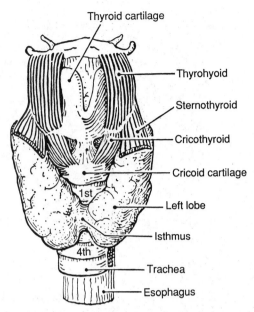

Figure 7.37. The thyroid gland (anterior view).

Labels on figure: Thyroid cartilage; Thyrohyoid; Sternothyroid; Cricothyroid; Cricoid cartilage; Left lobe; Isthmus; Trachea; Esophagus; 1st; 4th

serve its characteristic colloid structure. Preserve the posterior aspect of the lobe, where the parathyroid glands may be found.

Parathyroid Glands (*Atlas*, 8.41, 8.68). These small but vital glands lie along the posterior border of the thyroid gland between its capsule and its sheath. On the posterior aspect of the removed thyroid lobe, look for small brownish bodies, measuring about 5 mm in diameter. Usually, there are two parathyroid glands on each side. However, the total number may vary from 2 to 6.

Physicians must be fully aware of the close relationship between thyroid gland, parathyroids, and the recurrent laryngeal nerves. If, during thyroidectomy (removal of thyroid gland), one or both recurrent laryngeal nerves are injured, paralysis of the laryngeal muscles will occur. Note how intimately the recurrent laryngeal nerve is related to the thyroid gland (*Atlas*, 8.41, 8.68). Understand that a malignant tumor of the thyroid may easily lead to destruction of the recurrent laryngeal nerve or nerves.

The parathyroids play a vital role in the regulation of calcium and phosphorus metabolism. During thyroidectomy, these small endocrine glands are in danger of being damaged or of being removed. Appreciate this fact by studying the close relations between thyroid and parathyroid glands (*Atlas*, 8.68).

separate the digastrics from each other and expose the floor of the submental triangle.

Cervical Viscera

The superior parts of the digestive tract (pharynx and esophagus) and the respiratory tract (larynx and trachea) will be dealt with in special assignments. The thyroid gland can be conveniently explored at this time.

Thyroid Gland (Fig. 7.37; *Atlas*, 8.38B). The infrahyoid and the sternocleidomastoid muscles were reflected earlier. Therefore, the thyroid gland lies exposed. Verify that it extends between the carotid sheaths of the two sides (*Atlas*, 8.40). Identify the **right and left lobes.** The two lobes are connected by the **isthmus,** which usually covers the 2nd to 4th tracheal rings. In 50% of all cases, the gland has a **pyramidal lobe** that ascends from the isthmus superiorly, sometimes as high as the hyoid bone. Expect to find variations (*Atlas*, 8.42).

Being an endocrine organ, the thyroid gland has a rich blood supply and drainage. Once again, identify the **superior thyroid artery** (*Atlas*, 8.39). Demonstrate the **three veins** that drain the thyroid gland: **superior, middle,** and **inferior thyroid veins** (*Atlas*, 8.38A). To find the **inferior thyroid artery,** on the respective side, pull the lobe of the thyroid gland anteriorly. Observe the origin of the artery from the thyrocervical trunk (*Atlas*, 8.41, 8.46).

Cut the isthmus of the gland and turn the lobes laterally. Define and then sever the fascial band that attaches the capsule of the gland to the 1st tracheal ring (*Atlas*, 8.39). With a probe, display the **recurrent laryngeal nerve** that ascends just posterior to the gland on the side of the trachea.

On the left side only, cut all blood vessels leading to or from the left lobe of the thyroid gland. Then, enucleate this lobe. Cut into the substance of the gland. Ob-

Root of the Neck

The sternocleidomastoid, sternohyoid, sternothyroid, and the superior belly of the omohyoid were reflected earlier. If not already done, remove the fascia (loop) that binds the intermediate tendon of the omohyoid to the clavicle (*Atlas*, 8.34). Now, the root of the neck lies exposed, particularly on the left side, where the left lobe of the thyroid gland was resected (*Atlas*, 8.49).

To clarify the dissection field, cut the **common carotid artery** and the **internal jugular vein** (but not the vagus) about 2 cm superior to the clavicular level. Reflect the large vessels superiorly. Fix them in the reflected position with needles or a hemostat.

The next objective is to find the **thoracic duct.** The duct opens at (or near) the angle between the **left subclavian vein** and the **left internal jugular vein** (*Atlas*, 8.41, 8.49). The duct has approximately the same diameter as the superior thyroid vein. Usually, it is pale, collapsed, inconspicuous, and very easily torn.

To find the **thoracic duct,** proceed as follows (Fig. 7.38; *Atlas*, 8.50): pull the inferior portions of the severed common carotid artery and internal jugular vein anteriorly. Now, the duct lies exposed as it arches from the side of the esophagus laterally to the angle between internal jugular and subclavian veins. To clarify the dissection field, remove the vertebral vein. Usually, this vein descends posterior to the thoracic duct to empty dorsally into the brachiocephalic vein (*Atlas*, 8.49).

Realize that delicate **lymphatic trunks** empty into the *right* subclavian and jugular veins (*Atlas*, 1.81). You are not required to search for these lymph vessels.

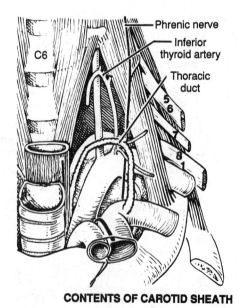

CONTENTS OF CAROTID SHEATH

Figure 7.38. Root of the neck: drainage of the thoracic duct.

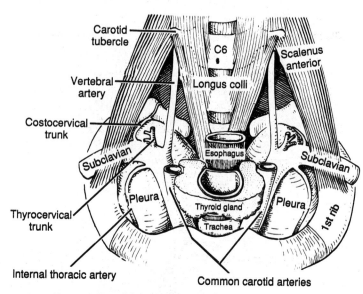

Figure 7.39. Root of the neck: triangle of the vertebral artery; branches of the subclavian artery.

Clean the vagus nerve and the phrenic nerve and follow these structures into the thorax. Once again, note that the phrenic nerve is intimately applied to the ventral surface of the scalenus anterior. The **transverse cervical and suprascapular arteries** pass directly anterior to the nerve and muscle (*Atlas*, 8.46, 8.49). Trace these two arteries back to their origin from the **thyrocervical trunk.** This arterial trunk arises near the medial border of the scalenus anterior (*Atlas*, 8.15). Identify a third branch of the thyrocervical trunk, the **inferior thyroid artery.** It passes posterior to the carotid sheath to enter the inferior pole of the thyroid gland (*Atlas*, 8.16). Expect to find variations: often the thyrocervical trunk does not give rise to all three arteries. On occasion, the arteries arise separately from the subclavian artery.

Inferior to the origin of the thyrocervical trunk, notice the origin of the **internal thoracic artery** (Fig. 7.39; *Atlas*, 8.15, 8.49).

The next objective is to find and partially trace the **vertebral artery.** It is the first and largest branch of the subclavian artery (Fig. 7.39; *Atlas*, 8.15). Identify this deeply running vessel in relation to two muscles, the scalenus anterior and the longus colli. These muscles form the two sides of the "**triangle of the vertebral artery.**" The **apex** of this triangle is the **transverse process of C6.** The anterior tubercle of this transverse process is an important landmark. The common carotid artery passes anterior to the tubercle and may be compressed against it ("carotid tubercle"; Fig. 7.39). Trace the vertebral artery to the apex of the triangle where it enters the transverse foramen of C6. Review the course of the vertebral artery (*Atlas*, 8.12).

The **sympathetic trunk and its ganglia** may be examined now (*Atlas*, 8.7, 8.8). However, these structures can be more conveniently studied in the prevertebral region, after removal of the head.

Parotid Region

Bony Landmarks

Refer to a bony skull and study the following pertinent **landmarks:**

1. On the **temporal bone** (*Atlas*, 7.2), identify: the **styloid process,** the **mastoid process,** the **external acoustic meatus,** and the **mandibular fossa** for the head of the mandible;
2. On the **mandible** (*Atlas*, 7.2), identify: the **head,** the **neck,** and the posterior border of the **ramus;**
3. On the exterior of the **base of the skull** (*Atlas*, 8.52, 8.53), identify: the **stylomastoid foramen,** located between the base of the styloid process and the mastoid process (the important facial nerve or cranial nerve VII passes through this foramen).

General Remarks

The parotid region is a restricted space occupied by the parotid gland and certain soft structures associated with it. Refer to a skull and define the bony space that forms the boundaries for the parotid bed (*Atlas*, 7.2):

1. Posteriorly, the mastoid process;
2. Anteriorly, the ramus of mandible;
3. Superiorly, the floor of external acoustic meatus;
4. Medially, the styloid process.

The posterior wall of the parotid region extends between the mastoid and styloid processes. Therefore, the muscles

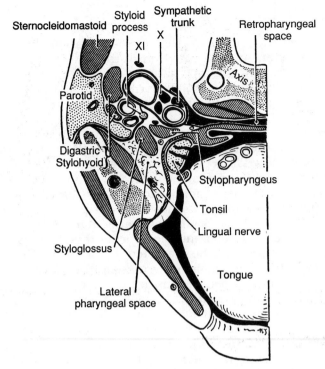

Figure 7.40. Transverse section of the head at the level of the parotid gland.

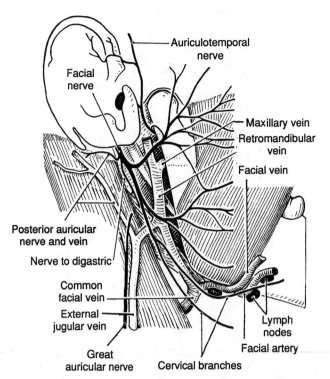

Figure 7.41. The facial nerve and veins in the parotid bed.

attached to these processes (sternocleidomastoid; posterior belly of digastric; stylohyoid) are closely related to the gland (Fig. 7.40; *Atlas*, 7.61, 7.65). The anterior wall of the parotid region is formed by the ramus of the mandible and the two muscles (masseter; medial pterygoid) applied to it (Fig. 7.40; *Atlas*, 7.85).

The parotid gland is traversed by branches of the facial nerve, arteries, and veins. This fact must be appreciated during dissection and during surgery.

Dissection

Observe the superficial extent of the parotid gland and the structures radiating from its margin (*Atlas*, 7.12): the **parotid duct,** the transverse facial artery, and branches of the **facial nerve.** These structures have already been cleaned. Note that the parotid gland is enclosed within fascia, the **parotid sheath.**

The first objective is to find the **stem of the facial nerve (VII)** as it emerges from the stylomastoid foramen (Fig. 7.41; *Atlas*, 7.61). Proceed as follows: make sure that the sternocleidomastoid is well cleaned where it attaches to the mastoid process. Reflect the muscle. With the handle of the scalpel, ease the parotid sheath and the contained parotid gland anteriorly. Hold it in this position with a hemostat. Again, refer to a skull, and examine how you must aim the handle of the knife in order to reach the stylomastoid foramen. Push the handle upward, anteromedially to the mastoid process, until it catches between the mastoid and styloid processes. Using a probe in the

cadaver, reveal the facial nerve as it leaves the stylomastoid foramen to enter the parotid sheath.

Follow the **temporal branches of the facial nerve** posteriorly. Trace them through the glandular tissue (*Atlas*, 7.61). You may find two large communications with the **auriculotemporal nerve** (a branch of V³) that carry secretory fibers to the parotid gland (*Atlas*, 9.14C). Using blunt dissection, shell the gland out of its fascial bed. Follow facial nerve branches deep through the substance of the gland. Trace the auriculotemporal nerve toward the neck of the mandible. The nerve runs medial and deep to the parotid gland (*Atlas*, 7.65).

The next objective is to identify the vessels that traverse the tissue of the parotid gland. Use scissors to spread the tissue. Establish the course of the **retromandibular vein** (Fig. 7.41; *Atlas*, 7.61). Next, trace the **external carotid artery** through the gland. The artery is deeply placed and sheltered by the ramus of the mandible (*Atlas*, 7.65). Posterior to the neck of the mandible, the external carotid artery divides into its two terminal branches: the **maxillary artery** and the **superficial temporal artery** (*Atlas*, 7.74A).

Cut the parotid duct close to the gland. Pull the gland posteriorly and inferiorly. Sever the facial nerve about 2 to 3 cm distal to the stylomastoid foramen. Remove the parotid gland.

Now, examine the **parotid bed** (*Atlas*, 7.65). Identify the **posterior belly of the digastric** and the **stylohyoid.** Palpate the styloid process. Clean the auriculotemporal nerve posterior to the temporomandibular joint. Mark the severed facial nerve by tying a piece of thread to it.

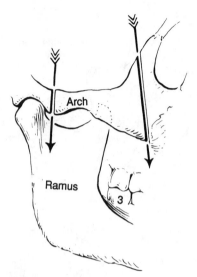

Figure 7.42.   Two saw cuts (*arrows*) through the zygomatic arch.

Appreciate the close relationship between the external ear canal and parotid gland (Gr., *para*, near; *otos*, = ear). A painful swelling of the parotid gland (e.g., as in mumps) characteristically pushes the ear lobe superiorly and laterally.

During parotidectomy (surgical excision of parotid gland), the facial nerve is in constant danger (*Atlas*, 7.13). In cases of benign parotid tumors, the stem of the facial nerve may be isolated at the stylomastoid foramen and the facial nerve branches may remain intact during removal of lobules of diseased parotid tissue. In malignant tumors, the facial nerve must be sacrificed. What will happen if the orbicularis oculi becomes nonfunctional as a result of facial nerve paralysis?

Temporal and Masseteric Regions

Bony Landmarks

Refer to a skull and study the following pertinent landmarks (*Atlas*, 7.2):

1. **Temporal lines,** curving backward from the frontal process of the zygomatic bone and indicating the margin of origin of the temporalis muscle; the temporal lines surround the **temporal fossa;** note that this fossa is formed by several bony components: *parietal* bone, *frontal* bone, squamous part of *temporal* bone, and greater wing of *sphenoid* bone;
2. **Zygomatic arch,** composed of the *zygomatic process* of the temporal bone and the *temporal process* of the zygomatic bone;
3. **Mandible** (*Atlas*, 7.2, 7.71A); identify the **ramus** and **angle;** the **mandibular notch** is located between the **head of mandible** and **coronoid process.**

Dissection

Remove the remains of the masseteric fascia and clean the **masseter** (*Atlas*, 7.62). Detach the posterior third of the muscle from the zygomatic arch. Turn the detached portion of the masseter anteriorly to display the **masseteric nerve and vessels** passing through the mandibular notch.

Next, the masseter must be reflected inferiorly together with its bone of origin. Proceed as follows (Fig. 7.42): pass a probe or closed forceps deep to the zygomatic arch to protect the underlying soft structures. Saw obliquely through the zygomatic bone as far anteriorly as possible. Then, saw through the zygoma as far posteriorly as possible. Reflect inferiorly the section of the zygomatic arch together with the attached masseter muscle. During this process, the nerve and vessels to the masseter will be torn. With the handle of a scalpel, detach the muscle fibers of the deep portion of the masseter from the superior portion of the ramus and from the lateral surface of the coronoid process. Detach the superficial portion of the muscle from the ramus of the mandible. Leave the masseter attached to the lower margin of the mandible (*Atlas*, 7.64).

Now, the **temporal fascia** is fully exposed. Review its attachment to the temporal line (it cannot be fully traced where the calvaria has been removed). Make a deep vertical cut through the fascia and evert it (*Atlas*, 7.62). Observe:

1. The muscle fibers of the temporalis partly arise from the fascia.
2. The temporalis inserts into the coronoid process of the mandible (*Atlas*, 7.64).
3. The anterior portion of the temporalis is thick. Its fibers take a vertical direction (important for closure of the jaw). The fibers of the smaller posterior portion take a posterior sweep from the coronoid process.

The temporal fascia splits to enclose a small fatpad between the temporalis and the lateral wall of the orbit. Notice that this fatty tissue is continuous with the buccal fatpad on the buccinator (*Atlas*, 7.6). Remove the fat. Realize that in the emaciated person, the loss of the continuous fatpads is responsible for the sunken cheeks and temples.

Infratemporal Region

General Remarks and Bony Landmarks

The infratemporal fossa contains two muscles of mastication: the mandibular nerve (V³), and the maxillary vessels. The fossa lies deep; its lateral wall is the ramus of the mandible. Therefore, access to the infratemporal fossa will necessitate partial removal of the ramus.

Profitable dissection of this region requires a thorough knowledge of the **pertinent bony features.** Refer to a skull

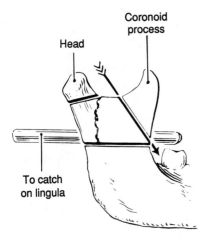

Head

Coronoid
process

To catch
on lingula

Figure 7.43. Three saw cuts through the mandible.

and identify on the **inner aspect of the mandible** (*Atlas*, 7.71B):

1. **Coronoid process;**
2. **Lingula** for the attachment of the sphenomandibular ligament;
3. **Mandibular foramen,** for the transmission of the inferior alveolar nerves and vessels;
4. **Mylohyoid groove,** for the nerve and vessels to the mylohyoid and anterior belly of the digastric.

Remove the mandible from the bony skull, thus gaining access to the bony landmarks of the infratemporal fossa. View this area inferolaterally (*Atlas*, 7.73) or from the **base of the skull** (*Atlas*, 8.52, 8.53). Identify:

1. **Lateral pterygoid plate** of the sphenoid bone;
2. **Infratemporal (posterior) surface of the maxilla;**
3. **Pterygopalatine fossa,** a wedge-shaped cleft that transmits blood vessels;
4. **Greater wing of the sphenoid,** with two important foramina: **foramen ovale** and **foramen spinosum.**

Now, identify the **walls of the infratemporal fossa** (*Atlas*, 7.70, 7.73):

1. Laterally, the ramus of the mandible;
2. Anteriorly, the posterior aspect of the maxilla; superiorly, it is limited by the inferior orbital fissure; medially, by the pterygopalatine fossa;
3. The **medial wall** is the lateral plate of the pterygoid process;
4. The **roof** of the infratemporal fossa is flat and formed by the greater wing of the sphenoid. The large foramen ovale transmits the mandibular nerve (V^3). The foramen spinosum is traversed by the middle meningeal vessels. The sphenomandibular ligament is attached near the spine of the sphenoid.

Dissection

First Saw Cut (Fig. 7.43).   To detach the coronoid process, proceed as follows: pass a probe or the blade of a forceps (*arrow* in Fig. 7.43) through the mandibular notch. Push the instrument obliquely inferiorly and anteriorly, in close contact with the mandible. Now, the soft structures deep to the coronoid process are protected from the saw blade. Cut obliquely through the **coronoid process.** Reflect it together with the insertion of the **temporalis muscle.**

Raise the anterior and posterior borders of the temporalis until the nerves to the muscle are seen lying on the bone. These nerves are accompanied by deep temporal arteries (*Atlas*, 7.76). Study the muscle. Subsequently, remove the temporalis muscle entirely and discard it.

Second Saw Cut (Fig. 7.43).   The objective of this procedure is to remove the superior part of the ramus of the mandible. However, the nerves and vessels just medial to the mandibular ramus must not be damaged. Proceed as follows: with a pencil, mark the approximate position of the **lingula** (center of ramus) on the lateral surface of the ramus. Below this pencil mark, the inferior alveolar nerve and vessels enter the mandible on its medial aspect (*Atlas*, 7.77). In order *not* to damage the inferior alveolar structures, the saw cut across the mandible must be made *superior* to the pencil mark. Pass the blade of an open forceps medial to the neck of the mandible. Keep in close contact with the bone. Work the instrument inferiorly until it is arrested by the lingula. Carefully make the prescribed saw cut and remove the bone fragment. Remaining bone, rough edges, or sharp spikes should be nibbled away with bone pliers. Guard your eyes against flying bone fragments.

Third Saw Cut (Fig. 7.43).   Cut through the neck of the mandible, just inferior to the **temporomandibular joint.** During the sawing procedure, protect the underlying soft structures with a probe or forceps.

Now, the **contents of the infratemporal fossa** lie exposed (*Atlas*, 7.76). Identify the **inferior alveolar nerve and artery** (the structures may be obscured by mandibular periosteum inadvertently left behind during bone removal). Trace the nerve inferiorly: it enters the mandibular foramen. Trace the nerve proximally (superiorly): it leads to the inferior border of the lateral pterygoid.

Follow the inferior alveolar nerve and vessels into the (bony) mandibular canal. With small bone pliers (or with a dental drill), open the canal. Note branches of the nerve and arteries to the teeth (*Atlas*, 9.11A). Finally, follow the distal portion of the inferior alveolar nerve through the mental foramen into the region of the chin and lower lip.

> **Mandibular block:** local anesthesia applied to the inferior alveolar nerve at the level of the mandibular foramen. Understand from your dissection that this block will not only anesthetize the mandibular teeth on the corresponding side, but also the lower lip and the chin inferior to it (*Atlas*, 9.11A).

Pick up the **lingual nerve,** which is closely applied to the ramus of the mandible (*Atlas*, 7.76). This large nerve runs

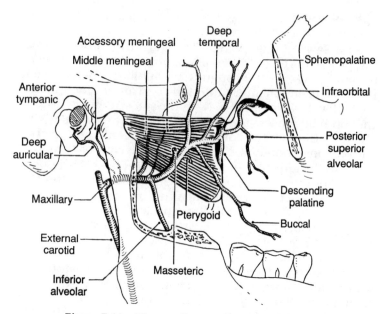

Figure 7.44. The maxillary artery and its branches.

anterior to the inferior alveolar nerve. Trace it to the inferior border of the lateral pterygoid, from whence it emerges. Posterior to the inferior alveolar nerve is the delicate **mylohyoid nerve.**

Maxillary Artery (Fig. 7.44; *Atlas*, 7.74A). Trace the artery through the infratemporal region. In most cases, it crosses superficial to the lateral pterygoid. However, in approximately one-third of all cases, it passes deep to the muscle (*Atlas*, 7.76, 7.77).

To obtain a complete and extensive view of the infratemporal region, the **lateral pterygoid muscle** must be removed. Notice that the muscle has two heads: one arises from the roof of the fossa, the other from the lateral pterygoid plate. With the handle of the scalpel, free the superior border of the lateral pterygoid from the roof. Next, define the inferior border of the muscle by inserting the handle into the interval between lateral and medial pterygoids. This interval is marked by the emergence of the lingual nerve and the inferior alveolar nerve. Work the handle anteriorly and superiorly and free the muscle from the lateral pterygoid plate. Finally, sever the muscle close to its pointed insertion into the neck of the mandible and into the articular disc (*Atlas*, 7.67). Remove the muscle completely. Do so in a piecemeal fashion to preserve superficially positioned nerves and vessels.

Now, the nerves and vessels in the infratemporal fossa can be examined in detail (*Atlas*, 7.77):

1. Identify the delicate **chorda tympani.** It joins the lingual nerve and it can be seen just posterior to the lingual nerve.
2. Follow the **inferior alveolar and lingual nerves** to the foramen ovale in the roof of the infratemporal fossa.
3. Push a thin probe through the **foramen ovale.** Locate the tip of the probe in the middle cranial fossa. Establish the continuity of nerve V³ with the trigeminal ganglion (*Atlas*, 7.36).

4. Identify and clean the **buccal nerve** (*Atlas*, 7.77). Its branches pierce the buccinator to supply the buccal mucosa with sensory fibers (*Atlas*, 7.8).
5. Identify the **auriculotemporal nerve** (*Atlas*, 7.77). Follow it to the foramen ovale.
6. Clean the **maxillary artery.** Identify two branches that pass through bony foramina:
   a. The **inferior alveolar artery;** follow it to the mandibular foramen; realize that it runs within the bony mandible to supply the mandibular teeth (*Atlas*, 7.74B);
   b. The **middle meningeal artery;** follow it to the foramen spinosum. Stick a needle through the **foramen spinosum.** Find the needle tip in the middle cranial fossa. Establish the continuity of the middle meningeal artery in the middle cranial fossa (*Atlas*, 7.23).
7. Notice **muscular branches** to the muscles of mastication. Most of these branches have been torn or cut during dissection.
8. Within the pterygopalatine fossa, the maxillary artery gives off several branches (Fig. 7.44; *Atlas*, 7.76, 7.77). Identify the **posterior superior alveolar artery.** The *infraorbital artery* and the *greater palatine artery* will be seen later.

Review the distribution of the mandibular division of the trigeminal nerve (*Atlas*, 9.11). Understand the importance of the delicate chorda tympani (*Atlas*, 9.12C).

Temporomandibular Joint

Refer to a skull and examine the following bony **landmarks** (*Atlas*, 7.67, 8.52, 8.53): the **mandibular fossa,** the **articular tubercle,** and the **articular condyle on the head of the mandible.**

Although the superior portion of the mandibular ramus has been removed, the head and neck of the mandible are still intact. The capsule of the temporomandibular joint is lax. It is thickened laterally to form the **temporomandibular ligament** (*Atlas*, 7.64). Manipulate the head of the mandible to verify the movements permitted at this joint: hinge movements, protraction, and retraction.

Enter the point of the scalpel into the mandibular fossa close to the bone. Open freely the superior cavity of the joint (*Atlas*, 7.67): remove the **articular disc** together with the head of the mandible.

In the isolated specimen (head and neck of mandible with articular disc), study the following:

1. Observe the insertion of the severed lateral pterygoid. The remains of the muscle are attached to the neck and articular disc.
2. Cut the disc anteroposteriorly and so open the inferior cavity of the joint. Observe the shape and varying thickness of the disc (*Atlas*, 7.67).

Axiom: In man, an articular disc implies two types of movements, one on each side of the disc. In the lower cavity, simple hinge move-

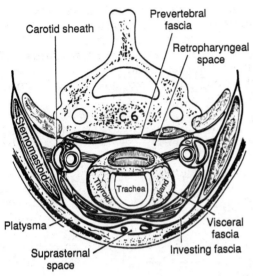

Figure 7.45. Transverse section through the neck at the level of C6. Retropharyngeal (retrovisceral) space.

ments between head and disc occur. In the upper cavity, the disc and head together glide on the articular tubercle during protraction of the mandible.

Place the little finger in the cartilaginous portion of your own external ear canal. Perform simple hinge movements of the mandible. Then protract and retract your lower jaw. By finger palpation, study the movements of the head of your own mandible.

Craniovertebral Joints and Removal of Head

General Remarks and Orientation

The head with the cervical viscera and the major nerves and vessels must be detached from the vertebral column and its associated musculature. This procedure will allow a posterior approach to the cervical viscera. Do not carry out any dissection at this time. Study a midsagittal section of the head and neck region (*Atlas*, 8.84), and understand:

1. The logical plane for separation is the **retropharyngeal (retrovisceral) space** that extends from the base of the skull into the superior part of the thorax.
2. The joints between cranium and vertebrae (craniovertebral joints) are the logical sites for separation between head and vertebral column. All ligaments holding these joints together must be severed in order to achieve separation.
3. In addition, the muscles connecting the vertebrae with the base of the skull must be severed.

Study a **transverse section of the neck** (Fig. 7.45; *Atlas*, 7.85). Identify the **retropharyngeal (retrovisceral) space.** Now, turn to the cadaver. Reflect the two sternocleidomastoids. On both sides at once, insert the fingers of

your right and left hands posterior to the carotid sheaths. Push your fingers medially until they meet posterior to the cervical viscera. Your fingers are now in the retrovisceral space. Work your fingers superiorly as high as the base of the skull; here is the superior limit of the retropharyngeal space. Work your fingers inferiorly toward the thorax; here, the space ends at the level of T3 where part of the prevertebral fascia fuses with the buccopharyngeal (visceral) fascia.

Before the head together with the cervical visera can be removed, the craniovertebral joints must be studied and, subsequently, disarticulated. Knowledge of pertinent bony reference points is essential.

Bony Landmarks

Refer to a skeleton (or skull and cervical vertebral column) and identify the following pertinent bony **landmarks:**

1. **Axis,** C2 (*Atlas*, 4.15). Note its **dens or odontoid process,** which is in apposition with the anterior arch of the atlas.
2. **Atlas,** C1 (*Atlas*, 4.15, 4.43). Identify: **posterior arch; anterior arch** with facet for dens; **transverse process; superior articular facet.** Understand that the dens of the axis is held tight to the anterior arch by the **transverse ligament,** which is bow-shaped and very strong.
3. On the **occipital bone,** identify (*Atlas*, 8.52, 8.53): anterior and lateral margins of **foramen magnum; occipital condyle.** The joint between the occipital condyle and the superior articular facet of the atlas is the **atlanto-occipital joint.**

Craniovertebral Joints

Turn the cadaver into the prone position (face down). A large wedge-shaped portion of the occipital bone was removed earlier. If not already done, resect the posterior arch of the atlas. Define the anterior border of the foramen magnum. Note the median knuckle-like eminence produced by the dens of the axis. Palpate the dens while rotating the head to the right and the left.

To expose the underlying ligaments, the **dura mater** and the **tectorial membrane** must be reflected (*Atlas*, 4.60B). First, excise the dura mater in the following fashion (Fig. 7.46; *Atlas*, 4.61): make a transverse incision through the dura, about 3 cm inferior to the dorsum sellae. From each end of this incision, carry an oblique vertical cut inferiorly to the point where the vertebral artery pierces the dura. This is just medial to the points of exit of the hypoglossal nerves. With a probe, ease the dura from the underlying membrana tectoria. Turn inferiorly the flap of dura as far as possible.

Next, examine the exposed **membrana tectoria.** Cut the membrane transversely above the anterior border of the foramen magnum. With the handle of a scalpel and a probe,

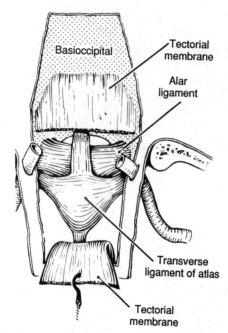

Basioccipital

Tectorial membrane

Alar ligament

Transverse ligament of atlas

Tectorial membrane

Figure 7.46. Removal of dura mater and tectorial membrane. Exposure of the ligaments of the craniovertebral region.

raise the membrane and reflect it downward as far as possible. Now, the major ligaments of the craniovertebral region are exposed.

Ligaments of Craniovertebral Region (Fig. 7.46; *Atlas*, 4.61A and B). Identify the **transverse ligament of the atlas.** It holds the dens of the axis firmly to the anterior arch of the atlas. The transverse ligament and the vertically oriented **superior** and **inferior bands** are collectively known as the **cruciform ligament.**

Next, identify the **alar ligaments** or **check ligaments** (*Atlas*, 4.61). They extend from the dens to the lateral margins of the foramen magnum. These strong paired ligaments are nearly as thick as a pencil. They check the lateral rotation and the side-to-side movements of the head. Observe the extent of rotation possible in the cadaver. Next, cut the alar ligaments close to the dens. Note that the rotation of the head is now very easy and extensive.

Removal of Head

With a scalpel, cut along the anterior border of the foramen magnum, thereby severing a fine median strand extending from the tip of the dens to the anterior border of the foramen. Next, cut close to the lateral margins of the foramen magnum, thereby cutting the attachments of the alar ligaments. Carry cuts close to the medial and posterior aspects of the occipital condyles; this procedure will open the atlanto-occipital joints. Force a chisel into the **atlanto-occipital joints** and disarticulate the joints as much as possible.

At this point, it is advantageous to turn the cadaver into the supine position (face up). Once again, place your hands into the already defined **retrovisceral space.** Pull the cervical viscera and the big vessels and nerves anteri-

orly. Thus, a convenient working space is created anterior to the prevertebral region. Now, proceed as follows:

1. Identify the **sympathetic trunk** and the large **superior cervical sympathetic ganglion** (*Atlas*, 8.51). Sever the sympathetic trunk on one side, just superior to the superior cervical ganglion, thus leaving it attached to the prevertebral region. On the other side, reflect the sympathetic trunk and its superior ganglion together with the cervical viscera.
2. Pull the cervical viscera anteriorly. Pass the knife between the transverse process of the atlas and the occipital bone. This procedure will sever the **rectus capitis lateralis** on each side (Fig. 7.47; *Atlas*, 8.51).
3. Next, carry the cut more medially. Cut the **rectus capitis anterior** and the thick **longus capitis.**
4. Carry the blade across the median plane just superior to the anterior arch of the atlas. This procedure will sever the **anterior atlanto-occipital membrane.** Safeguard cranial nerves IX, X, XI, and XII.

Now, detach the head and the cervical viscera with relative ease. At this point, you have *two options*:

1. Reflect the head and the attached cervical viscera inferiorly and anteriorly. This procedure will leave certain cervicothoracic relations intact. At the same time, it permits a posterior approach to the cervical viscera.
2. Or, isolate the head and the cervical viscera. In that case, mobilize the trachea and the esophagus. If not already done, cut the esophagus in the thorax. Sever the contents of the carotid sheaths. Remove the head together with the attached cervical viscera. Consult with your instructor.

Keep the cadaver moist at all times to make dissection possible.

Prevertebral and Lateral Vertebral Regions

The head has been detached at the atlanto-occipital joint. During this procedure, the muscles between transverse processes of atlas and occipital bone were cut and the superiormost portion of the longus capitis was severed.

Examine the deep investing fascia covering the lateral vertebral (scaleni) and prevertebral muscles. The fascia anterior to the vertebral column and extending between the transverse processes of the vertebrae is the **prevertebral fascia** (Fig. 7.45). It actually consists of two layers that are separated by loose connective tissue. With a forceps, pick up a fine fold of the more anterior layer (alar fascia). Insert a probe into the interval between the two layers of the prevertebral fascia. You are now in a space that has been termed by clinicians as the "danger space," since it

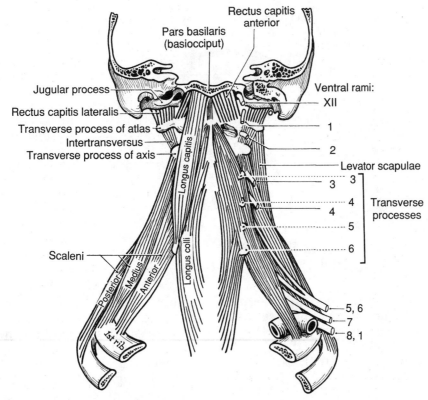

Figure 7.47. Prevertebral muscles. Ventral roots of the cervical spinal nerves.

constitutes a passageway for infections from the neck region all the way inferior into the posterior mediastinum.

On one side of the cadaver, the cervical part of the **sympathetic trunk** was left in place on the prevertebral muscles (*Atlas*, 8.51). Locate it. Identify the **superior, middle,** and **inferior cervical sympathetic ganglia.** The inferior cervical ganglion is positioned close to the anterior aspect of the head of rib 1. Frequently, the ganglion is fused with the **1st thoracic ganglion** to form the cervicothoracic or stellate ganglion (*Atlas*, 8.7, 8.8, 8.51). Observe the **rami communicantes** that connect the sympathetic ganglia with the cervical spinal nerves.

Identify the **longus colli, longus capitis,** and **scalenus anterior** (Fig. 7.47; *Atlas*, 8.51). Remove these muscles from the anterior tubercles of the transverse processes of C3 through C6. Now, the **cervical spinal nerves** are exposed. Trace a ventral ramus to the gutter-like end of the corresponding transverse process on which it rests (*Atlas*, 8.6). Review the contributions of ventral rami C5 to C8 to the brachial plexus (*Atlas*, 6.27, 8.51).

Follow the **vertebral artery** to the transverse foramen of C6. Be aware of possible variations (*Atlas*, 1.58).

Exterior of Base of Skull

Bony Landmarks

Refer to a bony skull and study pertinent features.

Anterior Transverse Line (Fig. 7.48). Pass a pencil or the handle of a probe through both mandibular notches across the base of the skull. The instrument marks a line that passes across the **foramen ovale** on each side.

Posterior Transverse Line (Fig. 7.48). This line stretches across the base of the skull between the mastoid and styloid processes of the two sides. Observe that the line crosses the **stylomastoid foramen, jugular foramen, hypoglossal canal, occipital condyles,** and the **foramen magnum.** Examine the **jugular foramen** more closely, and observe that **three compartments** may be distinguished (*Atlas* 7.31, 7.32**B**):

1. **Anterior compartment;** it transmits the inferior petrosal sinus; in the posterior cranial fossa, note the groove for this sinus running toward the anterior compartment of the jugular foramen; the inferior petrosal sinus joins the internal jugular vein;
2. **Intermediate compartment,** for the transmission of cranial nerves IX, X, and XI;
3. The large **posterior compartment;** it transmits mainly the sigmoid dural sinus, which here becomes the internal jugular vein.

Dissection

Examine the nerves and vessels at the exterior of the base of the skull (*Atlas*, 8.54 to 8.58). Pick up the cut end of the **common carotid artery.** Trace the **sympathetic**

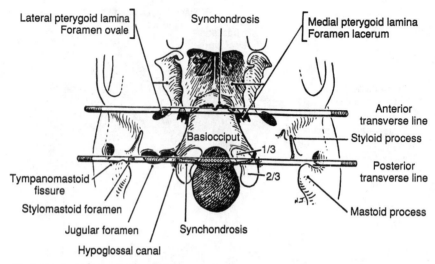

Figure 7.48. "Anterior transverse line" and "posterior transverse line" on the exterior of the base of the skull.

trunk (which lies posterior to the common and internal carotids) up to the carotid canal. Observe the long fusiform ganglion, the **superior cervical sympathetic ganglion** (*Atlas*, 8.57). The pharynx hangs from the pharyngeal tubercle, well anterior to the foramen magnum. The great vessels and nerves lie posterolateral to the posterior wall of the pharynx.

Identify the soft structures that traverse the foramina marked by the "posterior transverse line":

1. **Facial nerve,** emerging from the stylomastoid foramen;
2. **Internal jugular vein,** beginning at the posterior compartment of the jugular foramen, where it is continuous with the sigmoid sinus and the inferior petrosal sinus;
3. **Cranial nerves IX, X, and XI,** traversing the intermediate compartment of the jugular foramen; use bone pliers to remove the bone posterior to the jugular foramen; now, follow the nerves from the neck into the posterior cranial fossa;
4. **Cranial nerve XII,** emerging from the hypoglossal canal.

The **vagus (X) nerve** belongs to the digestive and respiratory tracts; therefore, it must proceed straight inferiorly. Trace the nerve between internal jugular vein and internal carotid artery (*Atlas*, 8.57). Just inferior to the jugular foramen, observe a 2-cm long swelling, the **inferior ganglion of the vagus** (nodose ganglion). The **superior laryngeal nerve** arises from the vagus about 2.5 cm inferior to the base of the skull. Trace this nerve to the larynx. The **pharyngeal branch of the vagus nerve** arises at a high level. Follow the branch between the internal and external carotid arteries to the pharyngeal wall. Here it joins the pharyngeal plexus. Review the vagus nerve and its essential branches (*Atlas*, 9.15B and C).

The **accessory nerve (XI)** supplies the sternocleidomastoid and the trapezius muscles. At the base of the skull, it lies immediately lateral to the vagus nerve. Follow nerve XI through the interval between internal jugular vein and internal carotid artery toward the substance of the sternocleidomastoid. The accessory nerve crosses anterior to the internal jugular vein in 70%, and posterior to it in about 30% of all cases. Review nerve XI (*Atlas*, 9.16).

The **hypoglossal nerve (XII)** supplies the muscles of the tongue. The quickest way to positively identify the nerve is to follow it proximally from the digastric triangle (*Atlas*, 8.54, 8.55). At the base of the skull, the hypoglossal nerve is closely adherent to the inferior ganglion of the vagus. Review nerve XII (*Atlas*, 9.17).

The **glossopharyngeal nerve (IX)** is destined for the pharynx and the back of the tongue; therefore, it must swing anteriorly (*Atlas*, 8.54, 8.55). In doing so, it passes between the internal and external carotid arteries. Separate the two carotid arteries. Observe a lumbrical-like muscle descending from the styloid process between the two arteries. This is the **stylopharyngeus.** The glossopharyngeal nerve is closely applied to its lateral side (*Atlas*, 8.57, 8.58). Review nerve IX (*Atlas*, 9.14).

Pharynx

General Remarks

The pharynx is the superior end of the respiratory and digestive tubes. It extends from the base of the skull to the inferior border of cricoid cartilage (vertebra C6). The **pharyngeal wall** consists of **five layers** or coats:

1. **Areolar coat or layer;** it is continuous with the areolar layer of the buccinator; therefore, it is called the **buccopharyngeal fascia;** this layer facilitates movements of the pharynx; it also contains the pharyngeal plexus of veins and nerves;
2. **Muscular layer;** it is composed of (a) an **outer circular part,** and (b) an **inner longitudinal part;**

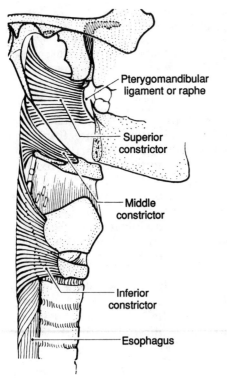

Figure 7.49. The three constrictors of the pharynx (lateral view).

3. **Fibrous layer or pharyngobasilar fascia**; it is especially strong where it anchors the pharynx to the base of the skull;
4. Submucous layer, the **submucosa**;
5. Mucous layer, the **mucous membrane.**

The outer circular part of the muscular layer consists of **three constrictors: superior, middle,** and **inferior** (Fig. 7.49; *Atlas*, 8.56). Each constrictor is fan shaped. The narrow ends of the fans are fixed anteriorly. Posteriorly, the fans of the opposite sides meet in a median raphe. Laterally, there are gaps between the constrictors. Through these spaces pass vessels, nerves, and muscles (*Atlas*, 8.55). The constrictors overlap each other to some degree.

External Aspect of Pharynx

Inspect and clean the posterior aspect of the pharyngeal constrictors (*Atlas*, 8.57). It is easiest to identify the **middle constrictor** first. Its fibers arise from the greater horn of the hyoid bone and from the inferior portion of the stylohyoid ligament (Fig. 7.50). Palpate the greater horn of the hyoid bone. Positively identify the middle constrictor.

The muscle fibers superior to the middle constrictor belong to the **superior constrictor.** This muscle arises from the pterygomandibular raphe or ligament and from the bone at either end of it.

The muscle fibers inferior to the middle constrictor belong to the **inferior constrictor.** Observe the continu-

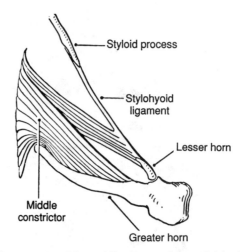

Figure 7.50. Origin of the middle pharyngeal constrictor from the hyoid bone and the stylohyoid ligament.

ous origin of this muscle from the thyroid and cricoid cartilages (Fig. 7.49). Demonstrate that the inferior constrictor overlaps the middle constrictor. Display the interval between the two muscles. Here, the **internal laryngeal nerve** and the superior laryngeal vessels pierce the thyrohyoid membrane (*Atlas*, 8.54, 8.55). Examine the free inferior border of the inferior constrictor. Here, the **recurrent laryngeal nerve** enters the pharyngeal wall. Note that the most inferior fibers of the inferior constrictor are continuous with the circular fibers of the esophagus (*Atlas*, 8.54).

Demonstrate the interval between the middle and superior constrictors (*Atlas*, 8.54, 8.55). The **stylopharyngeus** and the **glossopharyngeal nerve (IX)** pass through this gap. Verify this fact.

Internal Aspect of Pharynx

Incision. With scissors, slit open the posterior wall of the esophagus and the pharynx. Start at the cricoid cartilage and carry the median section all the way superiorly to the base of the skull (*Atlas*, 8.59).

The interior of the pharynx communicates anteriorly with three cavities: nose, mouth, and larynx (Fig. 7.51; *Atlas*, 8.59). Accordingly, the **pharynx is divided into three parts: nasal pharynx, oral pharynx, and laryngeal pharynx.** The soft palate, ending in the uvula, separates the nasopharynx superiorly from the oral pharynx inferiorly.

Nasal Pharynx or Nasopharynx. It lies superior to the soft palate. Verify that it is a posterior extension of the nasal cavities. Refer to a skull (*Atlas*, 8.52, 8.53) and identify the two posterior nasal apertures or **choanae**, which are separated by the bony **nasal septum.** Look through the choanae. Identify scroll-like bones projecting from the lateral wall of each nasal cavity. These are the **middle concha** and the **inferior concha.** Turn to the cadaver (*Atlas*, 8.59). Identify the nasal septum, choanae, and conchae.

On each side of the nasopharynx, 1 to 1.5 cm posterior to the inferior concha, is the **pharyngeal orifice of the auditory tube** (*Atlas*, 8.63). Place a probe into the opening.

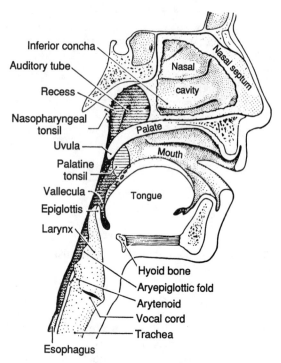

Figure 7.51.   Interior of pharynx.

Posterior to it, identify the **torus tubarius,** which is produced by the underlying cartilage of the auditory tube. Posterior to the torus, explore the **pharyngeal recess,** which extends laterally and posteriorly almost to the carotid canal.

The curved, bony roof of the nasopharynx is formed by the sphenoid and occipital bones. The mucous membrane on the roof and posterior wall contains a mass of lymphoid tissue, the so-called **pharyngeal (or nasopharyngeal) tonsil** (*Atlas,* 7.128, 8.84). Enlarged pharyngeal tonsils are known as "adenoids." Understand that large adenoids will obstruct the air passages from the nose through the nasopharynx, making mouth breathing necessary.

Examine the close relation of the nasopharyngeal tonsil to the orifice of the auditory tube. Understand that enlarged adenoids will obstruct the ostium, thus interfering with the air exchange between the nasopharynx and the middle ear cavity.

Oral Pharynx or Oropharynx (*Atlas,* 8.59).   The oral pharynx is bounded by the soft palate superiorly and the epiglottis of the larynx inferiorly. Push your finger anteriorly into the oral cavity. Palpate the posterior 1/3 of the tongue. Note two folds of mucous membrane that descend from the soft palate (*Atlas,* 8.63). The anterior fold, the **palatoglossal arch,** descends to the junction of the anterior 2/3 and the posterior 1/3 of the tongue. The palatoglossal arch forms a dividing line between the oral cavity and the oral pharynx. The posterior fold, the **palatopharyngeal arch,** descends along the lateral wall of the pharynx. Between the two arches lies the **palatine tonsil.** Examine the arches and the tonsil on a transverse section through the head (*Atlas,* 7.85). Identify the right and left palatine arches in the cadaver.

Examine the palatine arches in your fellow students. Notice the two prominent folds in subjects who have undergone tonsillectomy and observe the empty tonsillar beds. Study the palatine tonsil in several subjects. Note that the tonsils vary in size from person to person.

Laryngeal Pharynx or Laryngopharynx (*Atlas,* 8.59). This portion of the pharynx extends from the epiglottis to the lower border of the cricoid cartilage. Identify the epiglottis and the inlet (aditus) of the larynx. Palpate the cricoid cartilage through the mucous membrane. Place a probe into the right and left **piriform recesses.** Foreign bodies (bones; food particles) may become trapped here. Define the borders of the piriform recess (*Atlas,* 8.70): medially, the larynx; laterally, the thyroid cartilage and the thyrohyoid membrane; posteriorly, the inferior constrictor.

Carefully remove the mucosa of the piriform recess (*Atlas,* 8.70). Two nerves, which are submucous, are readily exposed. These are the **internal laryngeal nerve** and the **recurrent laryngeal nerve.** Identify the nerves. They will be studied more thoroughly during the dissection of the larynx.

Bisection of Head

General Remarks and Bony Landmarks

The nasal and oral cavities are not readily accessible in the undivided head. Therefore, the head must be bisected, close to the median plane. For practical purposes, it is best to carry the section just lateral to the nasal septum. Thus, one half of the head will have the nasal septum (*Atlas,* 8.84); the other half will have its nasal cavity fully opened (*Atlas,* 7.108).

Usually, the **nasal septum** deviates somewhat to one side. Thus, the nasal cavity is slightly wider on one side, slightly narrower on the side of septal deviation. Refer to one or several skulls and verify this fact. Logically, the section should be made on the less obstructed side, just lateral to the nasal septum.

Examine a skull and study the bones through which you must saw:

1. The saw cut must pass through the nasal bone and the remains of the frontal bone (*Atlas,* 7.1).
2. Subsequently, you must saw just lateral to the crista galli through one of the cribriform plates of the ethmoid bone (*Atlas,* 7.35). Then, the cut must be carried midsagittally through the body of the sphenoid bone and part of the occipital bone to the anterior margin of the foramen magnum (*Atlas,* 7.108, 8.84).
3. You must saw through the hard palate that forms the floor of the nasal cavities and the roof of the oral cavity.

Dissection and Bisection

In the midline, cut through the upper lip. Next, explore each nasal cavity with a probe. Decide on which side of the nasal septum the bisection should be carried out.

On the chosen side, carry out the following procedures:

1. Divide the uvula and the soft palate in the midsagittal plane.
2. Slit open the naris. Cut through the lateral portion of the septal cartilage all the way to the nasal bone (*Atlas*, 7.100).
3. If your instructors wish to use an electrical bandsaw for bisection, follow specific directions to be issued. Otherwise, insert a small saw into the nasal cavity. Keep the blade close to the septum. Cut superiorly through the nasal and frontal bones. Subsequently, saw through the cribriform plate, body of sphenoid, dorsum sellae, and basioccipital bone, until you reach the foramen magnum.
4. Saw in an inferior direction through the floor of the nasal cavity. Divide the hard palate close to the midsagittal plane.

Now, the two superior halves of the head will fall apart from each other. The tongue lies exposed. **Inspect the tongue.** Verify the following statements (*Atlas*, 7.83):

1. The anterior 2/3 of the tongue lies horizontally in the mouth. This is the **oral part.**
2. The posterior 1/3 of the tongue takes a curved vertical position and forms the anterior wall of the oral pharynx. This is the **pharyngeal part** of the tongue.
3. The boundary between the two parts is marked by the **sulcus terminalis.** This line has the shape of an inverted V (V). On each side, it runs from the palatoglossal arch posteriorly to a median pit, the **foramen cecum.**
4. Large and conspicuous **vallate papillae**, 7 to 12 in number, occupy a V-shaped row just anterior to the sulcus terminalis. (These papillae contain numerous taste buds.)
5. The anterior 2/3 of the tongue is covered with long **filiform papillae. Fungiform papillae** lie near the dorsum and margins of the tongue. (These papillae also contain taste buds.)
6. A median fold of mucous membrane, the **median glossoepiglottic fold,** runs from the dorsum of the tongue to the epiglottis. On each side of this fold are the **valleculae.**
7. The surface of the pharyngeal or posterior 1/3 of the tongue is conspicuously different from the oral part. It has no papillae. Its surface is uneven due to the presence of numerous lymphoid follicles. These encapsuled follicles are collectively called the **lingual tonsil.**
8. Realize that the tongue is supplied by five different cranial nerves (*Atlas*, 7.84).

The next objective is to bisect the mandible together with the floor of the mouth and the tongue. Proceed as follows: turn to the submental triangle between the anterior bellies of the digastrics (*Atlas*, 8.31, 8.32). Split the thin median raphe of the **mylohyoids** and separate the muscles. Identify the underlying paired **geniohyoids.** With probe and scissors, separate these muscles from each other. Clean their pointed mandibular origins. Next, saw through the mandible in the midsagittal plane, exactly between the geniohyoids.

Now, bisect the tongue in the midsagittal plane from the tip to the hyoid bone and to the epiglottis (*Atlas*, 7.81). Take care not to destroy the epiglottis. Do not bisect the hyoid bone and the larynx.

Nasal Cavities

Bony Landmarks

Refer to a skull and, in addition, to a bisected skull. Study the following pertinent features:

The **floor of the nasal cavity** (which is also the roof of the oral cavity) is formed by the **bony palate.** Study its inferior surface (*Atlas*, 7.86A). The anterior two-thirds of the bony palate consists of the **palatine processes of the maxilla.** The posterior one-third consists of the **horizontal plates of the palatine bones.** In the midline, immediately posterior to the incisor teeth, find the **incisive foramen.** Medial to the 3rd molar tooth, locate the **greater palatine foramen.** Gently push a thin, flexible wire through the greater palatine foramen into the **greater palatine canal.**

Examine the **vertical part** or **perpendicular plate of the palatine bone** that forms part of the lateral wall of the nasal cavity (*Atlas*, 7.102A, 7.110). The vertical plate has a **notch** on its superior border. This notch is in contact with the sphenoid bone; thus, the important **sphenopalatine (pterygopalatine) foramen** is formed. Identify the foramen in the bisected skull. Next, coming from the lateral aspect of the skull, look through the **pterygopalatine fossa** (*Atlas*, 7.73). Detect the **sphenopalatine foramen** in the depth of the fossa. Understand that the foramen is a passageway for vessels and nerves from the pterygopalatine fossa to the nasal cavity.

In the bisected skull, examine the body of the **sphenoid bone.** Locate the large **sphenoidal sinus** (*Atlas*, 7.108). Usually, the right and left sinuses differ in size. They are completely divided by a bony septum. Attempt to find the **posterior opening of the pterygoid canal.** This canal runs posteroanteriorly through the body of the sphenoid. Frequently, the canal causes a ridge on the floor of the sphenoid sinus. Pass a thin, flexible wire through the pterygoid canal. Note that the wire connects two foramina: **foramen lacerum** and **sphenopalatine foramen.** These relations are of importance. The greater petrosal nerve, carrying parasympathetic fibers, traverses the foramen lacerum and then the pterygoid canal to reach the pterygopalatine (sphenopalatine) ganglion (*Atlas*, 9.12C).

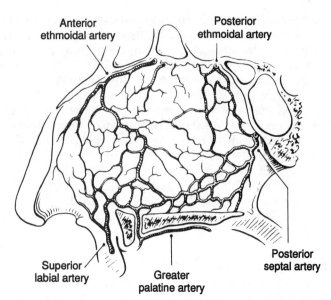

Figure 7.52. Arteries of nasal septum.

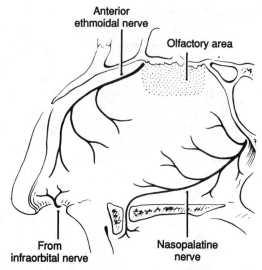

Figure 7.53. Nerves of nasal septum.

Preferably in the bisected skull, examine the **lateral wall of the nasal cavity**. Identify the following (*Atlas*, 7.102A):

1. **Frontal process of maxilla;**
2. **Vertical plate of palatine bone;**
3. **Inferior concha** (turbinate);
4. **Middle and superior conchae;** these structures are part of the ethmoid bone; they contain many small air cells; note the openings of some of these cells.

Just superior to the inferior concha, find an opening that leads to the large **maxillary sinus** (*Atlas*, 7.110, 7.119). Pass a wire through the **nasolacrimal canal,** and observe that the wire enters the nasal cavity under shelter of and lateral to the inferior concha. Pass a flexible wire from the **frontal sinus** into the nasal cavity.

Study the bony **roof of the nasal cavity** (*Atlas*, 7.102A). Observe: **nasal bone;** small part of frontal bone; **cribriform plate** of ethmoid bone; body of **sphenoid.**

Examine the **bony nasal septum** (*Atlas*, 7.102B). Identify the unpaired **vomer.** It articulates with the sphenoid and the bony palate. Identify the unpaired **perpendicular plate of the ethmoid.** Of course, the large septal cartilage is absent in the bony skull. Examine the two **choanae,** the posterior nasal apertures, and review their boundaries (*Atlas*, 8.59, 8.60). Review the complex **ethmoid bone** and its relations to the nasal cavity.

Nasal Septum

Turn to the cadaver. Examine the half of the head that contains the **nasal septum.** Strip the mucoperiosteum completely off and identify the three main components of the septum (*Atlas*, 7.102B): the **perpendicular plate of ethmoid,** the **vomer,** and the **septal cartilage.**

Next, carefully remove the bony and cartilaginous parts of the septum. However, leave intact the mucoperiosteum lateral to it. Now, the vessels and nerves running along the nasal septum can be examined in the remaining mucoperiosteal membrane.

Arteries. These vessels are difficult to trace, unless they are injected. You are not required to dissect these structures. However, realize that they exist. The arteries form a network that receives its blood supply from various sources (Fig. 7.52; *Atlas*, 7.106A).

Nerves (Fig. 7.53; *Atlas*, 7.107):

1. Close to the cribriform plate is the **olfactory area** that contains olfactory nerve fibers (*Atlas*, 9.3).
2. **Anterior ethmoidal nerve** (*Atlas*, 7.107); do not dissect this fine branch of V^1.
3. The **nasopalatine nerve** is a branch of V^2 via the pterygopalatine ganglion (*Atlas*, 9.10). From the palatine side, pierce and mark the incisive canal with a needle. Now, you have a reference point. Using a probe and forceps, trace the thin nasopalatine nerve toward the incisive canal.

Remove all remains of the nasal septum, including the mucoperiosteum. Expose the lateral wall of the nasal cavity. The lateral wall of the other side is already exposed.

Lateral Wall of Nasal Cavity

In the cadaver, inspect the **lateral wall of the nasal cavity** (Fig. 7.54; *Atlas*, 7.108). Identify:

1. **Inferior concha.** The space lateral to and inferior to it is the **inferior meatus.** Note that the free edge of the inferior concha is horizontal. About 1.5 cm posterior to the posterior limit of the inferior concha, identify the **pharyngeal orifice of the auditory tube.**

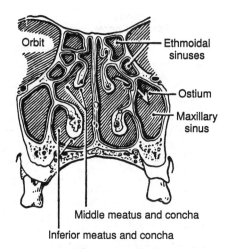

Figure 7.54. Nasal cavities and adjacent sinuses (coronal section).

2. **Middle concha.** The space lateral to and inferior to it is the **middle meatus.** Anteriorly, the free edge of the middle concha turns superiorly.
3. **Superior concha.** This small structure extends from the roof to the front of the sphenoid. Lateral to and inferior to it is the **superior meatus.** The space posterosuperior to the superior concha is the **sphenoethmoidal recess.**
4. **Vestibule.** It is located superior to the nostril and anterior to the inferior meatus. Note the presence of hairs on the mobile part.
5. **Atrium.** It is located superior to the vestibule and anterior to the middle meatus.

With scissors, cut away the **inferior concha** (*Atlas*, 7.109). Pass a stiff wire from the orbital cavity inferiorly through the **nasolacrimal duct** to the **inferior meatus.** Remove the mucoperiosteum from the lateral wall of the inferior meatus. Observe the opening of the bony **nasolacrimal canal** (which contains the nasolacrimal duct).

With scissors, cut away the **middle concha** (*Atlas*, 7.109). Identify a curved slit, the **hiatus semilunaris.** This hiatus has a sharp, inferior edge. Its more rounded superior edge is formed by the **ethmoidal bulla,** an elevation of the ethmoidal labyrinth.

Identify the **opened frontal sinus.** Pass a wire inferoposteriorly from the frontal sinus through the **frontonasal duct.** Usually, this duct opens into the upper portion of the **infundibulum.** The infundibulum is a narrow passage anterosuperior to the hiatus semilunaris. In frontal sinus infections, irrigation of the sinus may be necessary. This is done with a specially curved cannula that is passed through the infundibulum and through the frontonasal duct. Study these important relations in the cadaver.

Realize that the **ethmoidal cells** (or sinuses) are located lateral to the middle and superior conchae (Fig. 7.54). Stay above the hiatus semilunaris, and break into the **middle ethmoidal cells** of the ethmoidal bulla. Anteriorly, identify the **anterior ethmoidal cells.** Remove the superior concha

to display one or more of the **posterior ethmoidal cells** (*Atlas*, 7.113). Pick away the partitions between the ethmoidal cells until you reach the thin **orbital plate** (lamina papyracea) of the ethmoid bone (Fig. 7.54). If you break through this plate, you will enter the orbital cavity.

Explore the sphenoidal sinus. Find its orifice or ostium, which opens into the sphenoethmoidal recess. The size of the ostium may vary from 0.5 to 4.0 mm. Irrigation of an infected sphenoid sinus can be accomplished by inserting a special curved cannula through the ostium. Examine the orifice. Understand that it may not be accessible when the middle concha is too large or the septum is deviated. In that case, a trocar must be pushed directly through the anterior wall of the sphenoid into the sinus. Study these relations.

Explore the **hiatus semilunaris.** In it is the **ostium for the maxillary sinus** (Fig. 7.54; *Atlas*, 7.109). Pass a probe into the maxillary sinus. An infected maxillary sinus may be irrigated through its ostium. However, if difficulties are encountered, an artificial route of drainage is chosen. A curved trocar is pushed through the lateral wall of the inferior meatus into the maxillary sinus, close to its floor. With a probe, break through the thin lateral wall of the inferior meatus and create an artificial opening.

Now, with the aid of bone forceps, remove the medial wall of the maxillary sinus. Notice that it is a three-sided hollow pyramid. The average adult capacity is approximately 15 ml. Verify that the superior wall separates the sinus from the orbital cavity.

With forceps, remove the mucoperiosteum lining the maxillary sinus. Note a ridge on the orbital and anterior surfaces. This ridge is caused by the **infraorbital canal.** With a probe, break into the canal, open it along its length, and identify its contents: **infraorbital nerve and accompanying vessels** (*Atlas*, 7.105, 9.10A).

Examine the floor of the maxillary sinus. Look for the roots of teeth that may project into the sinus. Sometimes the roots are covered only with mucoperiosteum. Understand that an infection from a decaying tooth may readily spread into the sinus. During extraction of a molar or premolar tooth, the membrane superior to the projecting root may be torn. As a result, a fistula between mouth and sinus may occur.

Sphenopalatine Foramen and Pterygopalatine Fossa

Once again, review essential bony landmarks. Identify the sphenopalatine foramen and the pterygopalatine fossa. Gently push a thin, flexible wire through the greater palatine foramen into the greater palatine canal. Note that the wire emerges in the pterygopalatine fossa close to the sphenopalatine foramen. Review the course of the maxillary nerve V[2] (*Atlas*, 9.10). Once again, identify the pterygoid canal.

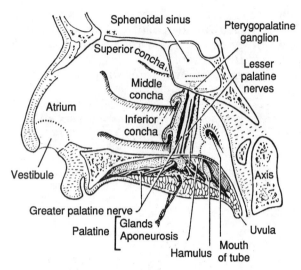

Figure 7.55. The greater palatine canal and the pterygopalatine ganglion.

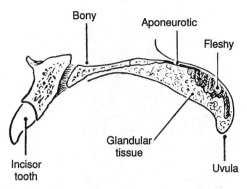

Figure 7.56. The hard palate and the soft palate on sagittal section.

The conchae and the medial wall of the maxillary sinus were removed earlier. The perpendicular plate of the palatine bone and the closely related greater palatine canal are still intact (*Atlas*, 7.102A). Now, strip the mucoperiosteum from the perpendicular plate of the palatine bone. In doing so, you will encounter the **posterior lateral nasal artery.** This artery is a branch of the **sphenopalatine artery** (*Atlas*, 7.106B). After traversing the sphenopalatine foramen, the sphenopalatine artery divides into a **posterior septal branch** (for the septum) and the posterior lateral nasal branch. Most of its small branches have been cut during removal of the conchae. Do not dissect the arterial network of the lateral nasal wall. However, realize that it exists.

The next objective is to **expose the sphenopalatine foramen and its contents.** The greater palatine canal leads to this foramen. Make use of this fact. Insert a needle (about 30 mm or 1¼ inches long) into the greater palatine foramen, just medial to the 3rd molar tooth (*Atlas*, 7.86A). Probe until you find the opening. Then, push the needle all the way through the greater palatine canal. The tip of the needle will be located anterior to the sphenoid bone and just lateral to the sphenopalatine foramen. Leave the needle in place. Now, use a probe and break down the medial wall of the greater palatine canal. This procedure will expose the contents of the canal: the **greater palatine nerve** (Fig. 7.55; *Atlas*, 7.107) and the **greater palatine artery,** a terminal branch of the maxillary artery (*Atlas*, 7.74A, 7.77).

Follow the greater palatine nerve superiorly to the sphenopalatine foramen. Here, find the **pterygopalatine (sphenopalatine) ganglion** (Fig. 7.55; *Atlas*, 7.107). If time permits, find the **nerve of the pterygoid canal.** Proceed as follows: Remove the mucoperiosteum from the sphenoid sinus. Find the ridge produced by the pterygoid canal. With a probe, open the canal. Follow the delicate nerve toward the pterygopalatine ganglion. Realize that the nerve of the pterygoid canal (Vidian nerve) consists of preganglionic parasympathetic fibers from the greater petrosal nerve, and postganglionic sympathetic fibers from the deep petrosal nerve (*Atlas*, 9.12C).

Next, turn the specimen over and approach it from its lateral aspect. Deep in the **pterygopalatine fossa,** identify the following pertinent structures (*Atlas*, 7.77):

1. **Maxillary artery,** giving off the **greater palatine artery** and the **sphenopalatine artery;** the sphenopalatine artery is the one passing through the sphenopalatine foramen;
2. **Maxillary nerve V²,** coursing from the foramen rotundum posteriorly to the inferior orbital fissure anteriorly;
3. **Pterygopalatine (sphenopalatine) ganglion.** It is attached to the maxillary nerve by two short stout medially running nerve branches (*Atlas*, 9.10A).

If you cannot satisfactorily see the ganglion in relation to nerve V², do not hesitate to remove the floor of the orbital cavity. Follow the infraorbital nerve posteriorly. Compare your field of dissection with the one depicted in *Atlas*, 7.105.

Palate, Tonsil, and Pharyngeal Wall

Hard Palate and Soft Palate

The palate consists of two portions: (a) the **hard palate,** comprising the anterior 2/3; and (b) the mobile **soft palate,** constituting the posterior 1/3 of the palate. Small mucous glands, the **palatine glands,** are abundant over the palate. The pinpoint orifices of their ducts are evident (*Atlas*, 7.86B).

Mark the greater palatine foramen by a needle, as described earlier. The **greater palatine nerve and vessels** emerge from this foramen to be distributed to the hard palate (Fig. 7.55; *Atlas*, 7.87, 7.88). To demonstrate nerve and vessels, proceed as follows: about 5 mm posterior to the marked greater palatine foramen, make a transverse cut through the thickness of the mucoperiosteum of the hard palate. With the rounded handle of the knife, ease the mucoperiosteum off the bony palate. Free the greater palatine nerve and vessels (*Atlas*, 7.87). Cut the reflected tissue close to the alveolar processes of the teeth.

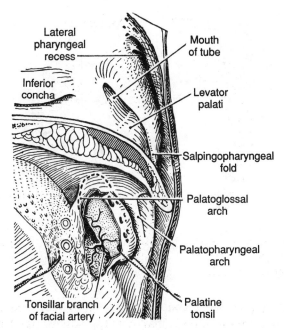

Figure 7.57. First step in removal of the palatine tonsil.

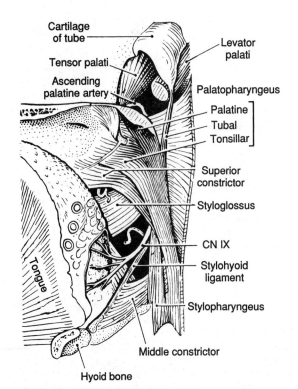

Figure 7.58. Bed of the palatine tonsil. Pharyngeal muscles.

Examine the soft palate, which had been cut earlier in the midsagittal plane. Observe (Fig. 7.56):

1. The thickness of the soft palate is due mainly to glands;
2. The strength of the soft palate depends on its aponeurosis situated in its anterior 1/3;
3. Its mobility is due to muscles situated in its posterior 2/3. These muscles will be studied later.

Palatine Tonsil

The right and left **palatine tonsils** lie on each side of the oropharynx. The tonsil is called "palatine" because its superior 1/3 extends into the soft palate, a matter of clinical importance. Each tonsil is located in the triangular interval between the **palatoglossal arch** and the **palatopharyngeal arch** (Fig. 7.57; *Atlas*, 7.85, 8.63). In older individuals, the palatine tonsil may be inconspicuous.

Enucleation. If the tonsil is present, remove it. Proceed as follows (Fig. 7.57; *Atlas*, 8.67): incise the mucous membrane along the palatoglossal arch. Using blunt dissection, free the anterior border and the superior part of the tonsil. This is easily done because the rounded lateral aspect of the tonsil has a fibrous capsule. This capsule is separated from the pharyngeal wall by a layer of loose areolar tissue. Work in the areolar space. Free the posterior part of the tonsil. Finally, detach the inferior part where the tonsil is most adherent. Note that the inferior pole of the palatine tonsil is continuous with the lymphoid tissue of the tongue, the so-called **lingual tonsil.**

Examine the enucleated palatine tonsil. Section it. Observe the **crypts** that extend from the free surface of the tonsil to almost the level of the capsule (*Atlas*, 8.62).

Examine the **bed of the palatine tonsil** (*Atlas*, 8.64). The thin fibrous sheet covering the bed of the tonsil is part of the **pharyngobasilar fascia.** Remove it, and expose two muscles: **palatopharyngeus** and **superior constrictor.** These muscles are part of the muscular coat of the pharynx. The superior constrictor has a delicate, free, arched inferior border, which does not reach the inferior third of the tonsil bed. If engorged, you may see the **paratonsillar vein.** This vein is often responsible for hemorrhage following tonsillectomy.

Push a probe inferior to the free inferior border of the superior constrictor. Using a probe as a protective guide, carefully remove a small part of the superior constrictor just anterior to the palatopharyngeus (Fig. 7.58; *Atlas*, 8.66). Now, the styloglossus and the glossopharyngeal nerve are exposed. Identify the **styloglossus.** It is a thick muscular band that passes from the tip of the styloid process to the lateral aspect of the tongue (*Atlas*, 8.29, 8.30). Find the **glossopharyngeal nerve (IX)** (*Atlas*, 8.66). It passes through the gap between the superior and the middle constrictors just lateral to the stylopharyngeus. The nerve spreads out to the mucosa of the posterior 1/3 of the tongue. Follow the nerve proximally to the base of the skull (*Atlas*, 8.57, 8.58). Review the distribution and functions of nerve IX (*Atlas*, 9.14).

Pharyngeal Wall

Carefully remove the mucous membrane from both surfaces of the soft palate, from the lateral pharyngeal wall, and from the nasopharynx. When removing the mucosa from the palatoglossal arch, the **palatoglossus** is displayed (*Atlas*, 8.64). After removal of the mucosa from the palatopharyngeal arch, the **palatopharyngeus** is exposed. This muscle is divided into three distinct parts (Fig. 7.58): *tubal*, several strands of muscle reaching the cartilage of the auditory tube; *palatine*, to the posterior portion of the soft palate; *tonsilar*, spreading toward the bed of the palatine tonsil. These parts of the palatopharyngeus and the stylopharyngeus form the **longitudinal musculature of the pharynx.**

The next objective is to display the **origin of the superior constrictor** from the **pterygomandibular raphe**. This raphe or ligament connects two bony landmarks: the **hamulus of the medial pterygoid plate** (*Atlas*, 7.86A), and an area of the **mandible** just posterior to the 3rd molar tooth. Observe these bony landmarks in the skull. Then, palpate the hamulus in the cadaver. Now, you can positively identify the fibrous pterygomandibular raphe (*Atlas*, 8.65). Verify that two muscles meet at the raphe: **superior constrictor** and **buccinator**. In addition, examine these relations from the lateral aspect of the head (*Atlas*, 8.54, 8.55).

Examine the free superior border of the superior constrictor. The gap between this border and the base of the skull is closed by the pharyngobasilar fascia. Passing through this gap are (Fig. 7.59; *Atlas*, 8.64): the **auditory tube**, the **levator palati**, and the **ascending pharyngeal artery.**

Auditory Tube (pharyngotympanic tube; Eustachian tube). It connects the nasopharynx with the tympanic cavity (*Atlas*, 7.132). It is about 36 mm long and consists of a cartilaginous and a bony portion. Refer to the base of a skull and look for the opening of the **osseous portion of the auditory tube** (*Atlas*, 8.52, 8.53). Pass a thin, flexible wire through the canal. Now, look into the external ear canal. You will see the wire in the middle ear cavity (in the cadaver, the external ear canal and the middle ear cavity are separated by the tympanic membrane).

The anterior 2/3 of the auditory tube is cartilaginous. Observe that the cartilage forms only the superior and medial walls of the tube (*Atlas*, 8.64). The inferior and lateral walls are membranous. The bony and the **cartilaginous portions of the auditory tube** meet at the **isthmus**. Here, the lumen of the tube is very narrow (Fig. 7.59). In the cadaver, pass a thin, flexible wire through the ostium of the auditory tube and push it into the tube for about 3 cm.

Levator Veli Palatini or Levator Palati (Fig. 7.58; *Atlas*, 8.64). At the base of the skull, it arises from the petrous bone and the medial portion of the cartilage of the auditory tube. The levator palati elevates and retracts the soft palate. Identify the muscle, which is slightly thicker than a pencil. Pass the handle of a scalpel between the levator and the floor of the auditory tube. Separate the two structures from each other. Cut the levator close to the base of the skull and reflect it.

Free the **auditory tube** from the medial pterygoid plate. Cut it and remove its anterior portion. Observe the collapsed, slit-like lumen of the tube. Note the cartilaginous and membranous walls.

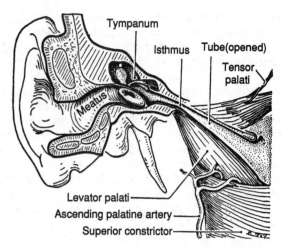

Figure 7.59. Auditory tube, levator palati, and ascending pharyngeal artery cross the superior border of the superior constrictor muscle.

Now, the **tensor veli palatini (tensor palati)** lies exposed (Fig. 7.58; *Atlas*, 8.64, 8.65). The muscle arises from the **scaphoid fossa.** Identify this bony landmark on the skull. Find the fossa at the superior end of the posterior border of the medial pterygoid plate (*Atlas*, 8.52, 8.53). Once again, identify the **hamulus** of the medial pterygoid plate, which serves as a pulley for the tensor palati. In order to render the soft palate "tense," the right and left tensors must pull it laterally. The thin, ribbon-like muscle ends in a tendon, which winds around the hamulus. In the cadaver, palpate the hamulus. Find the tendon of the tensor palati as it passes medialward to its insertion into the palatine aponeurosis (*Atlas*, 7.87).

Continue with the dissection of the specimen from its medial side (*Atlas*, 8.65). Retract the tensor palati superiorly, or remove its superoposterior portion. This procedure will expose the **mandibular nerve (V³)** as it emerges from the **foramen ovale.** Coming from the medial side, carefully pass the tip of a probe through the foramen. Immediately inferior to the foramen and on the medial aspect of V³ lies the small **otic ganglion** (*Atlas*, 7.79). The ganglion is difficult to find. Be aware of its functional importance (*Atlas*, 9.14C).

Mouth and Tongue

Inspection and Palpation

Vestibule of the Mouth (*Atlas*, 7.63, 7.130). It is the U-shaped space bounded externally by the lips and cheeks and, internally, by the teeth and gums. The teeth and gums separate the vestibule from the oral cavity proper. With a clean index or middle finger, explore the vestibule of your own mouth. Have a skull on hand for reference. Palpate the following structures:

1. **Mentalis,** passing from the incisive fossa of the mandible to the skin of the chin (*Atlas*, 7.6);

2. Inferior border of **zygomatic arch** (*Atlas*, 7.2B);
3. **Maxilla,** its anterior (facial) and infratemporal surfaces;
4. **Ramus** and **coronoid process of mandible; tendon of temporalis,** attached to the coronoid process (*Atlas*, 7.64);
5. **Masseter,** easily palpated when the teeth are clenched;
6. Posterior to the last molar tooth, the communication between vestibule and oral cavity proper;
7. **Frenulum** of upper lip and frenulum of lower lip; the two frenula (L. *frenum*, bridle) are folds of mucosa attaching the lips to the gums in the median plane;
8. **Orifice of the parotid duct;** a slightly elevated, whitish, constricted opening opposite the 2nd superior molar tooth; usually, this papilla can be readily palpated with the tip of the tongue; examine the right and left orifices.

Oral Cavity Proper. Define its **borders:** laterally and anteriorly the teeth and gums; superiorly, the hard palate (*Atlas*, 7.130); inferiorly, the tongue; posteriorly and laterally, the palatoglossal arch, marking the border between oral cavity and oropharynx. In the living, inspect or palpate the following **structures of the oral cavity proper:**

1. **Sublingual region;** this region is located inferior to the mobile portions of the tongue;
2. **Frenulum linguae;** connecting the tongue to the floor of the mouth; raise the tip of the tongue to see this median fold;
3. **Deep lingual veins,** easily seen on each side of the frenulum;
4. **Opening of submandibular duct;** observe it on each side of the root of the frenulum (*Atlas*, 7.78B);
5. **Plica sublingualis** (*Atlas*, 7.78B, 7.130), overlying the superior border of the sublingual salivary gland; several small sublingual ducts open onto this plica;
6. **Hamulus of medial pterygoid plate** (*Atlas*, 7.86A, 8.65).

Dissection of Sublingual Region

Refer to a bony mandible. Examine its medial aspect (*Atlas*, 7.71B) and identify two important bony landmarks:

1. **Mylohyoid line,** for attachment of mylohyoid muscle;
2. **Sublingual fossa,** for the sublingual gland and associated soft structures superior to the level of the mylohyoid muscle.

Turn to the bisected head of the cadaver. Examine the muscles of the floor of the mouth and of the tongue as they can be seen on median section (*Atlas*, 7.81): **mylohyoid, geniohyoid,** and the large, fan-shaped **genioglossus.**

The next objective is to expose the sublingual gland. Before dissecting, it is important that you understand the following (*Atlas*, 7.130):

1. Dissection of the lateral aspect of the gland is relatively simple, since no important structures intervene between gland and sublingual fossa of mandible.
2. Dissection medial to the gland will require great care. Important structures (nerve, duct, vessels) will be found in the space between gland and genioglossus muscle of the tongue.
3. The sublingual gland rests on the mylohyoid muscle.

With these facts in mind, proceed as follows: incise the mucous membrane between plica sublingualis and mandible. Start at the frenulum of the tongue. Carry the incision posteriorly, but not beyond the 2nd molar tooth. With a probe and handle of a scalpel, displace the **sublingual gland** medially. Identify the sublingual fossa of the mandible. Inferior to it, observe the origin of the mylohyoid (*Atlas*, 7.78B, 7.80).

Next, carefully incise the mucous membrane along the furrow between the **plica sublingualis** and the **tongue.** With a blunt instrument (probe or handle of scalpel), displace the gland laterally and the tongue medially. Identify the following (Fig. 7.60; *Atlas*, 7.78B).

1. **Sublingual salivary gland.** It is enveloped in a sheath of areolar tissue that fixes the gland to the floor of the mouth. Tease the tissue between superior border of sublingual gland and plica sublingualis and identify several very short and fine ducts. There are about 12 ducts that open on the summit of the plica.
2. **Submandibular duct.** It runs diagonally across the medial aspect of the sublingual gland. Follow the duct anteriorly to its papilla just lateral to the frenulum linguae. Then, follow the duct posteriorly to the substance of the **submandibular salivary gland.**
3. **Lingual nerve.** Pick up the nerve posterior to the last molar tooth. Once again, verify that the nerve runs between ramus of mandible and medial pterygoid (*Atlas*, 7.76, 7.78B). Trace the lingual nerve anteriorly. The nerve describes a spiral around the submandibular duct. In successive order, the relations of the nerve to the duct are: lateral and superior to; inferior to; inferior and medial to; and finally superior and medial to the duct. Observe that the nerve divides into several branches to the tongue. These branches lie in the submucosa of the anterior 2/3 of the tongue (Fig. 7.60; *Atlas*, 8.29).
4. **Submandibular ganglion** (Fig. 7.60; *Atlas*, 8.26). Far posterior, in the vicinity of the 3rd molar tooth, look for the submandibular ganglion. This small ganglion is suspended from the lingual nerve by two or more short branches. Carefully tease the inferior surface of the lingual nerve to reveal the ganglion. Understand the functional importance of the ganglion (*Atlas*, 9.12C).
5. **Hypoglossal nerve (XII).** Pick up the nerve as it runs anteriorly between submandibular gland and hyoglossus, well inferior to the lingual nerve (*Atlas*, 8.28, 9.17). Follow the nerve to the musculature of the tongue.

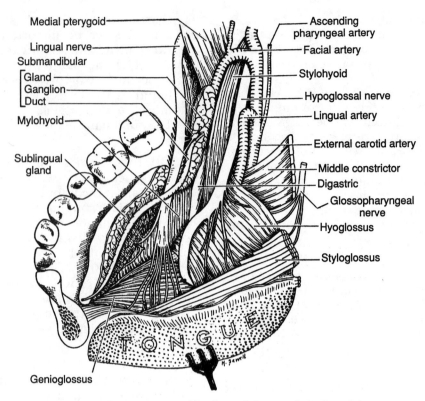

Figure 7.60. Dissection of the floor of the mouth (right side).

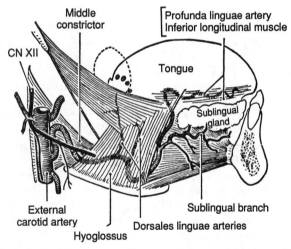

Figure 7.61. The tongue. The lingual artery and its branches.

Dissection of the Tongue

Approach the bisected head from its lateral aspect. With a probe, define the attachment of the **mylohyoid** to the hyoid bone (*Atlas*, 8.26). Subsequently detach the muscle from the hyoid bone and reflect it superiorly. Now, the **hyoglossus** is fully exposed (*Atlas*, 9.17). Observe the two important nerves that cross the hyoglossus laterally: **hypoglossal nerve** and, more superiorly, the **lingual nerve.**

With a probe, locate the origin of the **lingual artery** (Fig. 7.61; *Atlas*, 8.28, 8.30). Understand that this artery runs medial to the hyoglossus. To expose the course of the artery, this muscle must be reflected. Proceed as follows: pass a probe deep to the attachment of the hyoglossus to the hyoid bone. Cut the muscle, and reflect it superiorly.

Now the course of the **lingual artery** is exposed (*Atlas*, 8.29). Follow its branches to the musculature of the tongue. Search for fine branches to the sublingual gland.

Styloglossus (Fig. 7.61; *Atlas*, 8.29). Trace the muscle from the styloid process to the lateral aspect of the tongue. Note that its fibers interdigitate with those of the hyoglossus.

Genioglossus and Geniohyoid. Once again, examine these two muscles on median section (*Atlas*, 7.81). Separate the muscles with a probe. The geniohyoid is the one attached to the hyoid bone. Observe the large, fan-shaped genioglossus. With a probe, define its apical attachment to the genial tubercle of the mandible.

Next, cut the **genioglossus** close to the mandible. Observe that, as a result of this section, the tongue becomes quite mobile. Raise the tongue well posteriorly into the pharynx. Now, the underlying **geniohyoid** is exposed. Examine the attachments of this muscle to mandible and hyoid bone (*Atlas*, 7.80).

On one side of the bisected head only, make a **transverse section through the tongue.** Note the **intrinsic musculature of the tongue.** It consists of *vertical, transverse, and longitudinal fibers* (*Atlas*, 7.130). Review the hypoglossal nerve (*Atlas*, 9.17).

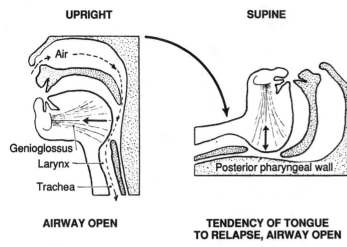

UPRIGHT **SUPINE**

AIRWAY OPEN **TENDENCY OF TONGUE TO RELAPSE, AIRWAY OPEN**

Figure 7.62. Maintenance of airway. As an individual moves from the upright to the supine position, the tongue has a tendency to relapse due to its own gravity (*downward arrow*). Normally, sufficient genioglossal muscle tone (*forward arrow*) prevents the tongue from falling completely posteriorly. However, if the base of the tongue reaches the posterior pharyngeal wall, the vital airway becomes occluded.

The **genioglossus** is a paired muscle that is fused in the midline. Its function is to protrude the tongue (move it anteriorly; stretch it out). If one-half of the muscle does not function (hypoglossal paralysis on that side), the tongue cannot be protruded in a straight fashion; rather the intact side is protruded more, and the damaged side is protruded less or not at all. As a result, the stretched-out tongue deviates to the side of the lesion.

The genioglossus is of great clinical importance. If paralyzed (bilateral hypoglossal paralysis; deep general anesthesia), the tongue cannot be protruded and, due to its own weight, will relapse posteriorly against the posterior pharyngeal wall when the patient is in the supine position. As a result, the vital airway will be occluded with the attendant risk of suffocation (Fig. 7.62). Recent research has shown that the muscular tone of the genioglossus is greatly diminished during certain phases of sleep, thus enhancing the risk of intermittent airway occlusion during sleep. Obese patients with substantial fatty infiltration into the tongue are particularly vulnerable.

Larynx

General Remarks

The **skeleton of the larynx** (*Atlas*, 8.71, 8.77) is responsible for maintaining the shape of this organ. It consists of a series of articulating cartilages that are united by membranes. The **cricoid cartilage** (Gk., *krikos*, ring) is shaped like a signet ring; its large plate or lamina is positioned posteriorly, its arch anteriorly.

The inferior horns or cornua of the **thyroid cartilage** articulate with the cricoid cartilage at special facets. At these facets, the thyroid cartilage can be tilted anteriorly or posteriorly in a visor-like manner.

On the superior border of the lamina of the cricoid are the articular facets for the paired **arytenoid cartilages**. These small pyramidal cartilages are capable of various movements:

1. Tilting anteriorly and posteriorly;
2. Sliding toward or away from another;
3. Rotary motion.

The posterior ends of the **vocal ligaments** are attached at the vocal processes of the arytenoid cartilages (*Atlas*, 8.77). The anterior ends of the vocal ligaments converge at the angle formed by the laminae of the thyroid cartilage.

The **epiglottic cartilage** lies posterior to the tongue and hyoid bone. The stalk of this cartilage is attached in the angle between the thyroid laminae, just superior to the vocal ligaments (*Atlas*, 8.77).

Laryngeal Muscles

The mucosa of the piriform recess was removed earlier, and the internal laryngeal and recurrent laryngeal nerves were already partially exposed (*Atlas*, 8.70).

Now, strip the mucosa from the entire pharyngeal aspect of the larynx. This procedure will expose the following **intrinsic laryngeal muscles:**

1. **Posterior cricoarytenoids** (*Atlas*, 8.70). This pair of muscles arises from the posterior lamina of the cricoid and inserts into the muscular processes of the arytenoid cartilages.
2. **Arytenoideus.** It unites the two arytenoid cartilages by transverse fibers. Some superficial oblique fibers cross to the opposite side and toward the epiglottis. This part of the muscle is known as the *aryepiglotticus*.

Define the **cricothyroid joint** (*Atlas*, 8.71, 8.72). Just posterior to the joint runs the recurrent laryngeal nerve. Cut through the ligamentous bands that hold the joint together. Disarticulate this synovial joint.

The next objective is to reflect a portion of the thyroid lamina in order to expose the remaining laryngeal muscles (*Atlas*, 8.72). Proceed as follows: saw or cut the lamina of the thyroid cartilage about 8 mm to the left of the midline. Reflect the thyroid lamina, which is attached to the cricoid by the cricothyroid muscle.

Now, the following **laryngeal muscles** can be identified and studied (*Atlas*, 8.72):

1. **Cricothyroid,** stretching from the surface of the cricoid to the inferior border and inferior horn of the thyroid cartilage;
2. **Lateral cricoarytenoid,** passing from the superior border of the cricoid and the cricothyroid ligament to the muscular process of the arytenoid cartilage;

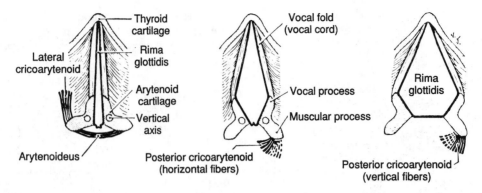

Figure 7.63. The rima glottidis (the interval between the vocal cords) is controlled by various laryngeal muscles.

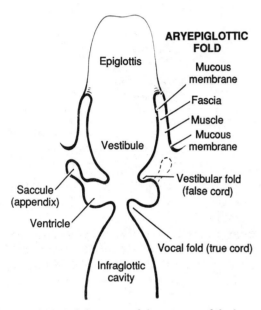

Figure 7.64. Subdivisions of the interior of the larynx.

3. **Thyroarytenoid,** positioned superior to the lateral cricoarytenoid; it passes from the thyroid cartilage anteriorly to the arytenoid cartilage posteriorly; its superior and most medial fibers are the *vocalis*;
4. **Vocalis,** applied lateral and inferior to the vocal ligament (*Atlas*, 8.74);
5. **Thyroepiglotticus,** from thyroid cartilage to epiglottis (*Atlas*, 8.72).

Manipulate the arytenoid cartilages. Understand their movements in response to the actions of various laryngeal muscles (Fig. 7.63; *Atlas*, 8.79). Only the **posterior cricoarytenoid** is capable of opening the **rima glottidis**, the interval between the true vocal cords. Thus, this muscle is vital in maintaining the respiratory airway. All other intrinsic laryngeal muscles close the rima glottidis. The cricothyroid muscle tilts the thyroid cartilage anteriorly and thus tenses the vocal cord (higher pitch of voice). Review the nerve supply to the laryngeal muscles (*Atlas*, 8.70, 8.72, 9.15**B**).

Interior of Larynx

The **cavity of the larynx** has **three compartments** (Fig. 7.64; *Atlas*, 8.75):

1. **Vestibule,** the compartment superior to the vestibular folds;
2. **Ventricle,** the middle compartment between vestibular and vocal folds;
3. **Infraglottic cavity,** inferior to the vocal folds and continuous with the trachea.

Inspect the interior of the larynx from its superior aspect (*Atlas*, 8.76). Observe the **vestibular folds** (ventricular folds; false cords) lying superolateral to the vocal cords (true cords).

The next objective is to expose the interior of the larynx. With heavy scissors, split the trachea, lamina of cricoid, and arytenoid muscle in the posterior median plane. In addition, cut the arch of the cricoid cartilage in the anterior median plane. Now, unfold the larynx (*Atlas*, 8.75).

Identify the **vestibular and vocal folds** (*Atlas*, 8.75, 8.76). On each side, the depression between the two folds is the ventricle. The ventricle may extend into a recess, the saccule (Fig. 7.64). With a probe, explore ventricles and recesses.

Remove the mucous membrane from one half of the interior of the larynx (Fig. 7.65; *Atlas*, 8.75). Start at the cricoid cartilage. Strip the mucosa from the triangular **cricothyroid ligament or conus elasticus.** Observe that this membrane is attached inferiorly to the superior border of the cricoid ring. Superiorly, the free edge of the conus elasticus is thickened as the **vocal ligament.** The vocal ligament forms the basis for the vocal fold.

Next, remove the mucosa from the epiglottis and expose the epiglottic cartilage. Examine its attachment to the thyroid lamina.

Peel the mucosa from the area extending between the lateral border of epiglottic cartilage and arytenoid cartilage (Fig. 7.65; *Atlas*, 8.75). The exposed membrane is the **quadrangular membrane.** Its free inferior border is the vestibular ligament, which supports the vestibular fold.

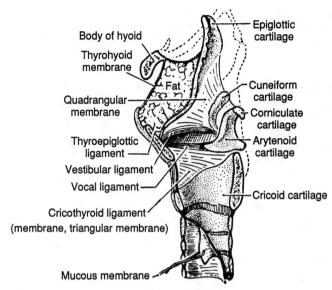

Figure 7.65. Interior of the larynx (after removal of mucous membrane).

Realize that the laryngeal mucosa superior to the vocal cords is supplied with sensory fibers by the **internal laryngeal nerve** (*Atlas*, 9.15B). Once again, trace this nerve through the thyrohyoid membrane toward the interior of the larynx.

Middle Ear

General Remarks

The middle ear cavity or **tympanic cavity** is an air space contained within the temporal bone. Refer to schematic diagrams of the middle ear (Fig. 7.66; *Atlas*, 7.132, 7.133, 7.138), and study its boundaries:

1. Laterally, the **tympanic membrane** (*Atlas*, 7.142); the small portion of tympanic cavity superior to the tympanic membrane is the **epitympanic recess**;
2. Posteriorly, the mastoid wall; the superior portion of the wall is open; here, the **aditus** leads to the **antrum** and **air cells of the mastoid process**;
3. Anteriorly, the **auditory tube** leads to the nasopharynx; just inferior to the auditory tube and anterior to the tympanic cavity is the **carotid canal** (Fig. 7.66; *Atlas*, 7.138A);
4. Medially, the structures of the inner ear are contained within the temporal bone;
5. Inferiorly, the floor of the tympanic cavity is closely related to the **jugular fossa** in which the superior jugular bulb is located (Fig. 7.66; *Atlas*, 7.142);
6. Superiorly, the roof or **tegmen tympani** is formed by a plate of the petrous portion of the temporal bone; the tegmen tympani separates the middle ear from the middle cranial fossa.

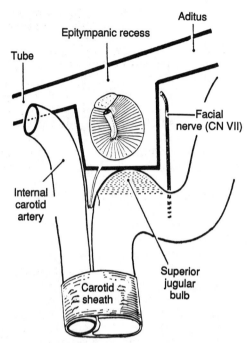

Figure 7.66. The tympanic cavity and its relations to major vessels and the facial nerve (VII).

Each tympanic cavity contains a chain of **three auditory ossicles** that connect the tympanic membrane with the inner ear (*Atlas*, 7.144, 7.145). The middle ear cavity and its associated recesses and air cells are covered with mucous membrane.

The **facial nerve** (VII) traverses the temporal bone. Its course is closely related to the inner and the middle ear. A branch of the facial nerve, the chorda tympani, passes between two of the auditory ossicles (*Atlas*, 7.142).

Bony Landmarks

Refer to a skull and identify the following pertinent bony **landmarks**:

1. **Mastoid process** (*Atlas*, 7.70);
2. **External acoustic meatus;**
3. **Suprameatal spine,** just posterior to the superior part of the external acoustic meatus;
4. **Internal acoustic meatus** (*Atlas*, 7.153);
5. **Hiatus** for greater petrosal nerve;
6. **Tegmen tympani,** a plate of the petrous part of the temporal bone, located in the middle cranial fossa (*Atlas*, 7.152);
7. **Jugular fossa** and jugular foramen (*Atlas*, 8.52, 8.53);
8. Bony portion of **auditory tube;**
9. **Carotid canal;**
10. **Stylomastoid foramen.**

Dissection

If separate decalcified temporal bones are provided, make the cuts described with a very sharp scalpel or a single-edge razor blade. If only your cadaver specimen is available, the hard temporal bone must be sawed. Carry this dissection out on one side only. The objectives of this dissection are: (a) to display the mastoid cells; (b) to expose the structures housed in the tympanic cavity; and (c) to explore the walls of the tympanic cavity.

First Saw Cut. Saw coronally through the temporal bone. Start the saw cut just posterior to the suprameatal spine (*Atlas*, 7.70). Carry the cut into the cranial cavity, dividing the bone into two pieces. Now, examine the **mastoid cells.** Find the **antrum.** From the antrum pass a fine nylon thread through the **aditus** into the tympanic cavity (*Atlas*, 7.147).

Identify certain soft structures that are relevant to this dissection. In the **middle cranial fossa,** remove the trigeminal ganglion and its three divisions. Define the **internal carotid artery** and the **middle meningeal artery** (or the foramen spinosum). In the **posterior cranial fossa,** identify the **facial nerve (VII)** and the **vestibulocochlear nerve (VIII)** as they pass through the internal acoustic meatus. Pass a probe into the meatus to gauge its length (approximately 19 mm). Then, remove the roof of the meatus. The bone is very hard. Use fine bone pliers. Protect your eyes against flying chips of bone. Observe the course of the **facial nerve** (*Atlas*, 7.150). Identify the **geniculate ganglion** and the **greater petrosal nerve.** Review these nervous structures (*Atlas*, 9.12C).

Next, carefully remove the tegmen tympani. With sharp, pointed forceps, remove the incus. The incus is the strongest and the intermediate of the three auditory ossicles. Leave the malleus attached to the tympanic membrane (*Atlas*, 7.144, 7.145).

Second Saw Cut. Stabilize the temporal bone as much as possible. Insert a fine saw into the gap created by the removal of the incus. The saw cut is slightly oblique and parallel to the slope of the tympanic membrane. Anteriorly, the cut passes between the internal carotid artery and middle meningeal artery (foramen spinosum). Carefully split the bone into a medial and lateral piece. With skill, the auditory tube will also be split longitudinally (*Atlas* 7.148, 7.149).

Remove the lateral piece. On it, examine the **lateral wall** of the tympanic cavity (*Atlas*, 7.142). Note the **tympanic membrane** with the attached handle of the **malleus.** The head of the malleus rises into the epitympanic recess. The **chorda tympani** is covered with mucous membrane. Identify it as it crosses the handle of the malleus medially. On the isolated piece, break down the anterior and inferior walls of the bony **external acoustic meatus** (*Atlas*, 7.134). Now, examine the lateral aspect of the tympanic membrane. Note that the membrane faces laterally, inferiorly, and anteriorly.

Anteriorly, the tympanic cavity leads to the **auditory tube.** Posteriorly, it leads to the **aditus ad antrum** (*Atlas*, 7.139, 7.147). Verify these facts in the cadaver.

Examine the **medial wall** of the cavity (*Atlas*, 7.143, 7.148). The features verge on the microscopic. Therefore, a magnifying lens is of great assistance. Observe at least the following features:

1. **Promontory,** a gentle elevation on the medial wall, facing the tympanic membrane;
2. **Stapes,** still in position in the **fenestra vestibuli** (oval window); you may be able to make out the delicate **stapedius tendon,** about 1 mm long, passing from the pyramid to the stapes;
3. **Fenestra cochleae** (round window), at the bottom of a depression posteroinferior to the promontory (*Atlas*, 7.154);
4. **Semicircular canals;** remove the mucosa from the medial wall of the tympanic cavity; with a probe, break into one of the three semicircular canals (*Atlas*, 7.153);
5. **Tensor tympani** (*Atlas*, 7.149); it passes in a mucous fold from the medial wall to the superior part of the handle of the malleus (its tendon was divided by the saw cut);
6. **Facial nerve** in the facial canal (*Atlas*, 7.148); follow the nerve proximally from the stylomastoid foramen; use a probe to force the canal open.

If you wish to dissect the inner ear in detail, utilize a decalcified temporal bone. Refer to the following figures: *Atlas*, 7.150, 9.13. The details of the inner ear can be studied by carefully cutting, with a single-edge razor blade, thin slices of the temporal bone to expose the canals, chambers, and nerve pathways.

LUMBAR APPROACH TO KIDNEY

General Remarks and Orientation

The **lumbar renal approach or retroperitoneal approach** to the kidney is an efficient surgical procedure. The lumbar approach does *not* involve the peritoneal cavity. Thus, contamination of the peritoneal cavity during surgery is avoided. The lumbar renal approach is indicated in a variety of renal disorders (inflammatory renal disease; renal cystic disease; tumors; calculi).

Level of Kidneys (Fig. A.1; *Atlas*, 2.1D).   In the recumbent position, the kidneys are at the level of vertebrae T12 to L3. Usually, the right kidney is slightly more inferior (1 cm) than the left one. The kidneys may move superiorly or inferiorly, depending on changes in posture and on respi-

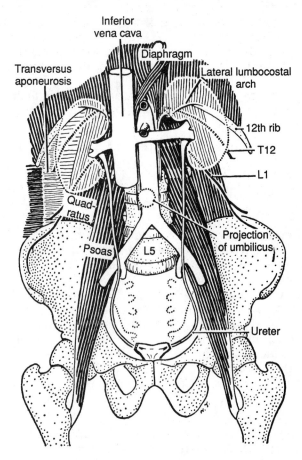

Figure A.1. Posterior relations of kidneys.

ratory movements. Also, there are individual variations in the precise positions of the kidneys.

Essential Posterior Relations (Fig. A.1; *Atlas*, 2.1D). These relations must be understood before attempting the lumbar approach. The **superior pole of the right kidney** rises to the level of **rib 12**. The **superior pole of the left kidney** may be positioned as high as **rib 11**. The superior parts of the kidneys (with the attached suprarenal glands) are separated from the pleural cavities by the diaphragm. The medial aspect of the posterior surface of the kidney is in contact with the **quadratus lumborum**. The lateral aspect of the posterior surface is in contact with the **aponeurosis of the transversus abdominis**. The lumbar renal approach is greatly facilitated by the fact that the quadratus lumborum has an *oblique lateral border*. Appreciate this fact. (If the quadratus lumborum were square and if it were running from the iliac crest to the entire length of rib 12, this thick muscle would greatly impede the lumbar renal approach.)

Two nerves, which must not be cut during surgery, are in close relation to the posterior surface of the kidney (Fig. A.1): **subcostal nerve** (T12), just below rib 12; and **iliohypogastric nerve** (L1), crossing obliquely the inferior pole of the kidney.

Important topographic knowledge can be gained by studying a transverse section through the kidneys (*Atlas*, 2.108). Again, note that the posterior surface of the kidney is related to the quadratus lumborum and the aponeurosis of the transversus abdominis. The psoas muscle lies medial to the kidney. Correlate these anatomical observations with magnetic resonance images (MRIs) of the abdomen (*Atlas*, 2.112, 2.113).

Review the tissues surrounding the kidney (*Atlas*, 2.108):

1. **Fatty renal capsule** (adipose capsule; perinephric fatty tissue). This perirenal fat surrounds the kidney. It is thickest at the margins of the kidney. At the hilus, the renal vessels and the ureter are embedded in the fatty tissue (*Atlas*, 2.112B).
2. **Renal fascia** (of Gerota). It encloses both the kidney and its fatty capsule (*Atlas*, 2.108). Note the two parts of the renal fascia: anterior layer and posterior layer. It will be obvious that the renal fascia must be incised in order to gain access to the kidney. Dorsal to the renal fascia is the **paranephric fat** (pararenal fat).

Dissection

Place the cadaver into the prone or the lateral position. If not already done, remove the skin superior to the iliac crest as indicated in *Atlas*, 2.107. Identify the **lumbar fascia**, the **latissimus dorsi,** and the **external oblique** of the abdominal wall.

Now, incise the latissimus dorsi along the course of rib 12. Reflect the muscle. Palpate rib 12. Identify the thin **serratus posterior inferior.**

Next, incise the **external oblique** just inferior to the tip of rib 12, and turn it laterally (*Atlas*, 2.109). Make an incision through the **internal oblique** parallel to the free posterior border of the external oblique. Carry the cut all the way to the iliac crest. Reflect the internal oblique medially. Now, the **aponeurosis of the transversus abdominis** is exposed. Note that the aponeurosis is pierced by the **subcostal and iliohypogastric nerves.** These nerves must not be cut. Accordingly, the aponeurosis of the transversus must be incised between the two nerves (*Atlas*, 2.110).

Divide the aponeurosis of the transversus abdominis (*Atlas*, 2.110). Reflect the aponeurosis medially and expose the **quadratus lumborum.** Extend the incision superiorly. If necessary, detach the serratus posterior inferior from rib 12. Using blunt dissection, remove any fat you may encounter. This is the **paranephric fat** outside the renal fascia (compare *Atlas*, 2.108).

Now, the **renal fascia** is exposed (*Atlas*, 2.110). Incise it. Palpate the kidney. Remove the **fatty renal capsule** posterior to the kidney. The structures of the hilus (renal artery, vein, renal pelvis, and ureter) lie just anterior to the quadratus lumborum (Fig. A.1). Gain access to these structures by retracting the quadratus lumborum medially and gently pulling the kidney laterally. Understand that the right kidney is less freely movable than the left one, since the right renal vein is much shorter than the left renal vein. Identify the **renal pelvis.** Realize that the actual surgical approach must be more delicate than the gross anatomical exposure of the kidney.

On occasion, it is advantageous to reach the kidneys and their vessels via the transabdominal route (e.g., in kidney transplant procedures).

JOINTS

Joints of the Lower Limb

Sacroiliac Joint

The synovial sacroiliac joint (articulation) is formed between the auricular surfaces of the **sacrum** and the **ilium** (*Atlas*, 4.28). Obtain an isolated hip bone (os coxae), and observe the **articular auricular surface of the ilium.** Note the corresponding **auricular surface in the isolated sacrum.** Note that each bone has a **tuberosity** dorsal to its auricular surface. Procure an articulated pelvis and observe:

1. The auricular surfaces are in apposition (*Atlas*, 3.1, 3.2).
2. The tuberosities are separated by a deep cleft (Fig. A.2).

Turn to the cadaver, which should be in the prone position (face down). Clean the following ligaments:

1. **Sacrotuberous ligament** (Figs. A.3, A.4). Scrape the remainders of the gluteus maximus from it. Define the attachments of the ligament and clean its superior extension to the posterior iliac spines.
2. **Sacrospinous ligament.** Define its attachments (Figs. A.3, A.4).
3. **Posterior (dorsal) sacroiliac ligaments** (Fig. A.3; *Atlas*, 4.27). Observe long and short fasciculi that pass between the sacrum and the ilium in various directions.
4. **Interosseous sacroiliac ligament** (Figs. A.2, A.4; *Atlas*, 4.27). It is exceedingly strong. It is the essential ligament of the joint. The interosseous sacroiliac ligament binds together the sacral and iliac tuberosities. This fact is best appreciated on transverse section (Fig. A.2) or coronal section (*Atlas*, 4.27). To expose the ligament, you must remove the posterior (dorsal) sacroiliac ligaments.

Anteriorly, identify the thin **ventral sacroiliac ligament** (*Atlas*, 3.4). Cut through this ligament that forms the ventral part of the joint capsule. Forcibly separate ilium and

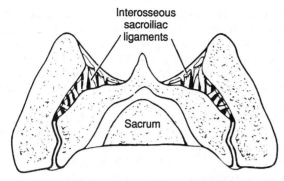

Figure A.2. Sacroiliac joint on transverse section. Note the interosseous sacroiliac ligaments anchoring the sacrum to the right ilium and left ilium.

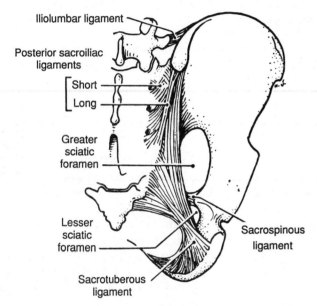

Figure A.3. Ligaments of the pelvis (posterior view).

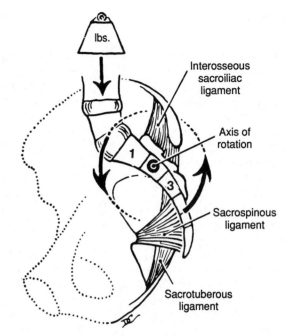

Figure A.4. Ligaments resisting rotation of the sacrum. The axis of rotation passes through S2.

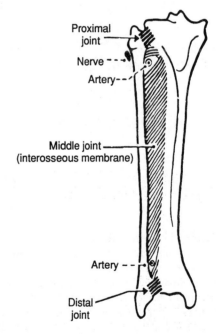

Figure A.5. Tibiofibular articulations. Note the unity of direction of the ligamentous fibers of the interosseous membrane.

sacrum. Examine the cartilage-covered auricular surfaces of the joint (*Atlas*, 4.28).

Understand: Considerable weight is transmitted to the sacrum by the superimposed vertebral column. This force causes a tendency of the superior end of the sacrum to rotate anteriorly and of the inferior end of the sacrum to rotate posteriorly (Fig. A.4). The anterior rotation of the sacrum is mainly resisted by the interosseous sacroiliac ligaments and the posterior sacroiliac ligaments. The posterior rotation of the sacrum is resisted by the sacrospinous and sacrotuberous ligaments (Fig. A.4). On occasion, you will find synostosis (bony fusion) of the joint.

Hip Joint (see Chapter 5).

Knee Joint (see Chapter 5)

Ankle Joint (see Chapter 5)

Tibiofibular Joints

Tibiofibular Joints (Fig. A.5; *Atlas*, 5.81). The fibula is moored to the tibia at its superior end, along its shaft, and at its inferior end at proximal, middle, and distal joints.

Examine an isolated fibula and a tibia. Note (*Atlas*, 5.74C) a small, flat, round facet on the head of the fibula; a similar facet on the posterolateral aspect of the lateral condyle of the tibia.

In the cadaver, remove the popliteus tendon and the popliteus bursa posterior to the **proximal tibiofibular joint** (*Atlas*, 5.81). Note that the joint capsule is strengthened by strong anterior and weak posterior fibers. Open the capsule and observe the small synovial cavity of this gliding joint.

The *middle* and *distal tibiofibular joints* are *syndesmoses*. The **interosseous membrane** (middle joint) extends along the respective sides of tibia and fibula, producing a sharp line on each bone. Strip the muscles from the anterior and posterior aspect of the interosseous membrane. Note the oval aperture between the proximal tibiofibular joint and the superior free margin of interosseous membrane. The *anterior tibial artery* passes through this opening (Fig. A.5). Observe the gap between the distal tibiofibular joint and the inferior free margin of interosseous membrane. The *perforating branch of the peroneal artery* passes through this opening (Fig. A.5; *Atlas*, 5.6).

Clean the anterior and posterior ligaments of the *distal tibiofibular joint* (Fig. A.5; *Atlas*, 5.117, 5.118, 5.119). These are the strong **anterior inferior** and **posterior inferior tibiofibular ligaments**. Grasp tibia and fibula well superior to the ankle, alternately squeezing the bones together and relaxing them. Note the yielding of the distal tibiofibular joint.

Joints of Inversion and Eversion (see Chapter 5)

Joints Distal to the Transverse Tarsal Joint

Intertarsal, Tarsometatarsal, and Intermetatarsal Joints. Review the bones of the foot (*Atlas*, 5.83, 5.89, 5.120). Frequently refer to *Atlas*, 5.83 and 5.117. Observe the **dorsal cuneonavicular ligaments.** Cut through the ligaments and open the **cuneonavicular joint** from the dorsum of the foot. Carry the incision to the **cubonavicular joint.** Explore the extent of the joint: anteriorly, it is continuous with the **intercuneiform and cuneocuboid joints.**

Note the bursa deep to the insertion of the tibialis anterior. This bursa communicates with the **first cuneometatarsal joint** (*Atlas*, 5.83, 5.117). Open this joint from the dorsum of the foot. Leave the plantar ligaments (*Atlas*, 5.129) intact to act as hinges. Open the joints between the tarsal and metatarsal bones. Note the **intermetatarsal joints** (between metatarsal bones).

Metatarsophalangeal and Interphalangeal Joints (*Atlas*, 5.83). These are hinges, similar to the corresponding joints in the hand. Identify the **plantar ligaments** of the metatarsophalangeal joints. Observe the two sesamoid bones inferior to the head of the first metatarsal (*Atlas*, 5.113). Examine an **interphalangeal joint.** Observe that it possesses a plantar ligament and collateral ligaments.

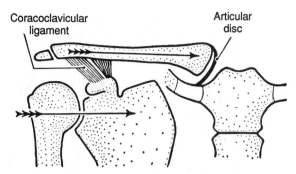

Figure A.6. Structures having unity of function: coracoclavicular ligament and articular disc of sternoclavicular joint.

Joints of the Upper Limb

Sternoclavicular Joint

In the articulated skeleton, observe the relations between **sternum** and **clavicle** (*Atlas*, 1.8B). Identify the **clavicular notch** of the manubrium sterni (*Atlas*, 1.11B). This notch and the adjacent parts of the first costal cartilage articulate with the enlarged sternal (medial) end of the clavicle.

Turn to the cadaver. Anterior to the **sternoclavicular joint** is the tendon of the sternomastoid. Remove it. Dorsal to the joint are the broad, fleshy, strap-like sternohyoid and sternothyroid muscles (*Atlas*, 8.41).

Note the superolateral direction of the dense, parallel fibers of the anterior part of the **joint capsule**. This is the anterior sternoclavicular ligament (*Atlas*, 1.12B, 8.41). The costoclavicular ligament runs obliquely from the first costal cartilage to the inferior surface of the clavicle near its medial end (*Atlas*, 1.12B). Clean the ligaments.

Cut through the anterior sternoclavicular ligament. In doing so, keep the blade of the scalpel close to the manubrium. Reflect the ligament. Now, the **articular disc** is exposed (*Atlas*, 8.41). Note that it divides the articular cavity into two parts. Observe that the articular disc is attached in such a manner as to resist medial displacement of the clavicle. Inferiorly, it is attached to the first costal cartilage; superiorly, it is attached to the clavicle (Fig. A.6; *Atlas*, 1.12B).

On yourself, palpate the **movements** at the sternoclavicular joint. Move the scapula and, with it, the clavicle. Observe that the sternoclavicular joint allows a limited amount of movement in nearly every direction.

Acromioclavicular Joint

Review the essential bony landmarks relevant to the acromioclavicular articulation and its associated ligaments (*Atlas*, 6.1A): **acromion** and **carocoid process** of scapula; **lateral end of clavicle**.

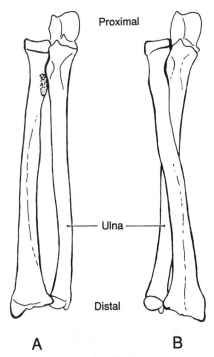

Figure A.7. Anterior view of right ulna and radius; **A**, in supination; **B**, in pronation. Note proximal and distal radioulnar joints.

Remove the deltoid and the trapezius from the acromion and the lateral end of the clavicle. Thus, expose the **acromioclavicular joint** (*Atlas*, 6.29, 6.48). The joint is subcutaneous; deep to it lies the subacromial bursa.

Identify the strong and important **coracoclavicular ligament** (Fig. A.6; *Atlas*, 6.46). Clean the two parts of the ligament, the conoid ligament and the trapezoid ligament.

Open the synovial acromioclavicular joint from its superior aspect. Remove the joint capsule completely; i.e., separate acromion from lateral end of calvicle.

Now, with the acromioclavicular joint disarticulated, the important functions of the coracoclavicular ligament can be studied. Realize that the ligament prevents the scapula from being driven medially (Fig. A.6; *Atlas*, 6.30).

On yourself, palpate the subcutaneous acromioclavicular joint. Observe that the joint enables the scapula to move vertically on the chest wall (as when shrugging the shoulders). The joint is essential to free elevation of the upper limb.

Shoulder Joint (see Chapter 6)

Elbow Joint (see Chapter 6)

Radioulnar Joints

The two bones of the forearm are united at the proximal, intermediate or middle, and distal radioulnar joints. The necessary rotary movements during supination and pronation take place in the proximal and distal radioulnar joints (Fig. A.7).

The **proximal radioulnar joint** (articulation) was considered with the elbow joint (see Chapter 6).

Intermediate (Middle) Radioulnar Joint (*Atlas*, 6.76C). The shafts of the radius and ulna are united by the **interosseous membrane.** Remove or reflect all muscles from the anterior and posterior forearm, and expose the interosseous membrane. Note the direction of its fibers. The general direction of the fibers of the membrane is such that an upward thrust to the radius is transmitted to the ulna. Understand: During an upward thrust (fall on the hand), the forces are transmitted from hand via wrist joint to radius, from radius via interosseous membrane to ulna, from ulna (and radius) to humerus.

Note that blood vessels are closely applied to the interosseous membrane, and that small vessels pierce the membrane (*Atlas*, 6.76C).

Distal Radioulnar Joint (Fig. A.7). Cut through the anular ligament and release the head of the radius. Cut the interosseous membrane. Pass the blade of the scalpel through a sac-like recess, the **sacciform recess** (*Atlas*, 6.133). Now, enter the distal radioulnar joint. Do *not* injure the triangular **articular disc** (*Atlas*, 6.133, 6.135, 6.136).

Swing the radius laterally and view the **articular disc.** Observe:

1. It is fibrocartilaginous. Its apex and its anterior and posterior margins are ligamentous.
2. The apex is attached to the styloid process of the ulna.
3. The base of the triangular disc is attached to the ulnar notch of the radius.
4. The ligamentous borders of the disc spread far laterally on the radius.
5. Commonly, the cartilaginous part of the disc is perforated (the disc is subjected to constant pressure and friction).

Wrist Joint (see Chapter 6)

Small Joints of the Hand

Review the bones of the hand (*Atlas*, 6.130). The osseofibrous **carpal tunnel** has already been opened (Chapter 6). Remove all contents from the carpal tunnel. Trace the tendon of the flexor carpi radialis through its special tunnel to the second metacarpal (*Atlas*, 6.99). Observe that the tubercle of the scaphoid acts as a pulley for the tendon. Note that the lunate bulges conspicuously into the carpal tunnel (*Atlas*, 6.128).

Clean the **intercarpal, carpometacarpal, and intermetacarpal ligaments.** Open all joints from the palmar aspect. First, open the **midcarpal joint (transverse carpal joint)** by entering the scalpel between tubercle of scaphoid and tubercle of trapezium (*Atlas*, 6.137). Observe the sinuous surfaces of the opposed bones. Note that synovial folds project into the joint.

Next, open the **carpometacarpal joints** (*Atlas*, 6.139). Observe that the carpometacarpal joint of the thumb (digit

1) has a loose capsule with parallel fibers. Manipulate the metacarpal bones. Observe the hinge movements at the bases of the 4th and 5th carpometacarpal joints. The flexion possible at these two joints allows the grip of the hand to be more secure (*Atlas*, 6.120)

Joints of the Digits

In the clefts between the fingers, the lumbrical muscles and the digital nerves and vessels pass anterior to the **deep transverse metacarpal ligaments.** The interossei pass dorsal to the ligaments (*Atlas*, 6.93, 6.99). On each side, the deep transverse metacarpal ligaments are continuous with the palmar ligaments that form the proximal limit of the posterior wall of the fibrous digital flexor sheath (*Atlas*, 6.99).

Metacarpophalangeal Joints (*Atlas*, 6.141).   Cut one or more of the deep transverse metacarpal ligaments. Remove the interossei and the dorsal extensor expansion. Clean a pair of collateral ligaments. They are triangular and important. A *cord-like part* passes to the base of the adjacent phalanx; a *fan-like part* passes to the side of the palmar ligament. Verify: the strong, cord-like parts of the collateral ligaments are eccentrically attached to the flat metacarpal heads. The ligaments are slack during extension and taut during flexion. Therefore, the fingers cannot be spread (abducted) unless the hand is opened.

Interphalangeal Joints (*Atlas*, 6.141).   Note the collateral ligaments of the interphalangeal joints. These are hinge joints. Explore the synovial cavity of the joints. Note the articular surfaces that are covered with smooth cartilage.

Finally, correlate the gross anatomical features of the bones of the hand with a radiograph and MRI scans of the wrist (*Atlas*, 6.131, 6.132).

APPENDIX III

DISSECTION OF EYEBALL OF BULL

General Remarks

The dissection of the *eyeball of the bull* is a convenient way to acquire a general knowledge of the gross anatomical features of the human eye.

The **eyeball or bulbus oculi has three concentric coats** (Fig. A.8; *Atlas*, 7.57A):

1. **External or fibrous coat:** *sclera* and *cornea;*
2. **Middle or vascular coat:** *choroid, ciliary body* and *iris;*
3. **Internal or retinal coat:**
   a. *Outer layer* of pigmented cells;
   b. *Inner layer;* the cells of this layer are nervous (visual) posterior to the ora serrata.

The **four refractive media** are (Fig. A.8):

1. **Cornea;**
2. **Aqueous humor;**
3. **Lens;**
4. **Vitreous body.**

Dissection

Clean the exterior of the eyeball or bulb by removing the adherent fat, muscles, and vessels. Leave the stump of the optic nerve intact. Anteriorly, sever the conjunctiva at the corneoscleral junction (margin) and remove it.

Divide the bulb into posterior and anterior halves by cutting with a sharp scalpel (new blade) around the equator. During this process, you will successively cut the sclera, choroid, retina, and the vitreous body.

Examination of Posterior Half, Inner Aspect.   The retina is dull and gray like an exposed photographic film and it is exceedingly friable. It is held in position and applied to the choroid by the vitreous body.

Gently scoop out the jelly-like **vitreous body** with the handle of a scalpel. Now, the **retina** is no longer firmly applied to the choroid. As a result, it falls into folds, except at the optic disc. The **optic disc** is the site where the fibers of the optic nerve pierce the sclera, choroid, and outer retinal layer to spread out into the inner (optic) layer of the retina. The disc is a blind spot (compare with the human eye; *Atlas*, 7.57).

The **choroid** is the thin and pigmented vascular middle coat (Fig. A.9). Generally, it is easily detached as a whole from the sclera. At several spots, however, the choroid is bound to the sclera of the posterior half of the bulb:

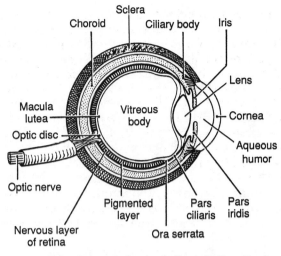

Figure A.8. Scheme of an eyeball (sagittal section).

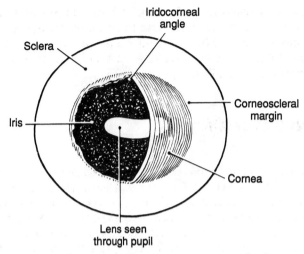

Figure A.10. Bull's eye; anterior approach—I.

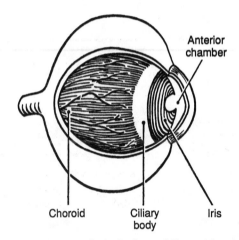

Figure A.9. Eyeball of a bull; the middle coat is exposed.

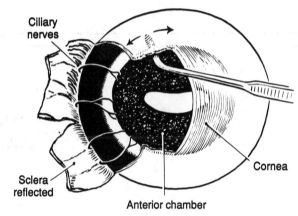

Figure A.11. Bull's eye; anterior approach—II.

1. Where it is pierced by the optic nerve;
2. Where the vorticose veins leave it near the equator to pierce the sclera (compare with the human eye; *Atlas*, 7.57B).

There are certain differences between the human eye and the bull's eye: the pupil of the bull's eye is not round. There is no macula in the eye of the bull. In the bull, but not in man, a wide triangular area of the choroid superior to the level of the optic disc has a greenish-blue metallic sheen. This is due to the presence of a fibrous sheet, the tapetum, between the layers of the choroid. In animals, this tapetum is responsible for the intense light reflections from the eyes at night.

Examination of Anterior Half, Inner Aspect. Observe the anterior part of the vitreous body. Gently remove it. The dull gray optic part of the retina ends well anterior to the equator in a slightly scalloped margin, the **ora serrata.**

Anterior to the ora serrata lies the ciliary zone. Here, about 70 black, finger-like ridges, the **ciliary processes,** converge on the equator of the **lens.** Note that the lens is

suspended by numerous **zonular fibers** (compare with the human eye; *Atlas*, 7.57A).

Dissection of the bull's eye; anterior approach (Fig. A.10). The sclera is white and tough. It is continuous with the transparent **cornea.** Through the cornea observe the dark **iris,** which surrounds the **pupil.** Posterior to the pupil is the lens.

With a sharp scalpel, incise the cornea vertically. With scissors, cut horizontally along the corneoscleral junction. Leave the right quarter of the cornea intact. You have now opened the **anterior chamber** which, in the living, is filled with aqueous humor. Place a probe into the angle between iris and cornea, the **iridocorneal angle** (Fig. A.11; compare with the human eye; *Atlas*, 7.57A). Pass the point of a probe through the pupil and into the space between the lens and the posterior surface of the iris. The probe is now in the **posterior chamber.**

Remove a section of the iris (Fig. A.12). Examine the exposed posterior chamber, which is triangular on transverse section. It is bounded anteriorly by the iris, posteriorly by the lens and zonular fibers, and laterally by the ends of the ciliary processes (compare with the human eye; *Atlas*, 7.57A).

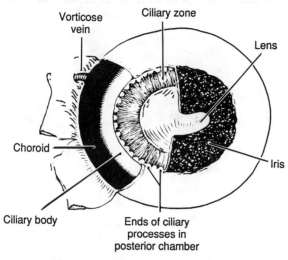

Figure A.12. Bull's eye; anterior approach—III.

Cut horizontally through the anterior portion of the capsule of the lens. The lens will pop out; if not, it can be easily extruded. Note that the anterior surface of the lens is less curved than the posterior surface.

Place the point of a probe in the iridocorneal angle (Fig. A.12). Break through the firm attachment of the ciliary muscle to the anterior limit of the sclera. Detach the ciliary muscle widely. Press the probe against the sclera in order not to damage the delicate choroidal coat. With strong scissors, cut a sector of sclera and reflect it posteriorly. Observe the following (Figs. A.11 and A.12):

1. A white circular band, about 4 mm in width; this is the outer surface of the **ciliary body;** the ciliary body contains the ciliary muscle and the ciliary processes;
2. Numerous white streaks; these are the **ciliary nerves;** they run toward the ciliary body and iris. Understand the function of these nerves (*Atlas*, 9.5**D**, **E**, and **F**).

INDEX

Page numbers in *italics* denote figures.